# Physical Therapy: Neurologic Interventions

# Physical Therapy: Neurologic Interventions

Editor: Camille Breen

STATES
ACADEMIC PRESS
www.statesacademicpress.com

**States Academic Press,**
109 South 5th Street,
Brooklyn, NY 11249, USA

Visit us on the World Wide Web at:
www.statesacademicpress.com



ISBN: 978-1-63989-415-4 (Hardback)



**Cataloging-in-Publication Data**

Physical therapy : neurologic interventions / edited by Camille Breen.
p. cm.
Includes bibliographical references and index.
ISBN 978-1-63989-415-4
1. Nervous system--Diseases--Physical therapy. 2. Physical therapy. 3. Nervous system--Wounds and injuries--Physical therapy. 4. Therapeutics, Physiological. I. Breen, Camille.
RC350.P48 P49 2022
616.804 62--dc23

# Table of Contents

# Preface

Physical therapy, also known as physiotherapy, is a healthcare specialty that deals with injuries or illnesses that limit functional mobility. It aims to ease pain and help function, move and live better. Physical therapy comprises trained professionals who evaluate and treat abnormalities using physical examination, diagnosis, prognosis, patient education, physical intervention, rehabilitation, disease prevention and health promotion. It is used to evaluate and treat various problems like stroke, fractures, spinal cord injuries, carpal tunnel syndrome, sports injuries, amputations and arthritis. Physical therapy can be a standalone treatment, or may support other treatment methods. Sports therapy is a sub discipline of physical therapy and helps athletes maximize their performance. This book unravels the recent studies on neurologic interventions in this field. It includes some of the vital pieces of work being conducted across the world, on various topics related to this field. This book contains contributions of experts and scientists which will provide innovative insights into physical therapy.

Various studies have approached the subject by analyzing it with a single perspective, but the present book provides diverse methodologies and techniques to address this field. This book contains theories and applications needed for understanding the subject from different perspectives. The aim is to keep the readers informed about the progresses in the field; therefore, the contributions were carefully examined to compile novel researches by specialists from across the globe.

Indeed, the job of the editor is the most crucial and challenging in compiling all chapters into a single book. In the end, I would extend my sincere thanks to the chapter authors for their profound work. I am also thankful for the support provided by my family and colleagues during the compilation of this book.

**Editor**

# 1

# The Effects of Motor Imagery after a Variety of Motor Learning Times on Excitability of Spinal Motor Neurons and Accurate Motion

Yuki Fukumoto and Yoshibumi Bunno

**Abstract**

**Purpose**: This study aimed to examine the effects of motor imagery on the excitability of spinal motor neurons and accurate motion. Subjects and Methods: About 30 healthy volunteers were recruited. F-waves were recorded at rest, while touching a sensor and motor imagery conditions. Also, the pinch force was measured before and after motor imagery. Furthermore, the subjects mastered the 50% MVC pinch force with learning times of 10 s, 30 s, 1 min, and 2 min beforehand. **Results:** Spinal motor neuron excitability with motor imagery after motor learning for 10 s, 30 s, 1 min, and 2 min was significantly increased as compared to other conditions. Accurate motion in the pinch task after motor imagery was better maintained than in the pinch task before motor imagery with motor learning times of 30 s and 1 min. However, with learning times of 10s and 2 min, the subject's ability to sustain accurate motion in the pinch task after motor imagery was significantly decreased as compared to that of the pinch task before motor imagery. **Conclusion**: Motor imagery increases spinal motor neuron excitability. To maximally improve accurate motion using motor imagery, it is important to practice and master motor learning beforehand

**Keywords:** F-waves, spinal motor neuron, motor imagery, motor learning, accurate motion

## 1. Introduction

Motor imagery is reproduced by memory. Motor imagery especially involves the activation of cognitive processes from working memory [1]. In addition, motor imagery and the preparation for motion reportedly had mechanisms similar to those of the processes of managing motion within the brain [2, 3]. Motor imagery might be applied to therapeutic exercise. Motor imagery may also serve as a therapeutic expedient for patients with restricted activities or in whom physical activity is contraindicated.

Effects of motor imagery on the central nervous system include the following: activations of the primary motor area, supplementary motor area, premotor area, primary somatosensory area, dorsolateral prefrontal area, cingulate cortex, and cerebellums occurred during motor imagery [4–7]. Accordingly, motor imagery increases the excitability of the central nervous system. Also, spinal motor neuron excitability was studied by using F-waves and the H-reflex. An F-wave is a compound action potential obtained as a result of re-excitation ("backfiring") of an antidromic impulse following distal electrical stimulation of motor nerve fibers in the anterior horn cells [8, 9] (**Figure 1**).

An F-wave is a compound action potential obtained as a result of re-excitation ("backfiring") of an antidromic impulse following distal electrical stimulation of motor nerve fibers in the anterior horn cells.

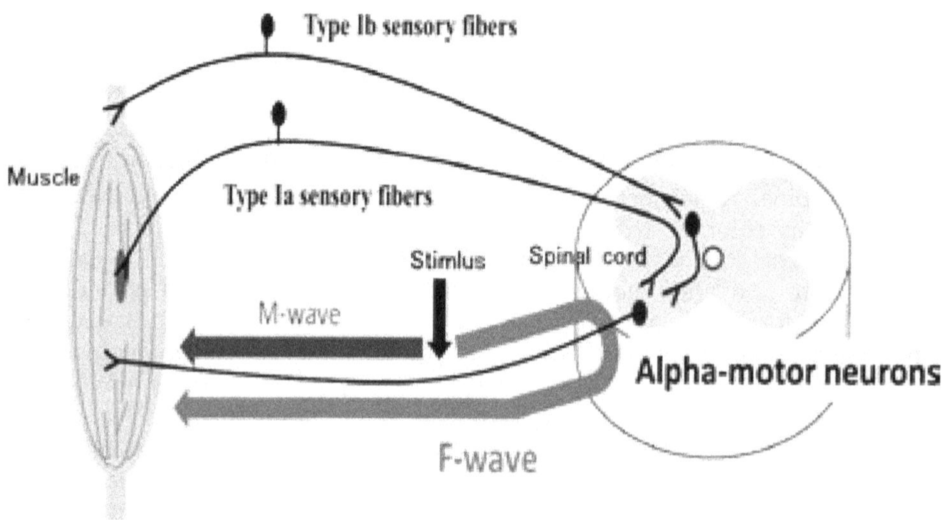


**Figure 1.** F-wave mechanism.

The H-reflex results from sub-maximal stimulation of type Ia sensory fibers. The potential enters the posterior horn of the spinal cord and passes through the synapses with alpha-motor neurons. Finally, a compound muscle action potential is generated and is recorded as H-waves [10]. F-waves and the H-reflex are generally used as an index of spinal motor neuron function. Suzuki et al. [11] reported that persistence and the F/M amplitude ratio during motor imagery at 50% maximum voluntary contraction (MVC) pinch action were significantly increased than those at rest. Taniguchi et al. [12] reported that persistence and the F/M amplitude ratio were significantly decreased after a sustained rest for 3 h as compared to the preresting condition. However, persistence and the F/M amplitude ratio were maintained, showing similar values, after the sustained rest as compared to the preresting condition when rest and motor imagery were combined. Kasai et al. [13] reported that no significant differences were observed in the H-reflex amplitude between the resting condition and motor imagery involving flexion-extension movements at the wrist joint.

Additionally, Oishi et al. [14] reported that the H-reflex amplitude was significantly increased, unchanged, or decreased with motor imagery involving skating, as compared to the resting condition, in a speed skater. Thus, studies have obtained a variety of results such as increased, unchanged, or decreased spinal motor neuron excitability during motor imagery. Given this wide range of observations, the only consistent result is an increase in activation of the central nervous system, while the excitability of spinal motor neurons may not always increase during motor imagery. To optimize improvement of motor function during physical therapy using motor imagery, it is necessary to enhance the excitability of spinal motor neurons as well as to activate the cerebellar cortex.

Next, we considered the effects of motor imagery on actual motion. Yue et al. [15] reported a comparison of muscular strengths after motor imagery of the little finger MVC abduction movement for 4 weeks among motor imagery, physical training, and control groups. They found that muscular strength was reinforced at 30% in the strength training group and at 22% in the motor imagery group. Guillot et al. [16] reported flexibility of the hamstrings and ankle joint muscles to be significantly improved in the postmotor imagery condition of stretching as compared to the premotor imagery condition in swimmers. Page et al. [17] reported that upper limb motor function was improved using a combination of physical therapy and motor imagery in poststroke hemiparesis patients. Dickstein et al. [18], likewise, reported gait speed to be improved using motor imagery in hemiparesis patients with cardiovascular disease. Thus, motor imagery improves muscular strength, range of motion, and motor function. However, it is unclear whether motor imagery affects the accuracy of motion. We use a tool and an object, manipulated by the upper limb, for activities of daily living. For example, buttoning and unbuttoning, using chopsticks, picking up coins, and so forth, are important motor activities. Therefore, the acquisition of accurate motion is crucial. Herein, we studied the effects of motor imagery after various motor learning times, that is, 10 s, 30 s, 1 min, and 2 min, on the accuracy of motion and the excitability of spinal motor neurons.

## 2. Subjects

We included 30 healthy subjects (males, 15; females, 15; mean age, 20.3 ± 1.0) in the group with a motor learning time of 10 s. This study was approved by the Research Ethics Committee at Kansai University of Health Sciences (Approval number: 15-04).

Next, we enrolled another 30 healthy subjects (males, 15; females, 15; mean age, 21.1 ± 1.2) in the group with a motor learning time of 30 s. This study was approved by the Research Ethics Committee at Kansai University of Health Sciences (Approval number: 16-25).

Then, we included 30 healthy subjects (males, 15; females, 15; mean age, 19.7 ± 1.3 years) in the group with a motor learning time of 1 min. This study was approved by the Research Ethics Committee at Kansai University of Health Sciences (Approval number: 16-26).

Finally, we enrolled 30 healthy subjects (males, 15; females, 15; mean age, 22.3 ± 3.0 years) in the group with a motor learning time of 2 min. This study was approved by the Research Ethics Committee at Kansai University of Health Sciences (Approval number: 16-47).

All subjects provided informed consent prior to study commencement. The experiments were conducted in accordance with the Declaration of Helsinki.

## 3. Methods

The study process required three conditions: resting, touching a sensor, and motor imagery. We recorded F-waves during isometric contraction of the thenar muscle. We also measured the pinch force before and after motor imagery. The process is described in detail in below text.

We recorded F-waves of the left thenar muscle and used the spinal motor neurons under the resting condition as an index. Suzuki et al. [11] reported that motor imagery is not simply a matter of carrying out an action, instead actually representing a combination involving maintenance of motion position. Accordingly, we recorded F-waves while the subjects not only simply touched the pinch meter sensor [Digital indicator F340A (Unipulse Inc.)] between the thumb and index finger (touching sensor condition) but also during the combination of touching the pinch meter sensor and performing motor imagery for 1 min (motor imagery condition). In advance, we determined the magnitude of MVC in subjects holding the pinch meter sensor while exerting maximum effort for 10 s. Furthermore, the subjects were required to learn 50% MVC beforehand with isometric contraction for the pinch action with various motor learning times, that is, 10 s, 30 s, 1 min, and 2 min. At this time, the subjects were instructed to maintain the 50% MVC while viewing the pinch meter display. Subsequently, the subjects were asked to subjectively determine the 50% MVC without using visual feedback before motor imagery. In addition, we measured the pinch force for 10 s (pinch task first trial). Again, the subjects were asked to subjectively estimate the 50% MVC without using visual feedback after motor imagery, and we measured pinch force for 10 s (pinch task second trial). On a different day, the control group, while not using motor imagery in a similar process in the motor imagery phase (without motor imagery condition), underwent F-wave recording. These tasks were performed randomly in the motor imagery and control groups (**Figure 2**).

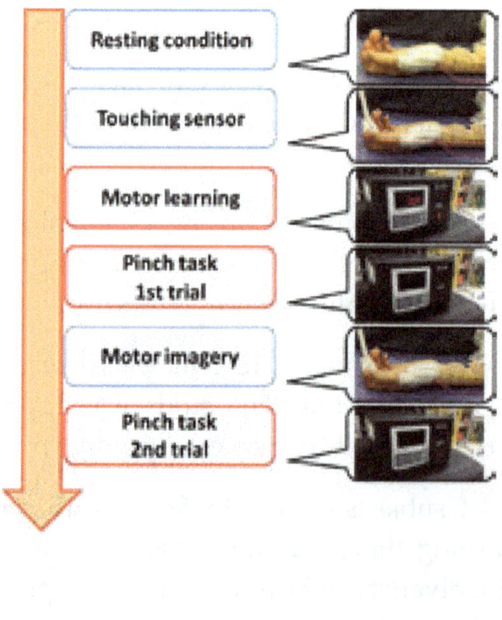


**Figure 2.** Study process.

We recorded F-waves under resting, touching a sensor, and motor imagery conditions. Also, the subjects were instructed to learn the 50% MVC with visual feedback prior to motor imagery. Furthermore, the subjects were asked to subjectively estimate the 50% MVC without using visual feedback before and after motor imagery.

The testing conditions for measurement of F-waves were as follows. A Viking Quest electromyography machine (Natus Medical Inc.) was used to record F-waves. The subjects were comfortably placed in the supine position. We recorded the F-waves by stimulating the left median nerve at the wrist. Supramaximal shocks (adjusted up to the value 20% higher than the maximal stimulus) were delivered at 0.5 Hz and 0.2 ms for F-wave acquisition. We recorded F-waves of the left thenar muscles using a pair of disks attached with collodion to the skin over the eminence of the thumb and the bones of the metacarpophalangeal joint of the thumb. The stimulating electrodes were composed of a cathode placed over the left median nerve 3 cm proximal to the palmar crease of the wrist joint and an anode placed 2 cm more proximally (**Figure 3**).

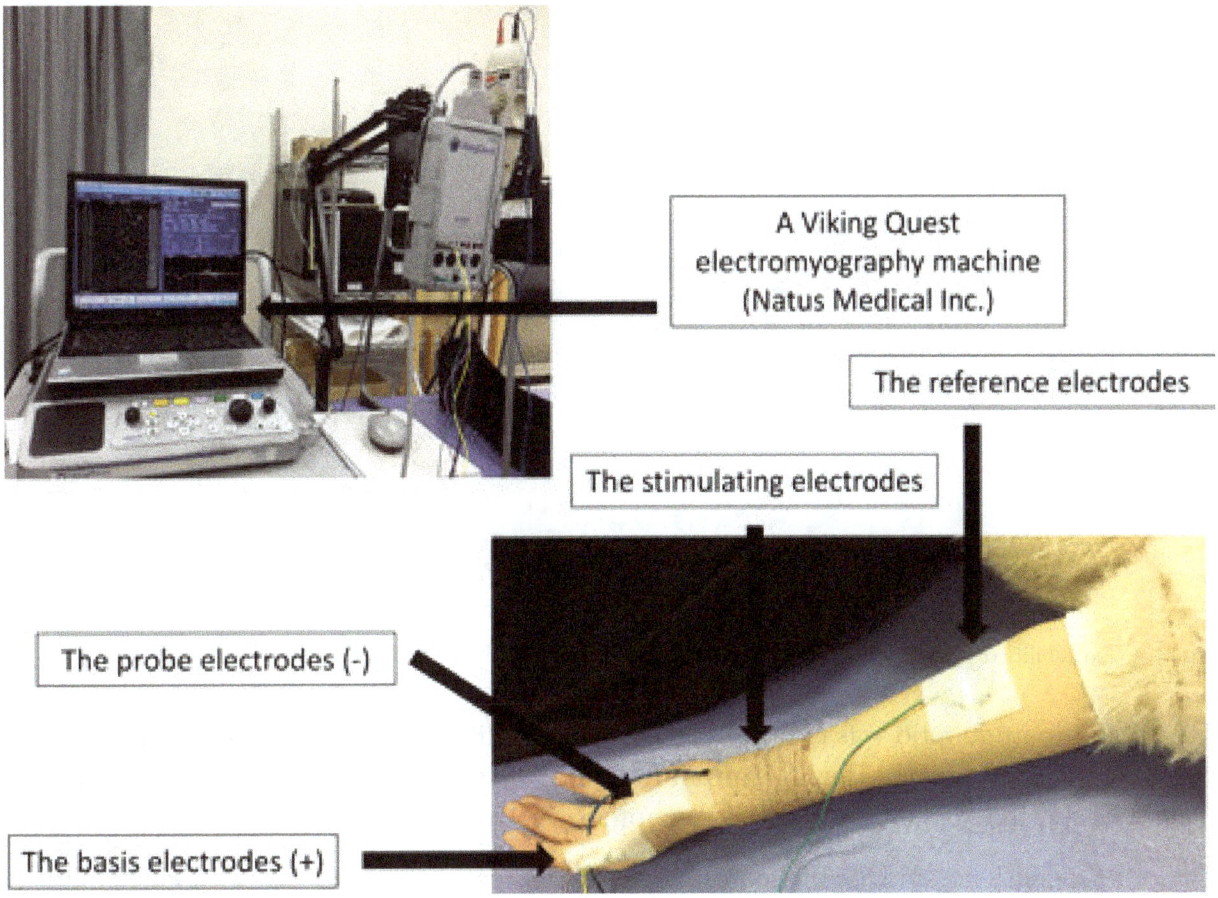


**Figure 3.** The F-wave testing conditions.

F-waves were analyzed with respect to persistence and the F/M amplitude ratio using 30 stimuli. Persistence was defined as the number of measurable F-wave responses divided by 30 supramaximal stimuli. Persistence reflects the number of backfiring anterior horn cells (**Figure 4**).

The F/M amplitude ratio was defined as the mean amplitude of all responses divided by the amplitude of the M-wave. The F/M amplitude ratio reflects the number of backfiring anterior horn cells and the excitability of individual anterior horn cells (**Figure 5**).

The number of measurable F-wave responses divided by 30 supramaximal stimuli. Persistence reflects the number of backfiring anterior horn cells. This case (17/30) × 100 = 56%

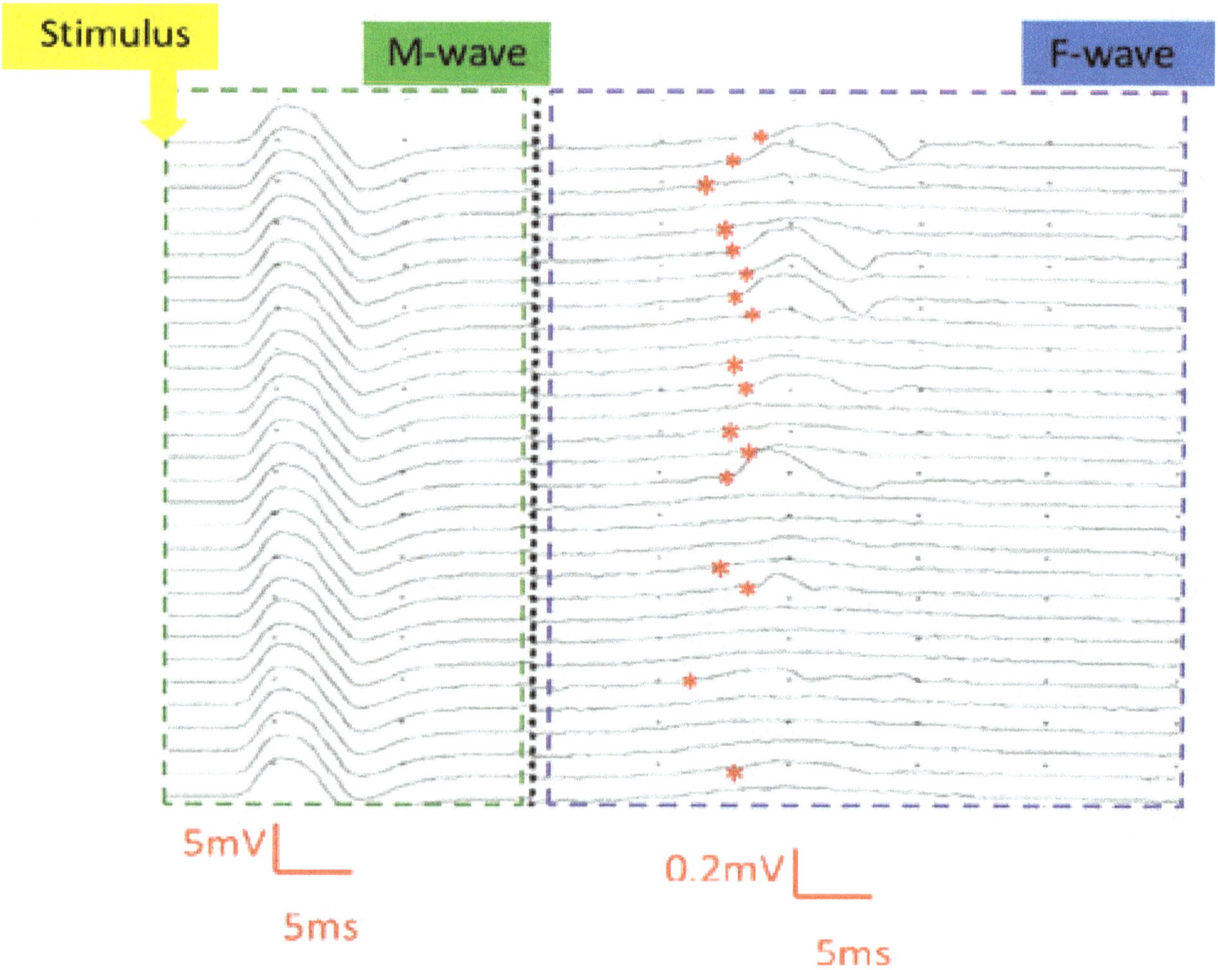


**Figure 4.** Excitability of spinal motor neurons examined for persistence.

The F/M amplitude ratio was defined as the mean amplitude of all responses divided by the amplitude of the M-wave. The F/M amplitude ratio reflects the number of backfiring anterior horn cells and the excitability of individual anterior horn cells.

Therefore, persistence and the F/M amplitude ratio are regarded as indices of the excitability of spinal motor neurons. In this study, provided that the excitability of spinal motor neurons in the motor imagery condition is significantly increased as compared to that in the touching a sensor condition, it may be improved by subjects performing motor imagery. Furthermore, we confirmed that no significant differences were observed in relative electromyogram integral values between the resting and touching a sensor conditions versus the motor imagery condition when using surface electromyography.

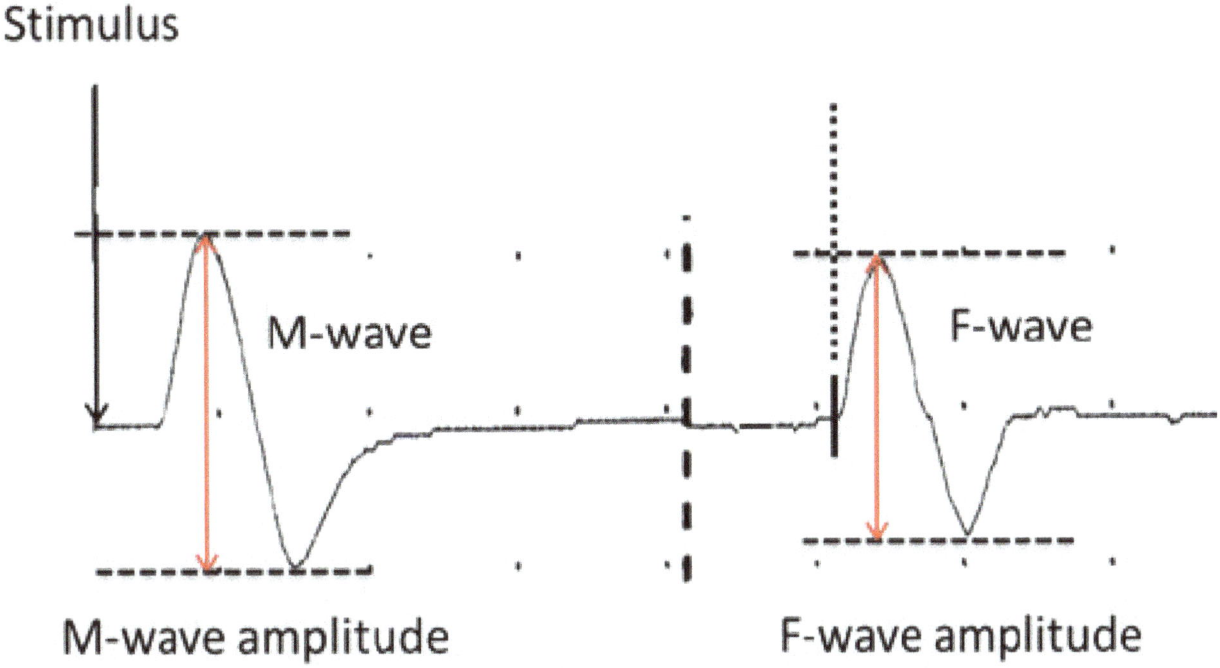


**Figure 5.** Excitability of spinal motor neurons examined for F/M amplitude ratio.

An index reflecting the accuracy of motion was applied, as follows. In this study, we defined two indexes representing the accuracy of motion (**Figure 6**). Since the index representing the accuracy of motion was not defined in the past literature, the first index used herein was correction time, which was the total time for 50 ± 5% MVC. Correction time reflects the ability to control the accuracy of muscle force in the pinch action. Blefari et al. [19] adopted an error range of ±5% as the index reflecting the accuracy of motion. Based on the aforementioned considerations, we adopted an error range of ±5%. We did this because our study and that of Blefari were similar in terms of adopting pinch action. The second index was the 50% MVC error, obtained by subtraction of the relative pinch force value at the 50% MVC from one. In addition, this index was converted to an absolute value, and then expressed as a percentage. The 50% MVC error reflects whether or not there is convergence on 50% MVC. The correction time and the 50% MVC error were calculated for the first trial and the second trial of the pinch task for the motor imagery and control groups. We measured the pinch force value using electromyogram recording software VitalRecorder2 (KISSEI COMTEC). We calculated two indexes reflecting the accuracy of motion using a versatile biological analysis system, the BIMUTAS-Video (KISSEI COMTEC). Provided that the index reflecting the accuracy of motion in the pinch task second trial is significantly improved as compared to that in the pinch task first trial, the effect of motor imagery is confirmed.

We defined two indexes reflecting the accuracy of motion. The first index was correction time (the total time of 50 ± 5% MVC). The second index was the 50% MVC error (derived by subtraction of the relative pinch force value at the 50% MVC from one, followed by conversion to an absolute value, and then expressed as a percentage).

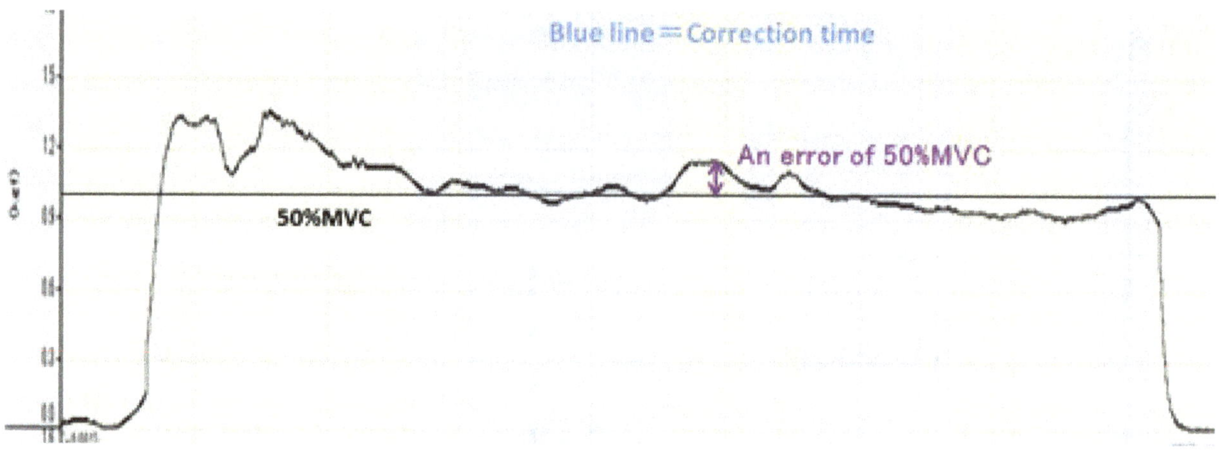


**Figure 6.** The index for the accuracy of motion.

Data analysis was carried out as follows. Statistical analysis for the normality of the distribution was performed using the Kolmogorov-Smirnov and Shapiro-Wilk tests. Because the data were not recognized as showing a normal distribution, the Friedman test was used to compare F-wave results among the resting, touching a sensor, motor imagery, and without motor imagery conditions. Thereafter, the Scheffe test was used to compare F-wave results across all conditions. Also, the Wilcoxon signed-rank test was used to compare correction time, the 50% MVC error between the first and second trials of the pinch task. The significance level was set at $p < 0.05$. We used SPSS ver. 19 for all statistical analyses.

## 4. Results

### 4.1. F-wave results

#### *4.1.1. F-wave results with a 10 s motor learning time*

In the motor imagery group when examined for persistence, the resting condition was 63.4 ± 22.7%, the touching a sensor condition was 78.1 ± 17.2%, and the motor imagery condition was 90.5 ± 9.6%. The persistence values under the touching a sensor and motor imagery conditions were significantly increased as compared to that of the resting condition. In addition, persistence was significantly increased in the motor imagery condition than in the touching a sensor condition (*$p < 0.05$, **$p < 0.01$, **Figure 7**). Accordingly, in the control group when examined for persistence, the resting condition was 47.4 ± 19.1%, the touching a sensor condition was 72.1 ± 16.5%, and in the condition without motor imagery was 67.5 ± 17.6%. The persistence values in the touching a sensor and without motor imagery conditions were significantly increased compared to that in the resting condition. However, no significant differences in persistence values were observed between the touching a sensor and without motor imagery conditions (*$p < 0.05$, **$p < 0.01$, **Figure 7**).

Next, in the motor imagery group when examined for the F/M amplitude ratio, the resting condition was 1.2 ± 0.6%, the touching a sensor condition was 1.8 ± 0.8% and the motor imagery condition was 2.2 ± 1.5%. The F/M amplitude ratio was significantly increased in the touching sensor and motor imagery conditions as compared to that in the resting condition. However, no significant differences in the F/M amplitude ratios were observed between the touching a sensor and the motor imagery conditions ($*p < 0.05$, $**p < 0.01$, **Figure 7**). Accordingly, in the control group when examined for the F/M amplitude ratio, the resting condition was 1.2 ± 0.5%, the touching a sensor condition was 1.9 ± 1.1%, and the condition without motor imagery was 1.8 ± 1.1%. The F/M amplitude ratio in the touching a sensor and without motor imagery conditions were significantly increased compared to that in the resting condition. However, no significant differences in the F/M amplitude ratios were observed between the touching a sensor and without motor imagery conditions ($*p < 0.05$, $**p < 0.01$, **Figure 7**).

In the motor imagery group, persistence values when examined in the touching the sensor and motor imagery conditions were significantly increased as compared to that in the resting condition. In addition, persistence was significantly increased in the motor imagery condition compared to that in the touching a sensor condition. The F/M amplitude ratio was significantly increased in the touching a sensor and motor imagery conditions than in the

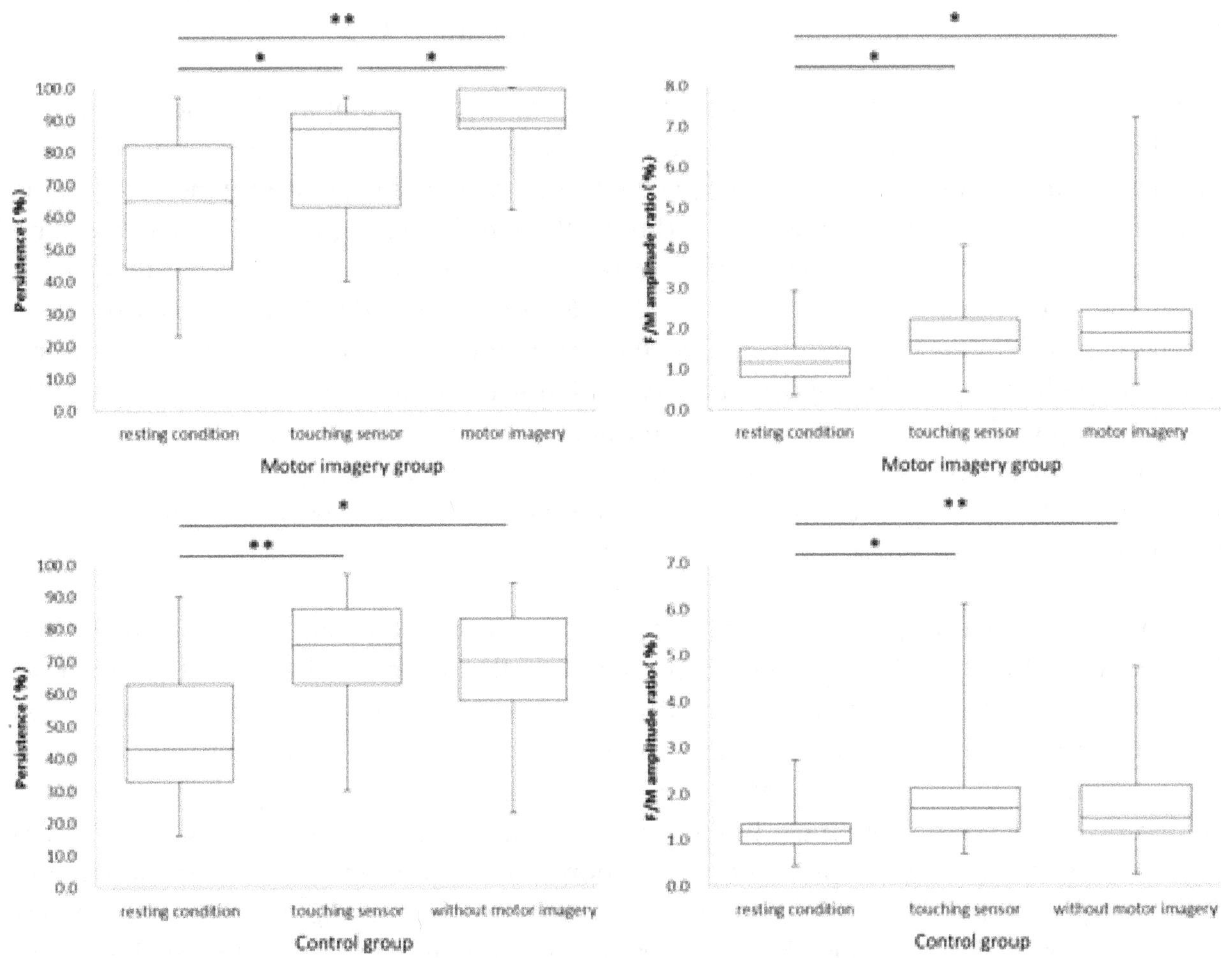


**Figure 7.** F-wave results.

resting condition. In the control group, the persistence values in the touching a sensor and without motor imagery conditions were significantly increased than that in the resting condition. The F/M amplitude ratios in the touching a sensor and without motor imagery conditions were shown to be significantly increased as compared to that in the resting condition.

#### *4.1.2. F-wave results with a 30 s motor learning time*

In the motor imagery group when examined for persistence, the resting condition was 55.6 ± 17.2%, the touching a sensor condition was 72.8 ± 14.3%, and the motor imagery condition was 84.5 ± 12.8%. The persistence values in the touching a sensor and motor imagery conditions were significantly increased as compared to that in the resting condition. In addition, the persistence value was significantly increased in the motor imagery condition than in the touching a sensor condition ($^{**}p < 0.01$, **Figure 8**). Accordingly, in the control group when examined for persistence, the resting condition was 54.3 ± 18.2%, the touching a sensor condition was 70.4 ± 14.4%, and the condition without motor imagery was 70.1 ± 17.7%. The persistence values in the touching a sensor and without motor imagery conditions were significantly increased as compared to that in the resting condition. However, no significant differences in the persistence values were observed between the touching a sensor and without motor imagery conditions ($^{**}p < 0.01$, **Figure 8**).

Next, in the motor imagery group when examined for the F/M amplitude ratio, the resting condition was 1.1 ± 0.7%, the touching a sensor condition was 1.5 ± 0.8%, and the motor imagery condition was 1.7 ± 0.8%. The F/M amplitude ratio was significantly increased in the touching a sensor and motor imagery conditions than in the resting condition. However, no significant differences in the F/M amplitude ratios were observed between the touching a sensor and motor imagery conditions ($^{**}p < 0.01$, **Figure 8**). Accordingly, in the control group when examined for the F/M amplitude ratio, the resting condition was 1.2 ± 0.7%, the touching a sensor condition was 1.5 ± 0.8%, and the condition without motor imagery was 1.6 ± 0.8%. The F/M amplitude ratios in the touching a sensor and without motor imagery conditions were significantly increased than that in the resting condition. However, no significant differences in the F/M amplitude ratios were observed between the touching a sensor and without motor imagery conditions ($^{*}p < 0.05$, $^{**}p < 0.01$, **Figure 8**).

In the motor imagery group, the persistence values in the touching a sensor and motor imagery conditions were significantly increased than that in the resting condition. In addition, the persistence value was significantly increased in the motor imagery condition as compared to that in the touching a sensor condition. The F/M amplitude ratio was observed to be significantly increased in the touching a sensor and motor imagery conditions as compared to the resting condition. In the control group, the persistence values in the touching a sensor and without motor imagery conditions were significantly increased than that in the resting condition. Next, the F/M amplitude ratios in the touching a sensor and without motor imagery conditions were observed to be significantly increased than that in the resting condition.

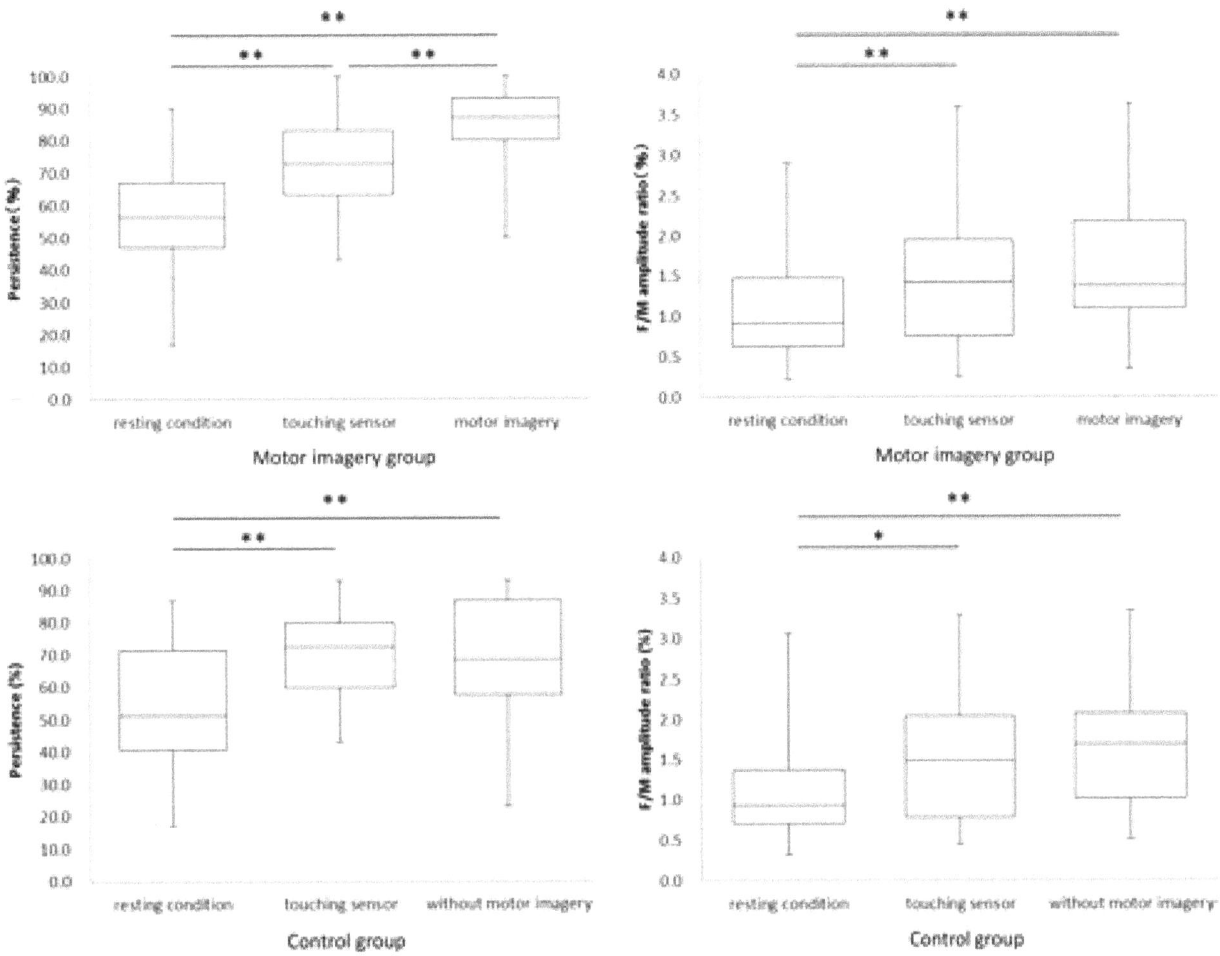


**Figure 8.** F-wave results.

### *4.1.3. F-wave results with a 1 min motor learning time*

In the motor imagery group when examined for persistence, the resting condition was 48.9 ± 20.3%, the touching a sensor condition was 69.1 ± 13.4%, and the motor imagery condition was 79.8 ± 10.4%. Persistence values in the touching a sensor and motor imagery conditions were significantly increased than that in the resting condition. In addition, persistence was significantly increased in the motor imagery condition as compared to the touching a sensor condition (**$p < 0.01$, $^{\#\#}p < 0.01$, **Figure 9**). Accordingly, in the control group when examined for persistence, the resting condition was 57.6 ± 20.5%, the touching a sensor condition was 74.5 ± 16.7%, and the condition without motor imagery was 68.2 ± 14.9%. Persistence values in the touching a sensor and without motor imagery conditions were significantly increased than that in the resting condition. No significant differences in the persistence values were observed between the touching a sensor and without motor imagery conditions (**$p < 0.01$, **Figure 9**).

Next, in the motor imagery group when examined for the F/M amplitude ratio, the resting condition was 1.8 ± 1.1%, the touching a sensor condition was 2.2 ± 1.2%, and the motor imagery condition was 2.6 ± 2.1%. The F/M amplitude ratio was significantly increased in the motor imagery than that in the resting condition (**$p < 0.01$, **Figure 9**). Accordingly, in the control group when examined for the F/M amplitude ratio, the resting condition was 1.5 ± 0.7%, the touching a sensor condition was 1.7 ± 0.9%, and the condition without motor imagery was 1.6 ± 0.9%. There were no significant differences in the F/M amplitude ratios among the three conditions (**Figure 9**).

In the motor imagery group, persistence values in the touching a sensor and motor imagery conditions were significantly increased as compared to that in the resting condition. In addition, persistence was significantly increased in the motor imagery condition as compared to the touching a sensor condition. The F/M amplitude ratio was observed to be significantly increased in the motor imagery condition as compared to that in the resting condition. In the control group, persistence values in the touching a sensor and without motor imagery conditions were significantly increased than that in the resting condition. There were no significant differences in the F/M amplitude ratios among the three conditions.

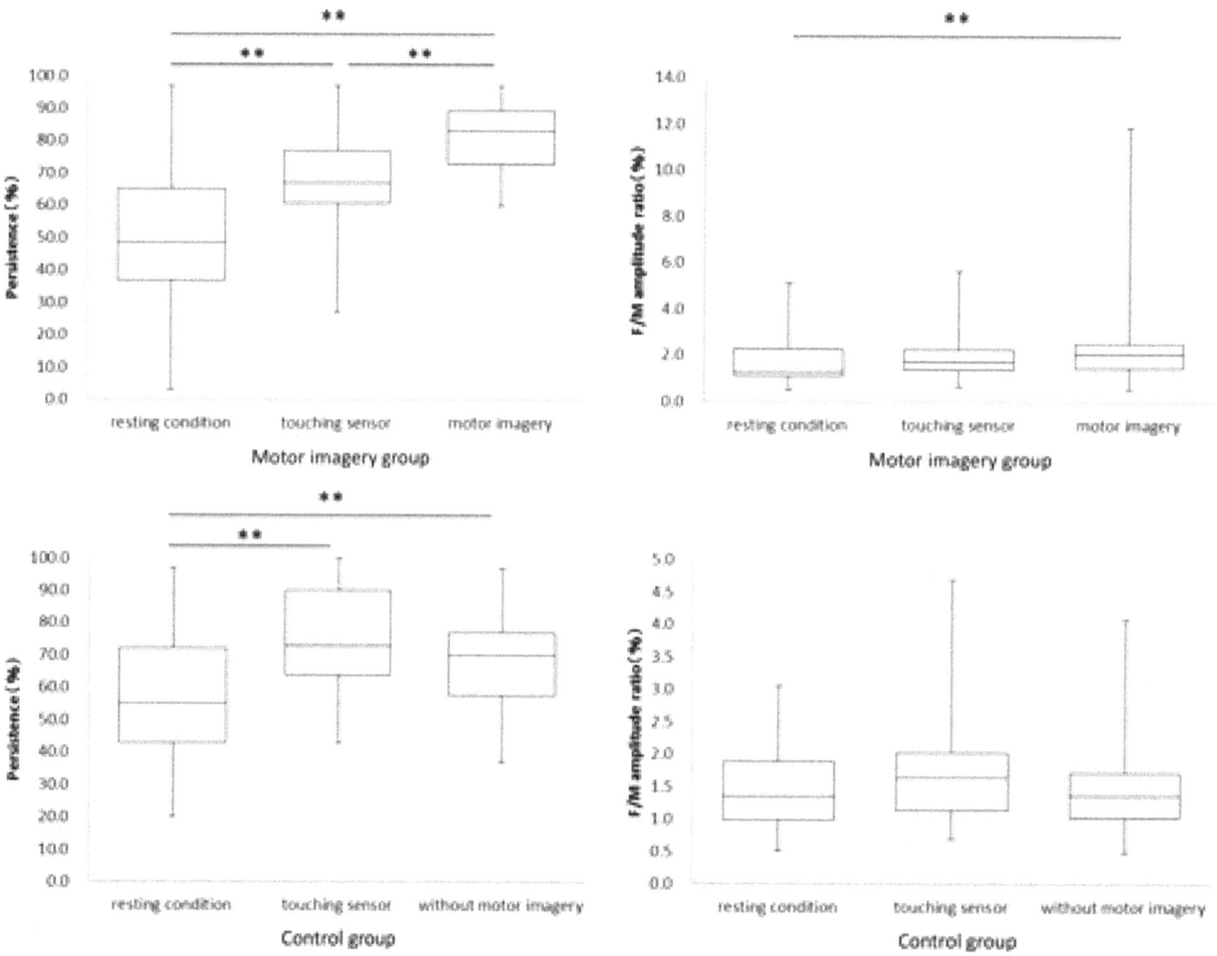


**Figure 9.** F-wave results.

*4.1.4. F-wave results with a 2 min motor learning time*

In the motor imagery group when examined for persistence, the resting condition was 63.7±14.2%, the touching a sensor condition was 72.8 ± 15.2%, and the motor imagery condition was 85.2 ± 14.1%. Persistence values in the touching a sensor and motor imagery conditions were significantly increased as compared to that in the resting condition. In addition, persistence was significantly increased in the motor imagery condition as compared to the touching a sensor condition ($^{**}p < 0.01$, $^{\#\#}\ p < 0.01$, **Figure 10**). Accordingly, in the control group when examined for persistence, the resting condition was 58.0 ± 19.9%, the touching a sensor condition was 75.7 ± 15.0% and the condition without motor imagery was 75.6 ± 15.2%. Persistence values in the touching a sensor and without motor imagery conditions were significantly increased than that in the resting condition. No significant differences in the

conditions ($^{**}p < 0.01$, **Figure 10**).

Next, in the motor imagery group when examined for the F/M amplitude ratio, the resting condition was 1.1 ± 0.5%, the touching a sensor condition was 1.3 ± 0.6%, and the motor imagery condition was 1.4 ± 0.6%. The F/M amplitude ratios were significantly increased in the touching a sensor and motor imagery conditions than that in the resting condition. However, no significant differences in the F/M amplitude ratios were observed between the touching a sensor and motor imagery conditions ($^{*}p < 0.05$, $^{**}p < 0.01$, **Figure 10**). Accordingly, in the control group when examined for the F/M amplitude ratio, the resting condition was 1.1 ± 0.7%, the touching a sensor condition was 1.3 ± 0.7%, and the condition without motor imagery was 1.4 ± 0.6%. The F/M amplitude ratios were significantly increased in the

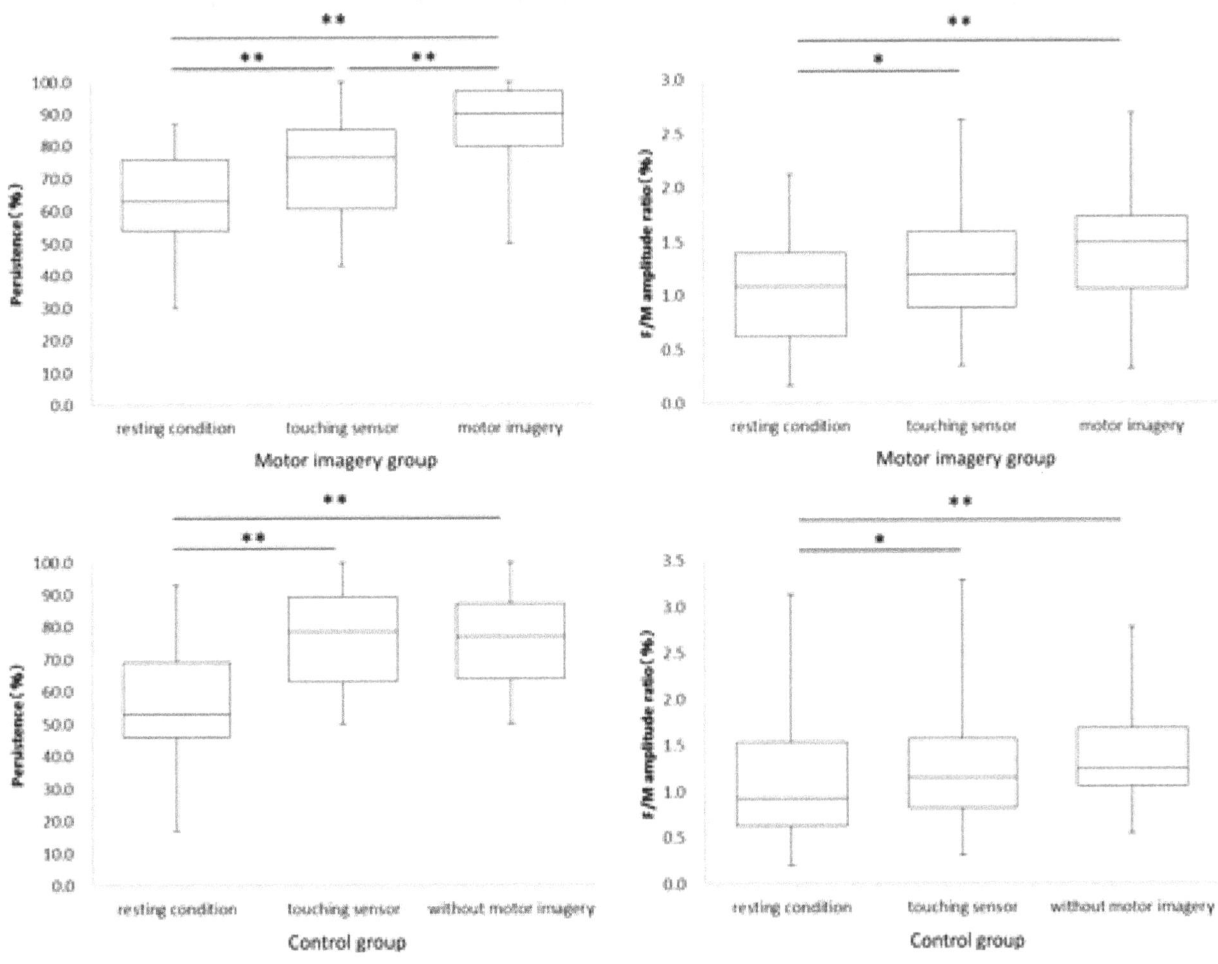


**Figure 10.** F-wave results.

touching a sensor and without motor imagery conditions than that in the resting condition. However, no significant differences in the F/M amplitude ratios were observed between the touching a sensor and without motor imagery conditions (*$p < 0.05$, **$p < 0.01$, **Figure 10**).

In the motor imagery group, persistence values in the touching a sensor and motor imagery conditions were significantly increased as compared to that in the resting condition. In addition, persistence was significantly increased in the motor imagery condition as compared to the touching a sensor condition. The F/M amplitude ratios were significantly increased in the touching a sensor and motor imagery conditions as compared to the resting condition. In the control group, persistence values in the touching a sensor and without motor imagery conditions were significantly increased as compared to that in the resting condition. The F/M amplitude ratios were significantly increased in the touching a sensor and without motor imagery conditions as compared to the resting condition.

## 4.2. The index for the accuracy of motion results

### *4.2.1. The index for the accuracy of motion results with a 10 s motor learning time*

In the motor imagery group when examined for the correction time, the pinch task first trial was 1.2 ± 1.5 s and the pinch task second trial was 0.7 ± 1.6 s. No significant differences were observed in the correction time between the first and second trials of the pinch task (**Figure 11**).

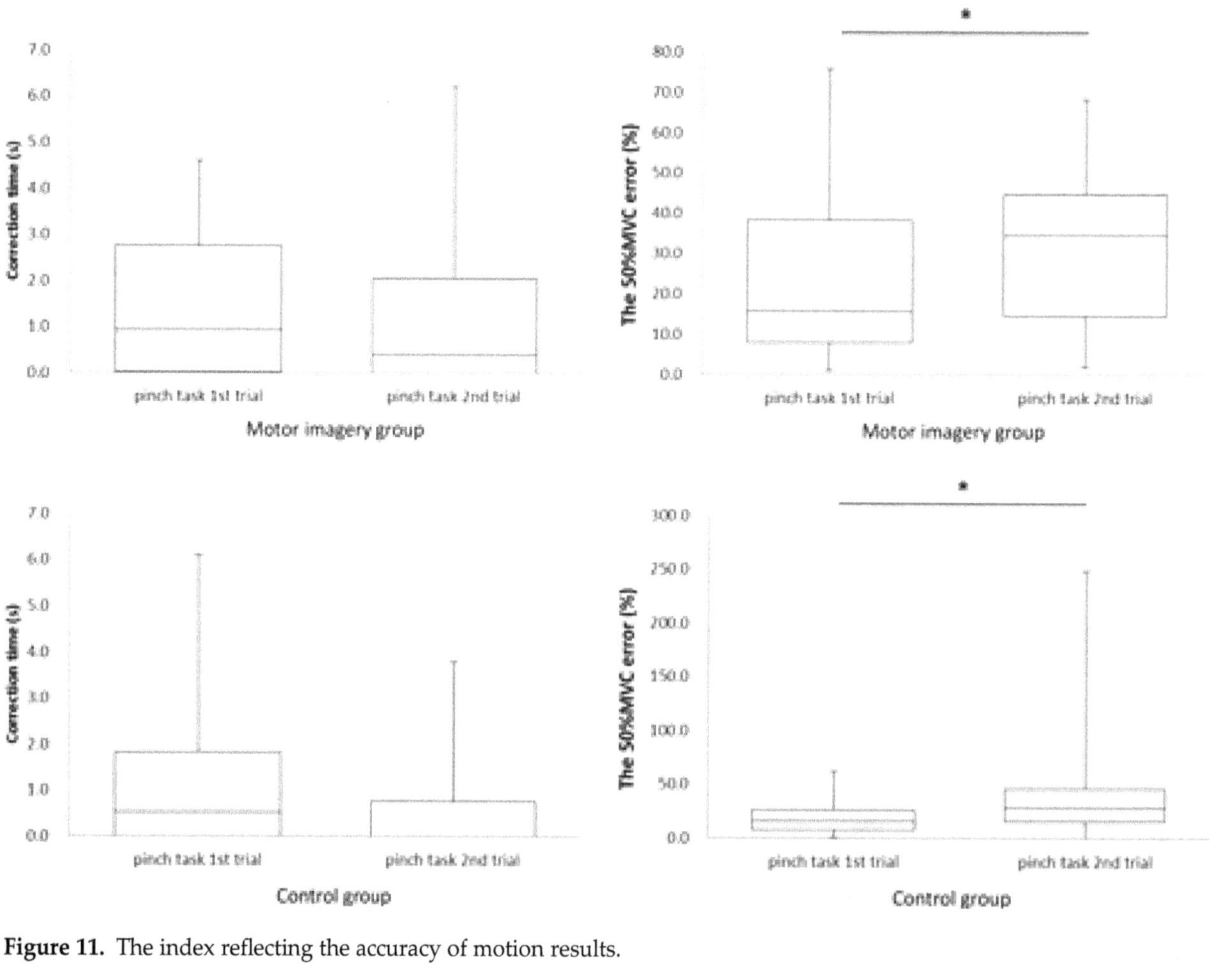


**Figure 11.** The index reflecting the accuracy of motion results.

Accordingly, in the control group when examined for the correction time, the pinch task first trial was 1.2 ± 1.7 s and the pinch task second trial was 0.7 ± 1.2 s. No significant differences were observed in the correction time between the first and second trials of the pinch task (**Figure 11**).

Next, in the motor imagery group at the 50% MVC error, the pinch task first trial was 25.7 ± 21.9% and the pinch task second trial was 32.3 ± 18.5%. The 50% MVC error was significantly increased in the second than in the first trial of the pinch task (*$p < 0.05$, **Figure 11**). Accordingly, in the control group at the 50% MVC error, the pinch task first trial was 20.9 ± 17.2% and the pinch task second trial was 36.3 ± 44.3%. The 50% MVC error was significantly increased in the second than in the first trial of the pinch task (*$p < 0.05$, **Figure 11**).

In the motor imagery group, no significant differences were observed in the correction time between the first and second trials of the pinch task. The 50% MVC error was significantly increased in the second as compared to the first trial of the pinch task. In the control group, no significant differences were observed in the correction time between the first and second trials of the pinch task. The 50% MVC error was significantly increased in the second than in the first trial of the pinch task.

#### *4.2.2. The index for the accuracy of motion results with a 30 s motor learning time*

In the motor imagery group when examined for the correction time, the pinch task first trial was 1.8 ± 1.9 s and the pinch task second trial was 1.8 ± 1.8 s. No significant differences were observed in the correction times between the first and second trials of the pinch task (**Figure 12**). Accordingly, in the control group when examined for the correction time, the pinch task first trial was 1.5 ± 1.6 s and the pinch task second trial was 0.9 ± 1.3 s. The correction time was significantly decreased in the second than in the first trial of the pinch task (*$p < 0.05$, **Figure 12**).

In the motor imagery group at the 50% MVC error, the pinch task first trial was 25.6 ± 18.8% and the pinch task second trial was 27.4 ± 22.3%. No significant differences were observed at the 50% MVC error between the first and second trials of the pinch task (**Figure 12**). Accordingly, in the control group at the 50% MVC error, the pinch task first trial was 21.1 ± 17.2% and the pinch task second trial was 31.9 ± 28.3%. The 50% MVC was significantly increased in the second than in the first trial of the pinch task (*$p < 0.05$, **Figure 12**).

In the motor imagery group, no significant differences were observed in the correction time or the 50% MVC error between the first and second trials of the pinch task. In the control group, the correction time was significantly decreased in the second than in the first trial of the pinch task. The 50% MVC error was significantly increased in the second than in the first trial of the pinch task.

#### *4.2.3. The index for the accuracy of motion results with a 1 min motor learning time*

In the motor imagery group when examined for the correction time, the pinch task first trial was 1.5 ± 1.6 s and the pinch task second trial was 1.3 ± 1.8 s. No significant differences were observed in correction time between the first and second trials of the pinch task (**Figure 13**). Accordingly, in the control group when examined for the correction time, the

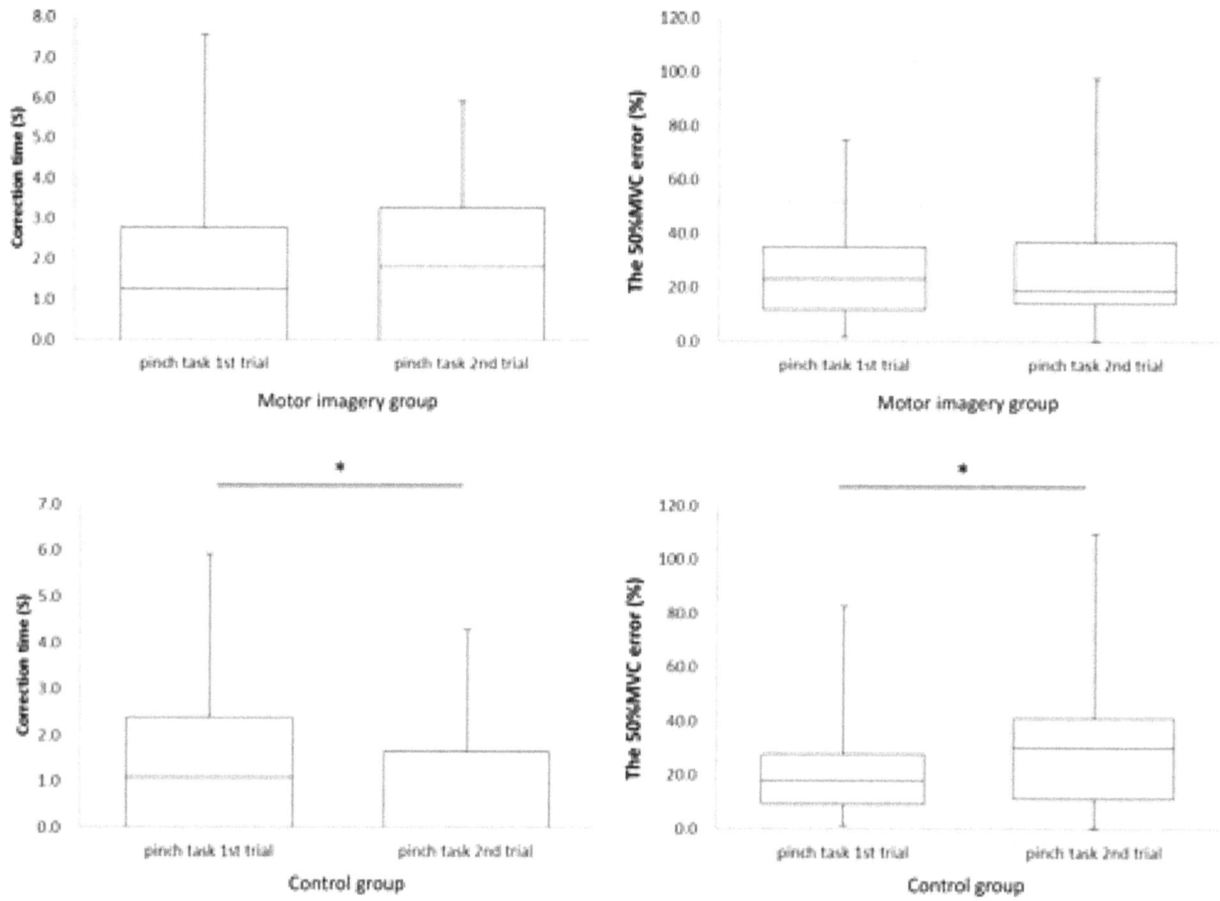


**Figure 12.** The index for the accuracy of motion results.

pinch task first trial was 1.5 ± 1.9 s and the pinch task second trial was 0.9 ± 1.3 s. Correction time was significantly decreased in the second as compared to the first trial of the pinch task. (**$p < 0.01$, **Figure 13**).

Next, in the motor imagery group at the 50% MVC error, the pinch task first trial was 21.5 ± 16.7% and the pinch task second trial was 24.7 ± 22.7%. No significant differences were observed in the 50% MVC error between the first and second trials of the pinch task (**Figure 13**). Accordingly, in the control group at the 50% MVC error, the pinch task first trial was 28.1 ± 29.1% and the pinch task second trial was 38.9 ± 40.4%. The 50% MVC error was significantly increased in the second than in the first trial of the pinch task (*$p < 0.05$, **Figure 13**).

In the motor imagery group, no significant differences were observed in correction time or the 50% MVC error between the first and second trials of the pinch task. In the control group, correction time was significantly decreased in the second than in the first trial of the pinch task. The 50% MVC error was significantly increased in the second than in the first trial of the pinch task.

#### *4.2.4. The index for the accuracy of motion results with a 2 min motor learning time*

In the motor imagery group when examined for the correction time, the pinch task first trial was 1.2 ± 1.7 s and the pinch task second trial was 1.3 ± 1.8 s. No significant differences were

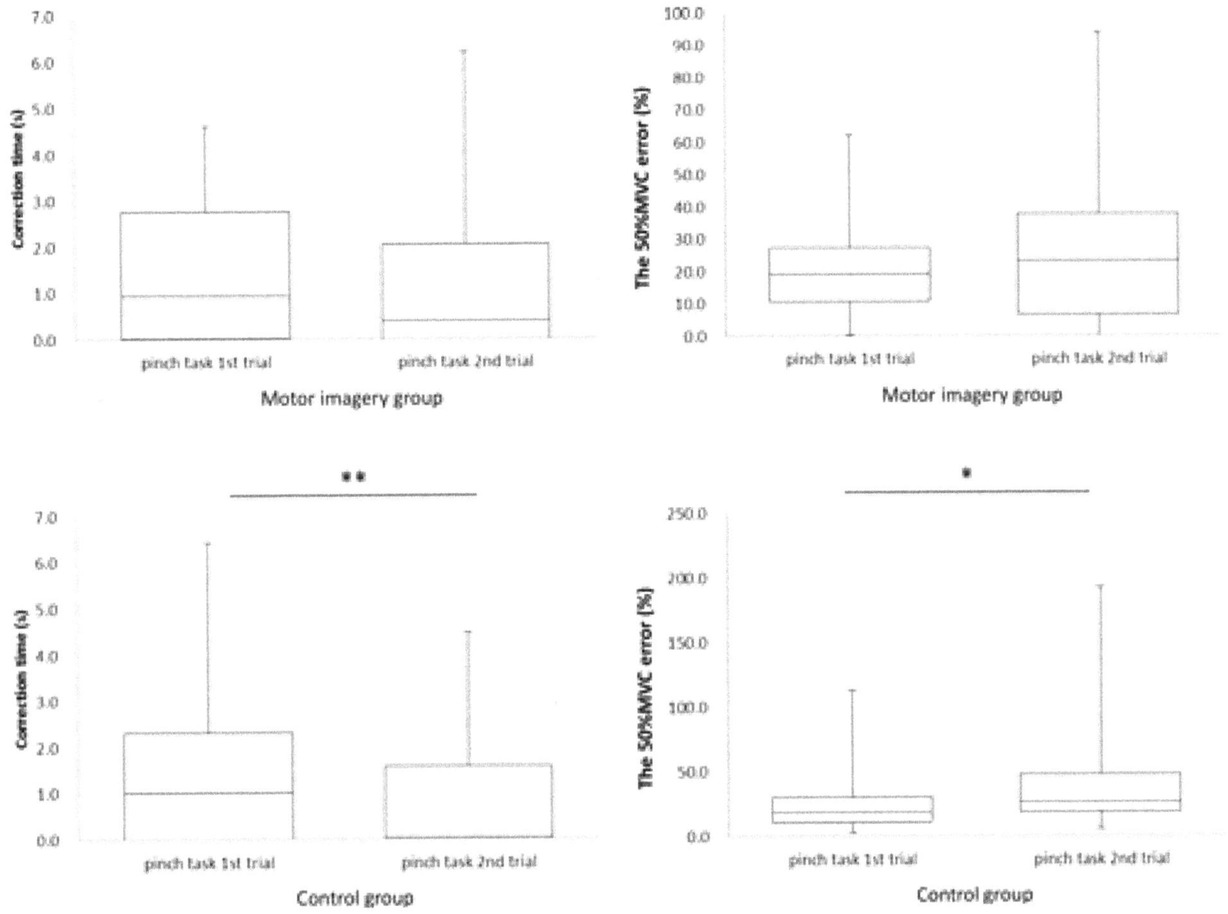


**Figure 13.** The index for the accuracy of motion results.

observed in correction time between the first and second trials of the pinch task (**Figure 14**). Accordingly, in the control group when examined for the correction time, the pinch task first trial was 1.6 ± 2.2 s and the pinch task second trial was 0.8 ± 1.2 s. Correction time was significantly decreased in the second than in the first trial of the pinch task ($*p < 0.05$, **Figure 14**).

In the motor imagery group at the 50% MVC error, the pinch task first trial was 25.3 ± 26.3% and the pinch task second trial was 36.8 ± 36.8%. The 50% MVC error was significantly increased in the second than that in the first trial of the pinch task ($*p < 0.05$, **Figure 14**). Accordingly, in the control group at the 50% MVC error, the pinch task first trial was 21.7 ± 17.4% and the pinch task second trial was 29.6 ± 25.7%. The 50% MVC error was significantly increased in the second as compared to that the first trial of the pinch task. ($*p < 0.05$, **Figure 14**).

In the motor imagery group, no significant differences were observed in correction time between the first and second trials of the pinch task. The 50% MVC error was significantly increased in the second than that in the first trial of the pinch task. In the control group, correction time was significantly decreased in the second as compared to that in the first trial of the pinch task. The 50% MVC error was significantly increased in the second than that in the first trial of the pinch task.

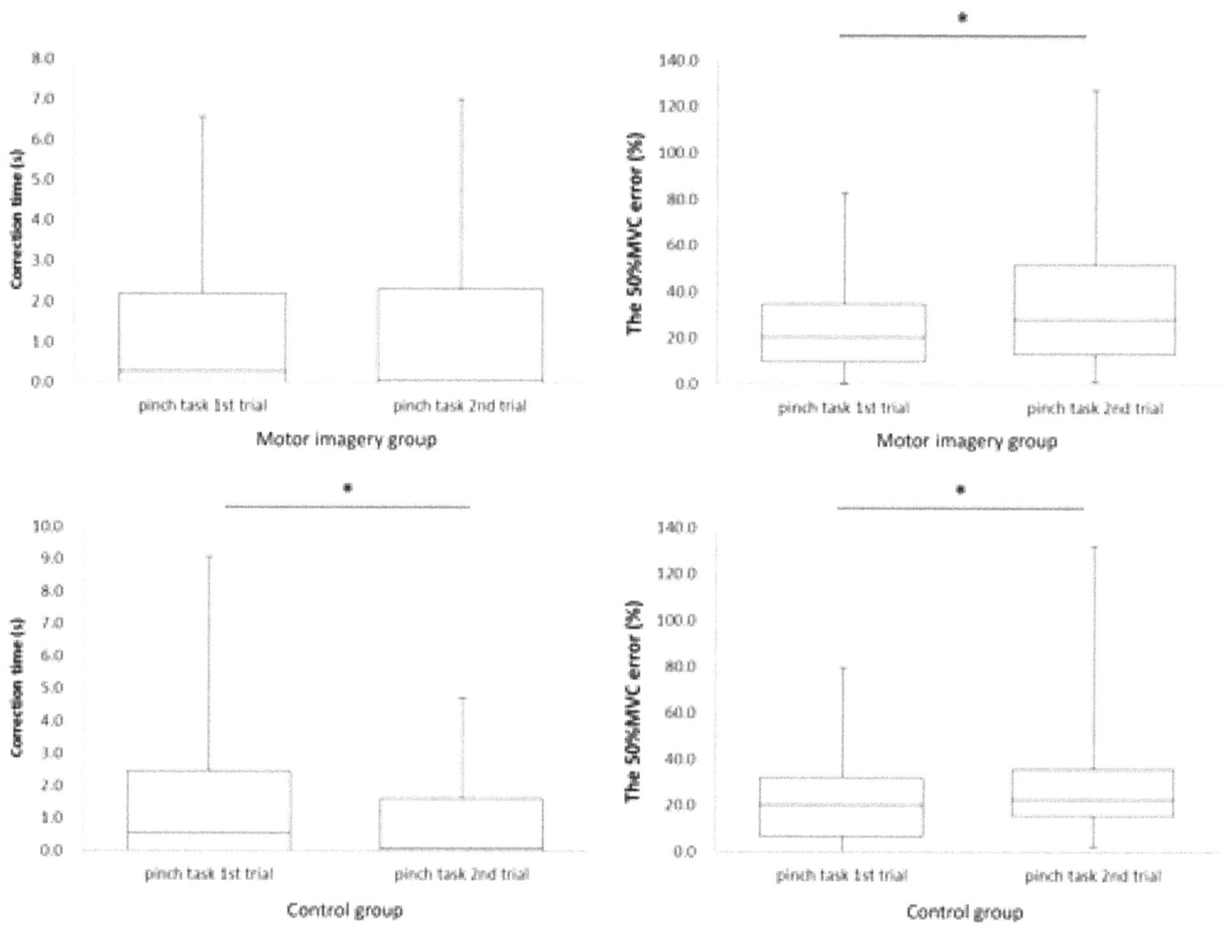


**Figure 14.** The index for the accuracy of motion results.

# 5. Discussion

## 5.1. The factor indicating increased spinal motor neuron excitability

The excitability of spinal motor neurons under the motor imagery condition was increased than that of spinal motor neurons at rest and in the touching a sensor condition. We attribute this to the influence of the descending pathways corresponding to the thenar muscle. In contrast, excitatory inputs travel through the corticospinal pathway and reticulospinal tract and from the corticospinal pathway and extrapyramidal tract to anterior horn cells. Suzuki et al. [11] reported the excitability of spinal motor neurons in the motor imagery condition to be influenced by the descending pathways from the cerebral nervous system. Furthermore, activation of the primary motor area, supplementary motor area, premotor area, primary somatosensory area, dorsolateral prefrontal area, cingulate cortex, and cerebellar regions occurred during motor imagery [4–7]. Therefore, activation of the cerebral cortex in the motor imagery condition presumably increased the excitability of spinal motor neurons via the corticospinal pathway and extrapyramidal tract. The subjects performed motor imagery while touching a pinch meter sensor. Therefore, the influences of tactile and proprioceptive inputs should be considered. Mizuguchi et al. [20, 21] reported that the responsiveness of afferent pathways to the primary somatosensory area during motor imagery while utilizing an object was modulated by a combination of tactile and proprioceptive inputs while touching the object. Tactile and proprioceptive inputs from the periphery are integrated after they have been hierarchically processed and then projected to the primary motor area. Furthermore, Suzuki et al. [11] reported that the excitability of spinalmotorneurons with motorimageryunderthe"with sensor" condition was increased than that of the spinal motor neurons with motor imagery under the "without sensor" condition. Thus, tactile and proprioceptive inputs while touching the pinch meter sensor would presumably increase the excitability of spinal motor neurons as part of a synergistic effect. Therefore, we hypothesized that our subjects might perform some form of motor imagery.

### 5.2. The effect of motor imagery on the accuracy of motion

With a motor learning time of 10 s, no significant differences were observed in the correction times between the first and second trials of the pinch task in either the motor imagery group or the control group. The correction time reflects the ability to control the accuracy of muscle force during the pinch action. We attributed this to numerous zero second correction times from the first trial and to the second trial of the pinch task. Surely, the subject could not be learning 50% MVC with a motor learning time of only 10 s. Accordingly, the correction time was not changed after versus before motor imagery or in the condition without motor imagery. The 50% MVC error was significantly increased in the second than that in the first trial of the pinch task in both the motor imagery and the control group. The error in 50% MVC reflects whether or not there is convergence on 50% MVC. Provided that the pinch value obtained represents convergence on 50% MVC, the 50% MVC error is decreased in the second trial as compared to the first trial of the pinch task. Conversely, provided that the pinch value obtained does not represent convergence on 50% MVC, the 50% MVC error is increased in the second than that in the first trial of the pinch task. Given these observations, our results suggest that motor imagery does not improve the ability to achieve accurate motion after motor learning for 10 s. Mulder et al. [22] reported that motor imagery improved the ability to achieve actual motion only in people with learning that corresponded to the motor imagery task. Accordingly, the subjects might not be able to learn the 50% MVC in only 10 s. Thus, it is necessary for the learning of subjects to correspond fully to the motor task. We conclude that adequate learning time should be provided in future studies.

With a motor learning time of 30 s, no significant differences were observed in the correction time between the first and second trials of the pinch task in the motor imagery group. Accordingly, the correction time was significantly decreased in the second than that in the first trial of the pinch task in the control group. These results suggest that the accuracy of motion was decreased in the control group. If the correction time is increased after motor imagery, the index of the accuracy of motion would be improved in the second trial as compared to the first trial of the pinch task. Conversely, the correction time should be decreased if there is no improvement in the accuracy of motion. Ronsse et al. [23] reported that the effectiveness of motor learning with the use of visual feedback was decreased over time with periodic flexion and extension at both wrist joints. Ohashi et al. [24] reported that the information pertaining to the intensity of force in an isometric contraction task was decreased over the course of time. In this study, the subjects carried out motor learning with isometric contraction and using visual feedback. Accordingly, if accurate motion was acquired with motor learning for 30 s, it was decreased over the course of time under inactive conditions. On the other hand, the accuracy of motion was not decreased between the first and second trials of the pinch task when performing motor imagery. Therefore, the accuracy of motion might be maintained by motor imagery after motor learning for 30 s. However, in our previous study, motor imagery after motor learning for 10 s failed to maintain accurate motion. It was concluded that a motor learning time of 10 s was insufficient, while 30 s was sufficient. In the motor imagery group, no significant differences were observed in the 50% MVC error between the first and second trials of the pinch task. However, in the control group, the 50% MVC error was significantly increased in the second than that in the first trial of the pinch task. Provided that the pinch value does not represent convergence on 50% MVC, the 50% MVC error would be increased in the second than that in the first trial of the pinch task. Consequently, the accuracy of motion was maintained only in the motor imagery group, results consistent with those for the correction time. Taken together, the present results suggest that motor imagery after 30 s of motor learning is found to be strongly involved in the accuracy of motion. In future studies, it will be necessary to extend the motor learning time before attempting motor imagery. Such a strategy will allow us to study the effects of motor imagery on the accuracy of motion.

With a motor learning time of 1 min, no significant differences were observed in correction time between the first and second trials of the pinch task in the motor imagery group. However, correction time was significantly decreased in the second than that in the first trial of the pinch task in the control group. We obtained the same result in our previous study. This study used isometric contraction and visual feedback at the time of motor learning. Accordingly, the effectiveness of motor learning was maintained only doing motor imagery. Moreover, we compared the pinch force in several pinch tasks between the motor imagery and control groups. In the motor imagery group, we found that the pinch force in the pinch task second trial generated a more authentic 50% MVC than the pinch task first trial in approximately half of all subjects. However, in the control group, the pinch force in the pinch task second trial generated a more authentic 50% MVC than the pinch task first trial in approximately 20% of all subjects. The motor imagery after motor learning for 1 min might show slight improvement in the accuracy of motion. No significant differences were observed at the 50% MVC error between the first and second trials of the pinch task in the motor imagery group. In the control group, however, the 50% MVC error was significantly increased in the second than that in the first trial of the pinch task. The same results were obtained in our previous study. Furthermore, these results were consistent with the correction time results. Taken together, these observations suggest the accuracy of motion to be maintained or even slightly improved by performing motor imagery after motor learning for 1 min. We believe that motor imagery can be adjusted for the variety and total number of mobilized motor units (recruitment), the firing rate of motor units (rate coding), the congruence of each motor unit activity timing (synchronization), the revision of motor programs, and so forth. In conclusion, for successful motor imagery, it is necessary for the subject to completely learn the corresponding motor task.

Finally, with a motor learning time of 2 min, no significant differences were observed in correction time between the first and second trials of the pinch task in the motor imagery group. In the control group, however, correction time was significantly decreased in the second than that in the first trial of the pinch task. The same result was obtained in our previous study. However, the 50% MVC error was significantly increased in the second than that in the first trial of the pinch task in both the motor imagery group and the control group. These results would appear to contradict the previously mentioned results for the correction time. This apparent contradiction is attributable to the correction time and the 50% MVC error differing slightly in meaning. Specifically, the 50% MVC error was increased in the second than in the first trial of the pinch task. Moreover, the aim of falling within 50 ± 5% MVC on both the first trial and the second trial of the pinch task was missed by many subjects. These subjects maintained accurate motion when viewing the correction time, but did not maintain an error 50% MVC without visualization. These subjects experienced muscle fatigue after motor learning for 2 min. Thus, we compared MVC of the pinch force after versus before motor learning. We found the MVC of the pinch force to be decreased after as compared to before motor learning in most of the subjects experiencing muscle fatigue. Vøllestad [25] reported that muscle fatigue was defined as a decrease in the ability to exert maximum muscle strength with some form of motion. In addition, Higashi et al. [26] reported that the 50% MVC isometric contraction task produced recognizable muscle fatigue over the course of time. In this study, the subjects may have been exerting 50% MVC pinch force for 2 min. In reality, however, the subjects might have gradually exerted 50% MVC with excessive pinch force influencing muscle fatigue. Accordingly, the subjects experiencing muscle fatigue were learning 50% MVC and exceeded the pinch value. Consequently, these subjects might not have been able to maintain accurate motion, because the motor imagery was not correct.

## 6. Conclusion

Motor imagery increases the excitability of spinal motor neurons. Furthermore, motor imagery may improve the accuracy of motion. In such an event, however, it is important to acquire memory corresponding to the motor imagery task in motor learning. Specifically, it is necessary to take account of the motor learning time. Motor learning times optimally range from 30 s to 1 min. In future studies, it will be important to apply a motor learning method with a motor learning time of 30 s to 1 min. Salmoni et al. [27] reported that motor learning may be impeded by excessive feedback information. It is necessary the concentration time focused on the internal information to be incorporated into a revision of the motor program. In this study, the subjects performed motor learning with continuous visual feedback. Winstein et al. [28] proposed that the learner should gradually be given decreased feedback (Faded Feedback). Also, Lavery et al. [29] proposed that the learner's experience should be combined with summarized feedback (Summary Feedback). Additionally, Sherwood et al. [30] proposed that the learner should be aware of when deviation from the constant bandwidth occurs (Bandwidth Feedback). Schmidt et al. [31] reported that learner paid attention to internal information based on these investigator's methods of motor learning. The above observations highlight the importance of the motor leaning method. We should thus study the effects of motor imagery on the accuracy of motion.

## Author details

Yuki Fukumoto[1]* and Yoshibumi Bunno[2]

*Address all correspondence to: fukumoto_3197@yahoo.co.jp

1 Graduate School of Health Sciences, Graduate School of Kansai University of Health Sciences, Osaka, Japan

2 Clinical Physical Therapy Laboratory, Faculty of Health Sciences, Kansai University of Health Sciences, Osaka, Japan

## References

[1] Farah MJ. The neural basis of mental imagery. Trends Neuroscience. 1989; 12(10): 395–399.

[2] Jeannerod M, Decety J, et al. Mental motor imagery: A window into the representational stage of action. Current Opinion in Neurobiology. 1995; 5(6): 727–732.

[3] Decety J. The neurophysiological basis of motor imagery. Behavioural Brain Research. 1996; 77(1–2): 45–52.

[4] Nakano H. Ueta K. Osumi M. et al. Brain activity during the observation, imagery, and execution of tool use: An fNIRS/EEG study. Journal of Novel Physiotherapy. 2012; S1-009: 1–7.

[5] Luft AR, Skalej M, Stefanou A, et al. Comparing motion- and imagery-related activation in the human cerebellum: A functional MRI study. Human Brain Mapping. 1998; 6(2): 105–113.

[6] Stephan KM, Fink GR, Passingham RE, et al. Functional anatomy of the mental representation of upper extremity movements in healthy subjects. Journal of Neurophysiology. 1995; 73(1): 373–386.

[7] Lotze M. Montoya P. Erb M. et al. Activation of cortical and cerebellar motor areas during executed and imagined hand movements: An fMRI study. Journal of Cognitive Neuroscience. 1999; 11(5): 491–501.

[8] Mesrati F, Vecchierini MF. F-waves neurophysiology and clinical value. Clinical Neurophysiology. 2004; 34(5): 217–243.

[9] Fisher MA. F-waves-physiology and clinical uses. Scientific World Journal. 2007; 7(1): 144–160.

[10] Palmieri RM. Ingersoll CD. Hoffman MA. The Hoffmann reflex: Methodologic considerations and applications for use in sports medicine and athletic training research. Journal of Athletic Training. 2004; 39(3): 268–277

[11] Suzuki T, Bunno Y, Onigata C, et al. Excitability of spinal neural function by motor imagery with isometric opponens pollicis activity: Influence of vision during motor imagery. Neuro Rehabilitation. 2014; 34(4): 725–729.

[12] Taniguchi S, Kimura J, Yamada T, et al. Effect of motion imagery to counter rest-induced suppression of F-wave as a measure of anterior horn cell excitability. Clinical Neurophysiology. 2008; 119(6): 1346–1352.

[13] Kasai T, Kawai S, Kawanishi M, et al. Evidence for facilitation of motor evoked potentials (MEPs) induced by motor imagery. Brain Research. 1997; 744(1): 147–150.

[14] Oishi K, Kimura M, Yasukawa M, et al. Amplitude reduction of H-reflex during mental movement simulation in elite athletes. Behavioural Brain Research. 1994; 62(1): 55–61.

[15] Yue G, Cole KJ. Strength increases from of motor program: Comparison of training with maximal voluntary and imagined muscle contractions. Journal of Neurophysiology. 1992; 67(5): 1114–1123.

[16] Guillot A, Tolleron C, Collet C. Does motor imagery enhance stretching and flexibility? Journal of Sports Science. 2010; 28(3): 291–298.

[17] Page SJ, Levine P, Sisto SA, et al. Mental practice combined with physical practice for upper-limb motor deficit in subacute stroke. Journal of Physical Therapy. 2001; 81(8): 1455–1462.

[18] Dickstein R, Dunsky A, Marcovitz E. Motor imagery for gait rehabilitation in post-stroke hemiparesis. Journal of Physical Therapy. 2004; 84(12): 1167–1177.

[19] Blefari ML, Sulzer J, Hepp-Reymond MC, et al. Improvement in precision grip force control with self-modulation of primary motor cortex during motor imagery. Frontiers in Behavioral Neuroscience. 2015; 18(9): 1–11.

[20] Mizuguchi N, Sakamoto M, Muraoka T, et al. Influence of touching an object on corticospinal excitability during motor imagery. Experimental Brain Research. 2009; 196 (4): 529–535.

[21] Mizuguchi N, Sakamoto M, Muraoka T, et al. The modulation of corticospinal excitability during motor imagery of actions with objects. PLoS ONE. 2011; 6(10): e26006.

[22] Mulder T, Zijlstra S, Zijlstra W, et al. The role of motor imagery in learning a totally novel movement. Experimental Brain Research. 2004; 154(2): 211–217.

[23] Ronsse R, Puttemans V, Coxon JP, et al. Motor learning with augmented feedback: Modality-dependent behavioral and neural consequences. Cerebral Cortex. 2010; 21(6): 1283–1294.

[24] Ohashi Y. A study for retention characteristics of iosometric force information. Journal of the Japanese Physical Therapy Association. 1993; 20(6): 355–359 (in Japanese).

[25] Vøllestad NK. Measurement of human muscle fatigue. Journal of Neuroscience Methods. 1997; 74(2): 219–227.

[26] Higashi T, Tsurusaki T, Funase K, et al. Effect of the elbow joint posture on elbow flexor fatigability and muscle strength during isometric contraction. Journal of Physical Therapy Science 19(2): 121–125 (in Japanese).

[27] Salmoni AW, Schmidt RA, Walter CB. Knowledge of results and motor learning: A review and critical reappraisal. Psychological Bulletin. 1984; 19(3): 355–386.

[28] Winstein CJ, Schmidt RA. Reduced frequency of knowledge of results enhances motor skill learning. Journal of Experimental Psychology Learning Memory and Cognition. 1990; 16(4): 677–691.

[29] Lavery JJ. Retention of simple motor skills as a function of type of knowledge of results. Journal of Psychology. 1962; 16(4): 300–311.

[30] Sherwood DE. Effect of bandwidth knowledge of results on movement consistency. Perceptual and Motor Skills. 1988; 66(2): 535–542.

[31] Schmidt RA. A Schema theory of discrete motor skill learning. Psychological Review. 1975; 82(4): 225–260.

# 2

# Neuroscience-Based Rehabilitation for Stroke Patients

Takayuki Kodama and Hideki Nakano

**Abstract**

Hitherto, physical therapy for rehabilitating patients with cerebral dysfunction has focused on acquiring and improving compensatory strategies by using the remaining functions; it has been presumed that once neural functions have been lost, they cannot be restored. However, neuroscience-based animal research and neuroimaging research since the 1980s have demonstrated that recovery arises from plastic changes in the central nervous system and reconstruction of neural networks; this research is ushering in a new age of neuroscience-based rehabilitation as a treatment for cerebral dysfunction (such as stroke). In this paper, in regard to mental practices using motor imagery and kinaesthetic illusion, we summarize basic discoveries and theories relating to motor function therapy based on neuroscientific theory; in particular, we outline a novel rehabilitation method using kinaesthetic illusion induced by vibrational stimulus, which the authors are currently attempting in stroke patients.

**Keywords:** stroke, kinaesthetic illusion, motor imagery, neuroscience-based rehabilitation

## 1. Introduction

Conventional physical therapy (PT) for the rehabilitation of patients with brain dysfunction focuses on the acquisition of function through alternative means by using and improving the patients' existing functions, and it is based on the assumption that once a neutral function is lost, it can never be recovered [1]. However, animal neuroscience studies [2–4] that were conducted after the 1980s and neuroimaging studies [5, 6] have shown that recovery can occur as a result of plastic changes in the nervous system or reorganization of the neural network, and rehabilitation (neuroscience-based rehabilitation, NBR) after cerebral dysfunction (e.g. stroke) has reached a new era in treatment. These observations suggest that the plasticity that is observed in patients is related to the characteristic that the more the patient receives therapy in specific parts of their body, the more that the brain areas that control these parts will be functionally as well as anatomically extended.

Functional recovery originally referred to a patient's recovery from limitations in their behavior, movements, and/or activity [7]. Therefore, the purpose of NBR is not only to induce the reorganization of brain functions through neural plasticity mechanisms but also recover comprehensive bodily motor functions and brain functions for autonomous and active social behavior. What type of treatment strategy is required so that patients feel positively engaged by it, gradually understand its effects, and work toward a goal? Previous studies have revealed important factors in the effects of NBR treatment, such as the amount of therapy [8, 9], rehabilitation implementation environment [10], and performance of neurocognitive rehabilitation [11] through mental practice techniques, such as motor imagery (MI) [12]. Among these factors, treatments involving MI are strongly recommended because MI contributes to the reorganization of neural functions. MI, which is an approach that is based on neuroscientific data and the motor learning theory, is defined as the capacity to internally mimic physical movements without any associated motor output [13]. The cognitive process that occurs during the imagination of movements involves various components, such as mutual understandings between oneself and others (environment), observations of movements, mental manipulations of objects, and psychological time and movement planning. Instead of repeating simple physical movements to receive feedback on outcome in the actual therapy, the practice of voluntary and skill-requiring movements that are geared toward task completion induces the functional recovery [14]. Thus, an important element of the patients' engagement in the therapy is that it occurs in an active and top-down fashion through the use of MI. However, because MI has a task-specific nature, cognitive functions and memories of motor experiences that equip the patients to perform the task are required. Patients with neurofunctional states that make motor execution (ME) difficulty may suffer not only from impairments in motor-related brain areas but also from modifications in their intracerebral body representations (e.g. somatoparaphrenia) [15, 16]. In such cases, the exploitation of kinaesthetic illusions [17–20], which can be induced in the brain by extraneous stimuli, such as vibratory stimulations, becomes important for inputting appropriate motor-sensory information into the brain in a passive and bottom-up fashion. Therefore, the implementation of a mental practice to determine the criteria for adequate treatment according to the states of the patient's cognitive functions and motor functions is important in order to select and implement the best therapy. Thus, this paper summarizes the basic understanding and theories of mental practices that use MI or kinaesthetic illusion and discusses, in particular, research results concerning kinaesthetic illusions that are induced by vibratory stimulations, which we are currently attempting on stroke patients.

## 2. What is neuroscience-based rehabilitation?

NBR involves a series of processes that are selected for the intervention according to the current brain function theories that have been revealed by neuroscience and other similar studies and verification of its outcomes. For example, the selection of a NBR strategy for a stroke patient requires a combination of deep clinical reasoning, the experience of the therapist, and a vast understanding of the evidence obtained by studies from wide-ranging academic fields on the factors that support recovery mechanisms and produce particular outcomes. First, the neural basis of brain cell reorganization will be presented.

### 2.1. Neural basis of brain cell reorganization

The current understanding of neural reorganization after dysfunction is not that the neurons themselves recover after their axons are damaged but rather that damaged functional networks recover due to several processes that induce the recovery of motor and cognitive functions. Cajal [1], who was a proponent of neuron theory, stated that the central nervous system (brain and spinal cord) of adult mammals would not recover once it is damaged. However, studies that have been conducted since the 1980s and that have shown that alterations in the peripheral nervous system, such as denervation and amputation, change somatic sensations and the representations of body parts while they are in motion have revealed that the brain has plasticity. In 1998, Eriksson et al. [21] reported the new formation of neurons in the central nervous system of human beings. These findings raised the question of whether the plastic changes and functional reorganization that occur in subjects with cranial nerve disorders originate from an ischemic state, such as a cerebrovascular disturbance. The underlying mechanisms of the plasticity that occurs after a cortical deficit are thought to involve (i) the redundancy of neuronal connections in the central nervous system, (ii) morphological changes in the neurons, and (iii) changes in synaptic information transmission [22]. If neurons are damaged, astrocytes begin to divide due to the activity of microglia. These glial cells then reinforce the areas that have been damaged by brain lesions and release neurotrophic factors, such as nerve growth factor, to promote neuronal sprouting (it takes around two weeks for synapses to grow after nerve damage [23]). The sprouted neurons are then connected to an existing neural network, which forms a new network. In other words, if neurons are damaged, new neurons begin to reorganize themselves in order to compensate for it. Adequate NBR stimulates the neural network with the neurofunction that is most similar to the predamaged functional state of the neural network, even though the new network is not located in the damaged region. If strong inputs enter the network multiple times, the synaptic connections will be reinforced. However, plasticity will not be induced in synapses with little information (input specificity), and the synapses will be excluded from the network formation [24, 25].

These findings have been confirmed by several famous studies. Nudo et al. [8] caused artificial cerebral infarcts in monkeys in the region of the primary motor cortex (M1) that corresponds to fingers and then forced the monkeys to use fingers with motor deficits. Thus, they reported that the brain region that previously controlled the shoulders and elbows prior to the therapy then controlled the fingers and more distal body parts (**Figure 1**). Merzenich et al. [26] surgically sutured the fingers of monkeys and then compared the pre- and post-surgical somatotopies of Brodmann area (BA) 3b, which corresponds to the sensorimotor area (SMA). Microelectrodes were used to record the responses in BA3b to finger stimuli. The third and fourth fingers were then surgically sutured, and the responses were recorded again a month later. Thus, the boundary between the third and fourth fingers became unclear. In addition, the results of a study that was conducted in human beings suggested that the plasticity of brain cells depends on sensory input. The results of a magnetoencephalography study that compared the somatotopies of the

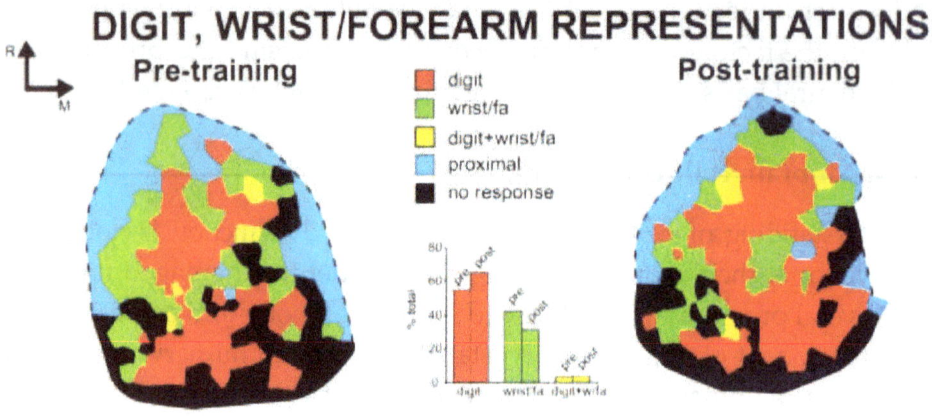


**Figure 1.** Representation of the distal forelimb in cortical area 4 derived from pre- and post-training mapping procedures [8].

first and fifth fingers of string players to normal controls showed that a broader cerebral cortical area was activated for string players compared to the controls [6].

These findings suggest that the size of the intracerebral somatotopic representation, which is vital to ME, is determined by the degree of use of the region. If you try to induce plasticity in specific parts of the bodies of stroke patients, as mentioned above, the induction of neural plasticity in a pathway that allows highly efficient information processing by repeating movements in a pattern like the normal pattern should be possible, provided the patient has retained their motor functions to a certain degree. However, if a patient has the functional level of almost not able to perform movement or is only able to perform the movement in an abnormal pattern, the stimulation of the plasticity for the formation of a neural network that is required to be able to regain normal motor function may not be possible. Ward et al. [27] chronologically examined the relationships between motor function recovery scores and task-related brain activities for approximately 12 months after the onset of stroke with functional magnetic resonance imaging. They found a negative correlation between motor function recovery scores and a decline in the hyperactivity of brain areas in the damaged and undamaged hemispheres (M1, premotor cortex; PMC, supplementary motor cortex; SMC, cerebellum). These findings suggest that a better recovery of motor function is associated with better connectivity between the functional systems of multiple brain regions and that a continuous and long-term approach is required to study the changes in the morphologies and networks of neurons. Thus, a qualitative and continuous approach [28] is required in studies of the recovery of the entire neural system (e.g. transcortical network, M1-PMC neural network [29]) in order to be able to perform movement rather than merely establishing quantitative interventions of movement. Thus, next, we will discuss the current understanding of what is required in interventions for stroke patients.

## 3. Interventions for stroke

The establishment of a series of tripartite relationships between actual physical movement, a sense of ownership or agency, and imaging of physical exercise is an important component of

NBR, rather than only involving actual physical movement for patients with motor or sensory disturbances or patients who lost their sense of body presence. Recently, decreased grey matter has been shown in multiple motor areas, and it affects the prognosis of motor function recovery [30]. The similar results of a study of monkeys that developed brain infarcts in their M1 area showed that the fiber connections between M1 and the hand brain area of the ventral premotor cortex (PMv) were altered [31]. The observations were conducted prior to and 5 months after the induction of the infarct. Prior to the infarct, M1 was observed to be connected with the SMC, PMv, the dorsal premotor cortex, primary somatosensory cortex, and secondary somatosensory cortex by fibers, and these connections with M1 ceased to exist 5 months later. In contrast, the PMv was connected with M1 and the frontal rostral area prior to the infarct, and these connections with M1 ceased to exist after 5 months. However, a new network was formed between PMv and the primary somatosensory cortex. The results of these studies demonstrate that a cortical somatotopic representation is not a simple schema of the projection of one point to another point but rather a pervasive pattern in a broader range of the cortex, and a network that is based on the functional connectivity between areas is dynamically reconfigured by experience in order to reorganize the representation. These findings not only confirm the hypothesis that ME involves a large number of cerebral areas, including the motor areas but also implies that a simple movement treatment is not sufficient for functional recovery and that an intervention of a brain function network, including the relevant brain areas, is required.

Sharma et al. [32] classified the intervention components of previous studies that positively affected motor function recovery after a brain infarct into three concepts of approach: (i) sensory feedback, (ii) discharge through the corticospinal tract to produce movement, and (iii) motor processes that precede movement. The first concept, sensory feedback, is an approach that uses feedback from visual and auditory perception as well as somatosensory information to promote the recovery of motor functions. Sensory feedback implies that an enhancement of the nervous activity in the M1 4p area through somatosensory input is related to the recovery of motor functions. The human M1 consists of two distinct areas: 4a and 4p [33]. The 4a and 4p areas have different cellular structures and different receptor densities. 4a is located in the anterior (rostral) part of M1, and it is called old M1 because it is a phylogenetically old area. Output from the old M1 controls physical movement through the corticospinal tract and spinal interneurons. In contrast, 4p is located in the posterior (caudal) part of the primary motor cortex, and it is called new M1 because it is a relatively new motor cortex. New M1 contains motor cortical neuronal cells that will be directly connected with spinal motor neurons through synapses. These synaptic connections are not mediated by spinal interneurons, and they are involved in the formation of highly skilled and complex movements [34]. Besides the structural difference, a functional difference in somatosensory afferent information processing has been found between 4a and 4p. A study of the differences in the neural activities of 4a and 4b in the motor area of monkeys in response to the inputs of different sensory modalities [35] showed that 4a is rich in cells that respond to the proprioceptive sensory inputs of muscles and joints, and 4p is rich in cells that respond to cutaneous sensory input. These findings suggested that paralyzed limbs need to be given cutaneous sensory input in order to enhance the excitability of 4p. In addition, 4p is affected by active attention. In order to enhance the neural activity of 4p, it is important to attract the active attention of the target subject toward the PT, in addition to simply providing him or her sensory stimuli. The second concept of discharge through the corticospinal tract to produce movement is an approach that requires the utilization of the corticospinal tract through the positive and intense production of movements. Task-oriented training can be produce by a typical intervention. This training, which consists of several components, is considered an intervention with a high evidence level [36]. The components include the provision of sufficient amounts of movement stress, gradual adjustment of the task difficulty, and feedback utilization. Sufficient amounts of repetitive training and training time need to be provided while rigorously setting up purposive tasks rather than having them repeat simple movements without purpose. Moreover, the most important point is that the intervention should not be a simple increase in the repetition of a movement but rather a step-by-step adjustment in task difficulty [37]. Therapists must be able to appropriately set and adjust the task difficulty according to the functional state of the patients.

Interventions that are based on concept (i) and (ii) stated thus far must involve proper physical movements so that patients do not learn wrong movements while processing actual sensorimotor information. The performance of skilled movement learning tasks is the most important component in PT. The learning of motor skills has been revealed to occur not only during movement practice (online learning) but also during sessions in which a subject is not practicing movement (offline learning) [38]. It is important to consider how offline learning should be implemented in an intervention. The third concept of motor processes that precede movement sheds light on this. Motor processes that precede movement represent the process of simulating a movement. Several mental practices have been developed to explicitly activate this process. However, while some stroke patients are in a brain functional state in which they are able to perform mental practice while actively imagining movements (top-down process), other stoke patients are not. If a top-down intervention is difficult, it is necessary to begin by intervening based on sensory information input (bottom-up process), reconstructing the body schema toward ME, and enhancing the intracerebral body representation capability. In addition, an important strategy of NBR is to ultimately maintain the coherency of the information that is processed and constructed in the brain by the top-down and bottom-up processes.

## 4. Therapy based on voluntary top-down processing

MI [39, 40] is a top-down process involving the active imagining of various states in the mind, rather than a bottom-up process of generating motion-related perceptions based on sensory input. Although the imagery in this context represents a mental image, MI is unlike visual imagery which is induced by the input of sensory information to the body in that MI is pragmatic, whereas visual imagery is semantic [41]. The intracerebral information processing in MI involves not only the formulation of a movement plan but also the cognitive manipulation of what has been imagined [13] as well as elements of self-image (first-person image) and images of others (third-person image) [42]. In addition, because imagery occurs by activating cognitive processing that utilizes working memory [43, 44], MI can also be defined as the mental motor representation that is reproduced by working memory.

Hétu et al. [45] reported that MI is produced in several brain areas, including the cerebellum, inferior/superior parietal lobule, precentral gyrus, inferior frontal gyrus, middle frontal gyrus, and SMC (**Figure 2**). Of these areas, the SMC is involved during the imagining of both motor images of the upper limbs and lower limbs, and the areas of the SMC that are active during MI and ME partially overlap [46]. The SMC is thought to be involved in the formation and manipulation of internal representations of movement in the brain when there are no extraneous stimuli or clues [47]. Because MI only lacks the actual movements and sensory feedback that occurs during ME, it can be considered functionally equivalent to ME except for these processes. Jeannerod et al. [48] stated that MI and ME are not distinct brain processes and that they differ only in the brain process concerning movement. Moreover, a study that examined and compared the brain activities of healthy subjects and stroke patients while they were performing ME, MI, passive movement, and movement observation [49] revealed that the MI brain activity of patients resembled the ME brain activity of healthy subjects and that MI is suited for sensorimotor system activation. In addition, the corticospinal tract is excited through its connection with MI. During transcranial magnetic

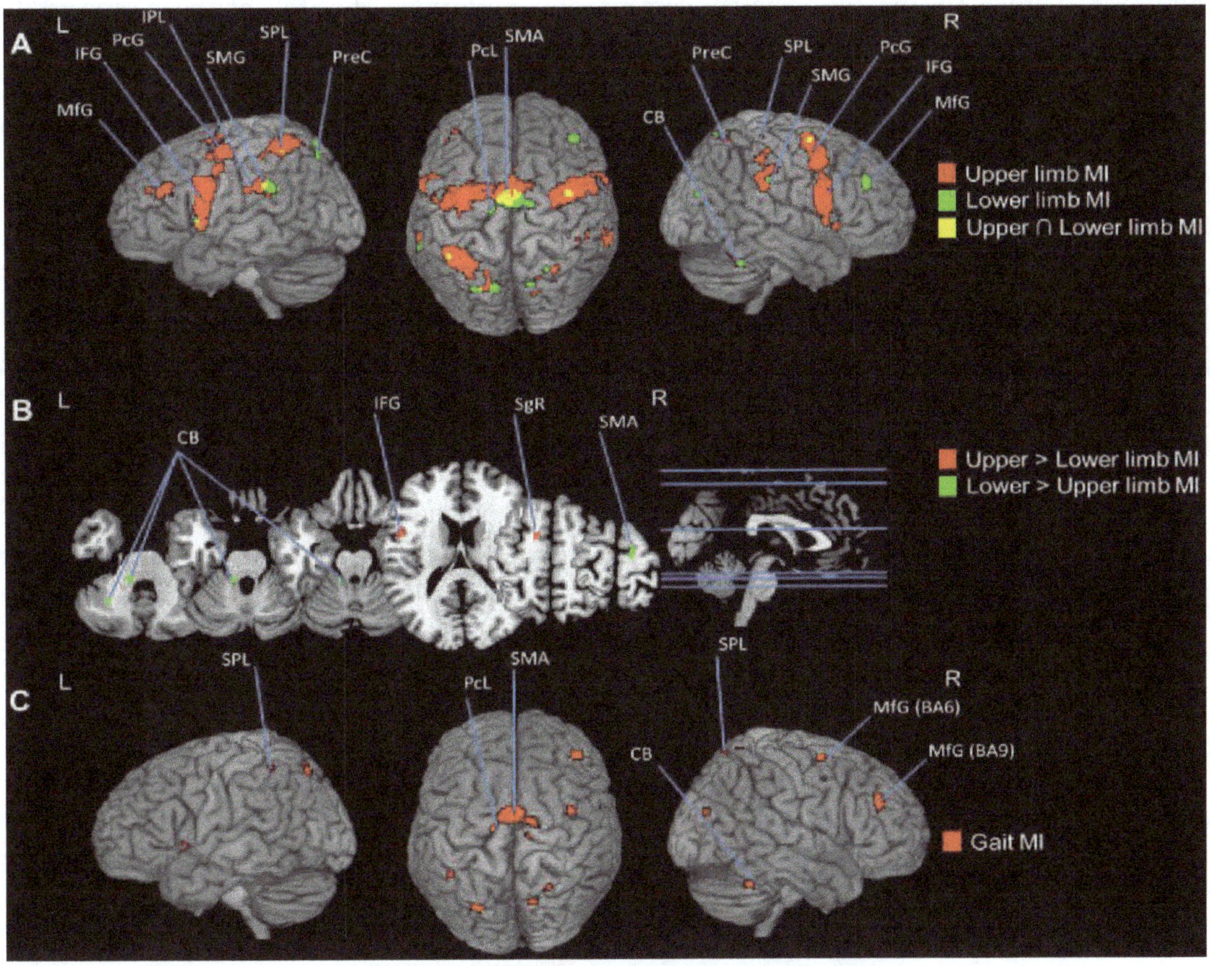


**Figure 2.** Regions consistently activated during motor imagery of the upper and lower limbs [45]. A: Maps of consistent activations while subjects imagined movements of the upper (red) or lower (green) limbs. Regions consistently activated by both types of movements are shown in yellow. B: Results of the subtraction analysis: regions with more consistent activity during motor imagery of upper limbs are shown in red and of lower limbs in green. C: Regions consistently activated while imagining gait movements. CB: cerebellum; IPL/SPL: inferior/superior parietal lobule; PcG: precentral gyrus; IFG: inferior frontal gyrus; MfG: middle frontal gyrus; SMA: supplementary motor area; SMG: supramarginal gyrus; PreC: precuneus; PcL: paracentral lobule; SgR: subgyral region.

stimulation, the threshold of motor-evoked potentials (MEP) and intracortical facilitation decrease, and a latent time reduction and amplitude increment are observed. In the neurotransmission test, a spinal H-reflex amplitude increment and increase in the F-wave frequency rate have been reported [50]. Electroencephalography (EEG) shows that the formation of MI, like ME, reduces the $\alpha$-wave (Mu-rhythm) amplitude in the SMA (Refer to Section Interventions based on extraneous bottom-up processes), which is called event-related desynchronization (ERD). The degree of change rate in ERD that is associated with MI correlates with the motor-evoked potential increment, intracortical inhibition reduction, and F-wave frequency rate, and ERD is thought to reflect the excitability of the corticospinal tract [51].

However, activity in M1, which is the final area of motor output, during MI is debatable (**Figure 3**) [45]. As reported by studies by Sharma et al. [52] and Ehrsson et al. [53], some studies report M1 neural activity during MI [54, 55], whereas others report that no activity was observed, and whether it is active or not varies according to each subject. MI is also thought to reflect a suppression process so that the actual movement is not performed The SMC has been reported to inhibit M1 activation during MI [48, 56], which then causes ME to cease [57]. Thus, the different reports on activation can be explained by the finding that the information that is processed during MI is supposed to be inhibited so that ME does not occur, which has sometimes been conveyed to M1 Through the contamination of an image by muscle activity [50].

Two components have been revealed to exist in the information processing system for generating MI in the brain: one is the simulation of motor parameters, which generates a concrete motor execution plan, such as which muscles should be moved and how in movement execution, and the other is the simulation of motor perception, which predictively generates a motor execution plan that is based on expected motor perceptions during the motor preparation phase. Because network activities in a number of areas, such as the frontal lobe, basal ganglia, and cerebellum, are involved in this system [58], it is considered necessary during PT to intervene and direct the patients by asking them to imagine the direction of a movement and the muscles that must be moved to perform the movement or imagine the motor perception that accompanies movement and the perception that forms between themselves and an object in order to leverage all these areas. Furthermore, the observation that MI changes intracerebral neural activities and the excitability of the corticospinal tract suggests the possibility that MI is a useful intervention method in PT. An intervention that has recently used ERD through MI is the brain machine interface (BMI).

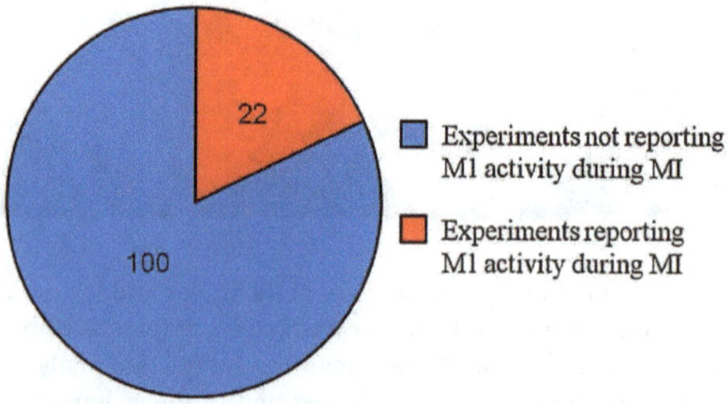


**Figure 3.** Proportion of neuroimaging experiments on motor imagery where activity in the primary motor cortex (M1) was found [45].

Among the rehabilitation therapies that use BMI, there is a functional compensation BMI that aims to compensate for the loss of function, and a functional recovery BMI that aims to recover functions. In particular, a strategy of functional recovery BMI that has been proposed is the use of robots to support near-normal movement and generate correct sensory inputs to induce plasticity in brain neurons [59]. A study by Ramos-Murguialday et al. [60] that examined the effects of functional recovery BMI and that utilized MI reported the results of a randomized comparison test that examined the effects of BMI training on 32 cases of chronic stroke patients who had difficulty extending the fingers on their paralyzed hand by dividing them into the BMI-trained group and the control group. In the BMI training, ERD during MI was analyzed, and the brain moved the upper limb robot and the finger orthosis in accordance with the changes (**Figure 4**). The control group moved their hands randomly. Because of an intervention that was performed for an average of 17.8 days, the paralyzed side of the upper limb functions improved significantly for the BMI-trained group compared to the control group. Furthermore, the improvements were reported to be related to an electromyographic amplitude value during voluntary muscle contraction as well as the degree of activity shift from the undamaged hemisphere to the damaged hemisphere on the functional MRI.

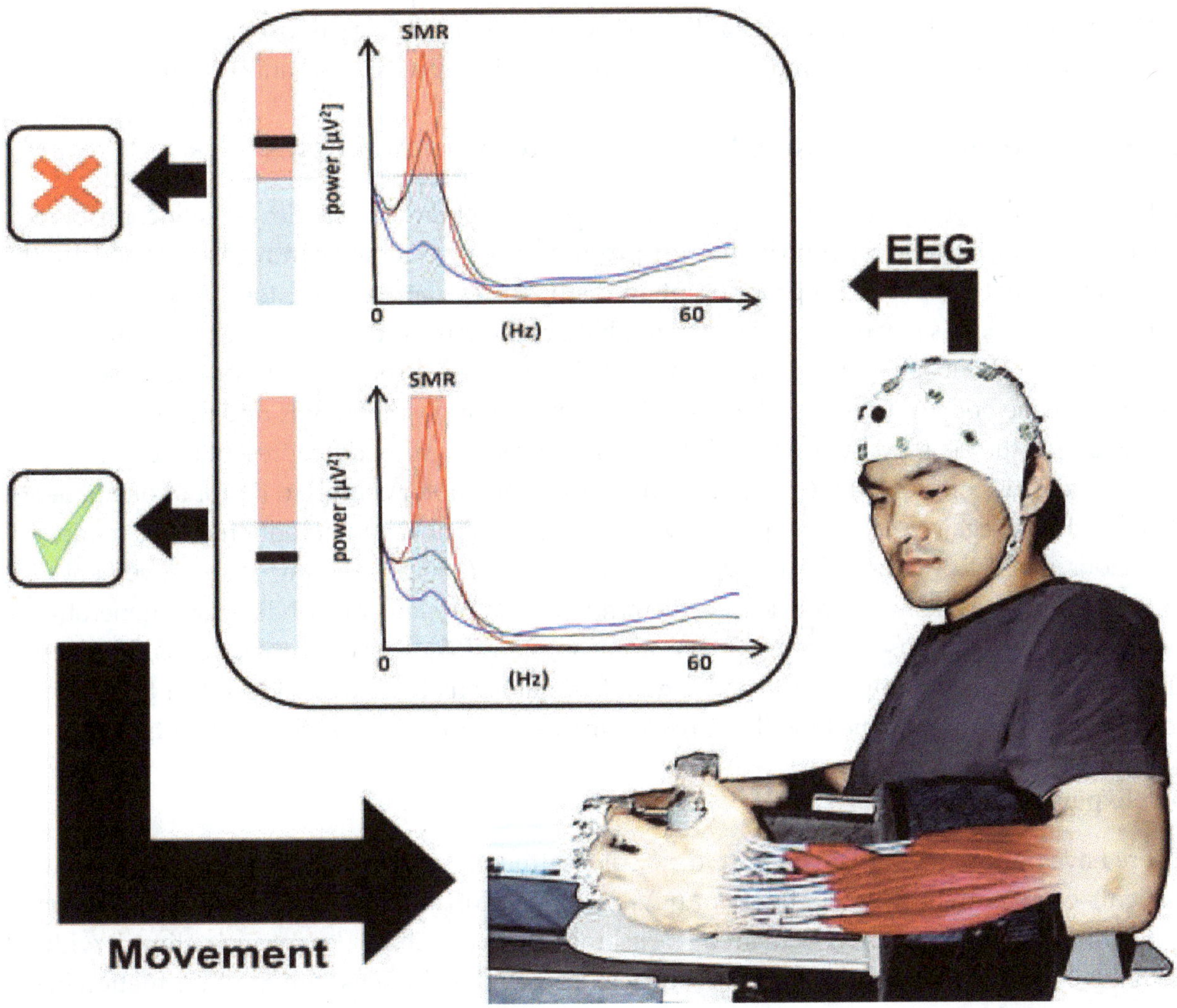


**Figure 4.** Brain-machine-interface in stroke [60].

With the recent development and advances in analysis and intervention tools, mental practice that utilizes MI is currently being established. However, because MI has problems that are related to vividness, controllability, immersion, and habitude, large individual differences in image recollection capabilities are suspected. The bottom-up–processed image that is based on visual information proceeds according to two distinct pathways: "the what pathway" (ventral stream), which processes shape and color and "the where pathway" (dorsal stream), which processes spatial locations and movements [61]. The processing occurs in a phased and hierarchical manner with the former processing object imagery and the latter processing spatial imagery. This enables us to understand image capability based on image capability assessments, such as the Object-Spatial Imagery Questionnaire [62]. However, a large number of studies have revealed that MI is processed in a top-down manner. An interesting study that shows this functional difference by Macrae and Troll et al. [63] reported that patients who could not imagine home and the way to go home nevertheless made no mistakes going home and exhibited no mistaken behavior at home. Because the recollection capability of MI involves memory that is related to one's own movements and movement experiences, it is possible that the body representation capability within the brain has largely declined in stroke patients who have suffered disturbances of their sensorimotor functions for an extended period of time since onset, which makes it impossible to recollect MI. For these cases, the motor sensory information input needs to occur in a bottom-up manner and the sense of ownership needs to reorganize itself.

## 5. Interventions based on extraneous bottom-up processes

When the brain controls bodily movements, the proprioceptors in muscles largely contribute to their realization. The great contribution of proprioception to motor control is revealed by the observation that patients with proprioception disturbances cannot move their fingers very well [64]. In addition, this perception is deeply involved in the intracerebral body representation. Two concepts of body image [65] and body schema [66] have been proposed for body representation. Of the two, the body schema, which is a model of one's own posture that is updated every second according to the sensory information input, is an intracerebral body representation before it is brought to consciousness. If the treatment goal is to regain motor control in PT for stroke patients, it is difficult to regain smooth and predictive motor control only by interventions in the manner of conscious control or control based on visual information. Because many limb movements are executed unconsciously, we considered them an important element in NBR for regenerating a body schema that is based on input from proprioception [65]. Based on these ideas, we present the details of a study [20] that utilized kinaesthetic illusions that were induced in the brain by tendon vibration to examine how they affected the neural functions of stroke patients.

### 5.1. Experiment

There have been many reports on the efficacy of treatment using illusory kinaesthesia for NBR in patients with a cerebrovascular accident (CVA). Illusory kinaesthesia is defined as an illusion in which the subject feels the movement of their limbs by extrinsic and/or intrinsic stimuli without actual voluntary movement [67]. Illusory kinaesthesia evoked by sensorimotor information in the brain activates brain nerve activity, and the neural activity can be considered as the neural basis of motor control and can be applied for motor learning [68]. When illusory kinaesthesia is used as a treatment, it is required to predict sensory information that would be inputted prior to the illusory movement and to simulate previous sensory movement experiences as the motor image [69]. Thus, it is important to assess whether this brain neural process observed in healthy adults can also occur in patients with a CVA to understand the efficacy of the approach as an intervention. In this experiment, to understand the functional brain status from the time when the motor imaging is started prior to the illusory kinaesthesia, we evaluated how illusory kinaesthesia influences brain neural activity in patients with CVAs using electroencephalography (EEG).

#### *5.1.1. Methods*

##### *5.1.1.1. Subjects*

Subjects were 12 healthy adults who did not have any orthopedic or neurological diseases and who were without motor and sensory disorders (healthy control group) and 13 patients with CVAs (CVA group). In the CVA group, subjects did not have any cognitive dysfunction and superficial and deep sensory tract disorders.

##### *5.1.1.2. Experimental conditions and neurophysiological outcomes*

For vibratory stimulation, vibration was applied to the tendon of the distal part of the right biceps, and the target movement of illusory kinaesthesia was elbow extension. As the neurophysiological outcome of the influence of illusory kinaesthesia on brain neural activity, we used mu-rhythm (μ-wave), which is one of the frequency components of the brain wave and is the same frequency band as the $\alpha$ wave band. The μ-wave decreases not only during actual movement but also during motor imaging [70, 71]; thus, it can be an outcome of brain neural activity, including the generation process, during illusory kinaesthesia around the sensorimotor area. For vibratory stimulation, a handheld massager (THRIVE MD-01, Thrive co., Ltd) was used. Since the vibratory stimulation was applied on the skin, it could stimulate not only the muscle spindles but also the superficial sensory receptors. The μ-wave, which changes depending on the sensorimotor information, can also be affected by sensory information from cutaneous stimulation [72]. To control these effects, we subtracted the EEG data obtained during the contact of the vibratory device on the right biceps tendon without vibratory stimulation from the EEG data when applying vibratory stimulation to evoke illusory kinaesthesia to obtain data for analysis. The frequency of the vibratory stimulation was set at 91.7 Hz [67, 73, 74].

##### *5.1.1.3. EEG analysis*

We used Neurofax (Nihon Koden) to record EEGs. The measurement site was based on the international 10–20 system, and EEGs were obtained from 18 electrodes with bilateral earlobes as reference electrodes. The recording time for each trial was 60 seconds [73].

In the EEG data that were controlled by sensory information in both the healthy control and CVA groups, to investigate brain activity in the μ-wave band area, we first divided the waves into epochs of 2 seconds (30 epochs in total) each. We analyzed the cumulative mean of the data using the three-dimensional filtering of brain neural activity, that is, standardized low resolution brain electromagnetic tomography (sLORETA) [75, 76], to identify brain neural activity in the μ-wave band area. For obtaining the results of the analysis, the brain neural activity area was calculated as the current density value simulated with 6234 voxels (MNI coordinates [77]) in the brain, and this was identified as the Brodmann area (BA). For comparison of the vibratory stimulation condition-specific differences in brain neural activity areas between the groups, we used sLORETA-based SnPM analysis [78].

*5.1.2. Results*

The brain neural activity in the μ-wave ($\alpha$ wave when it appears in the posterior lobe [79]) band area due to vibratory stimulation was significantly greater in the posterior lobe compared to the cerebral cortex area in both groups, while there was no significant neural activity in the sensorimotor area (**Figure 5a** and **b**). For group differences, the healthy control group

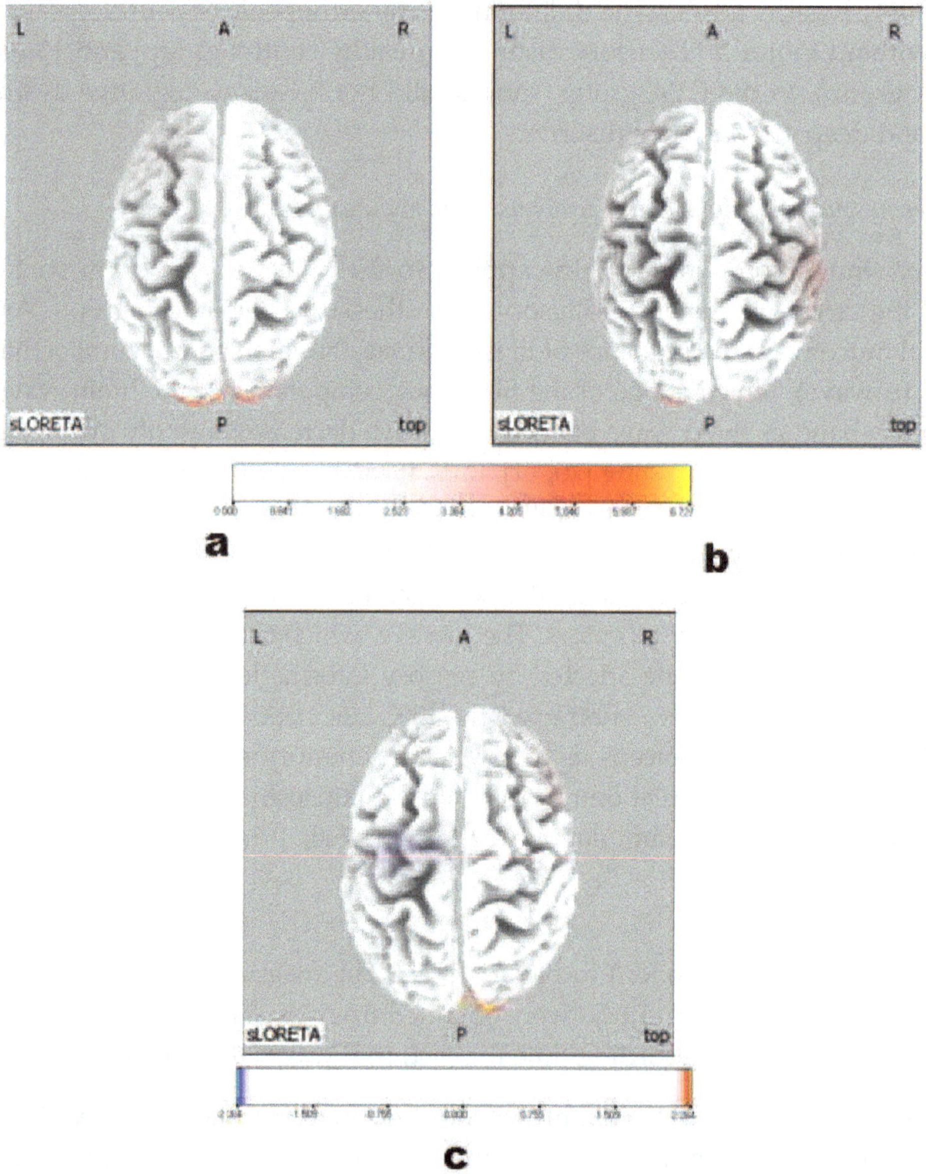


**Figure 5.** Brain neural activity in the μ-wave band area due to vibratory stimulation. (a) Brain neural activity in the μ-wave band area of the healthy control group, (b) brain neural activity in the μ-wave band area of the CVA group, (c) comparison of brain neural activity in the μ-wave band area between the healthy control and CVA groups. The neural activity in the SMC was significantly greater in the CVA group compared to the healthy control group. The color scale shown in the bottom of the image indicates the *t*-value ($t = 2.264$).

had a significantly greater increase in neural activity in the posterior lobe compared to the CVA group, while the CVA group had a significantly greater increase in the SMC (**Figure 5c**).

*5.1.3. Discussion*

This study assessed the influence of illusory kinaesthesia evoked by vibratory stimulation on brain neural activity in patients with CVAs, using the EEG μ-wave, which is a neurophysiological outcome.

As for the brain neural activity in the μ-wave band area due to vibratory stimulation, we did not find significant expression of the μ-wave in the sensorimotor area in both groups. This may be due to the increase in sensorimotor information in the bilateral sensorimotor-related area [80] causing event-related desynchronisation in neural activity, which decreased the μ-wave [70, 71]. Furthermore, the neural activity in the M1 area, which is the main sensorimotor area, is not only involved in the generation of functional connectivity with BA3b, which deals with sensory information processing from the muscle spindles, but is also related to the cause of illusory kinaesthesia itself [81]. Thus, it is believed that the amount of perception of illusory kinaesthesia is greater when excitability of the motor cortex is greater [68]. Therefore, illusory kinaesthesia was evoked also in the CVA group by enhancing neural activity in the sensorimotor area using vibratory stimulation.

Furthermore, for a significant increase in the SMC in the CVA group compared to the healthy control group, the SMC stores evoked motor images of not only the constant sensorimotor feedback information during movement execution, but also the sensorimotor information during passive movement input, such as illusory kinaesthesia [69]. This was deeply related to spatial cognitive processes [82] in brain representations [83, 84]. Therefore, it was presumed that, in patients with CVAs who had movement deficits, there were some functional differences in the simulation process of the motor image during generation of illusory kinaesthesia compared to healthy adults. Furthermore, information processing to generate the illusion and completeness of the generated motor image may be different.

The results of our study showed that there might be functional differences in the generation mechanism of illusory kinaesthesia between healthy adults and adults with CVAs, while illusory kinaesthesia can also be evoked in patients, which increases the neural activity in the sensorimotor area and SMC.

## 6. Toward a therapy that aims for unification

The utilization of kinaesthetic illusions allows for the induction of realistic motor perceptions, which constitutes the neural basis of ME, while activating the sensorimotor area. This therapy can be used to help patients be aware of physical movements that they perform as well recover a sense of ownership while triggering neural reorganization. To make kinaesthetic illusions more vivid and realistic, the combination of ME and MI is required with the intention of motion. Naito et al. [19] reported that kinaesthetic illusions and hand MI collectively utilized the motor areas of the SMA, dorsal premotor cortex, and cerebellum. Between the body schema of MI and the body schema of kinaesthetic illusion lies the common neural basis. If patients intentionally create an MI of quasi movement while experiencing a kinaesthetic illusion, the experience of the kinaesthetic illusion is enhanced, which allows them to experience a more realistic movement [19]. These findings revealed that there is an interference between kinaesthetic illusions and MI. In NBR, the focus is on eliciting voluntary and active movements from the patients themselves. kinaesthetic illusions, which reflect the processes of the sensorimotor area that converts signals from proprioception to motor commands, is itself a neural mechanism that is directly connected with motor control. This will be a useful strategy for PT for patients with impaired motor functions to create an intention of movement through the MI and elicit the ME while evoking kinaesthetic illusions.

## 7. Conclusion

This paper presented several theories of the reorganization of brain functions in stroke patients that were based on neuroscientific evidence and an outline of such attempts. A therapist's accurate understanding of the patient's state results in increased options for treatment strategies. In addition, therapists have greater options for patients to have the possibility of an autonomous social life. However, we must understand the limitations and individual differences in functional recovery [85, 86]. Thus, the application of the same therapy may not cause the same level of recovery. Furthermore, the induction of network reinforcement and fixation by the simple input of stimuli into neurons is difficult because mental acts by the patient are vital. PT becomes most effective when adequate interventions that induce neural network reorganization and positive states of mind are combined.

## Acknowledgements

This study was part of a research program funded by the JSPS (research grant 15K01439). The funding source had no role in study design/concept, data collection/analysis/interpretation, and manuscript preparation/submission.

## Author details

Takayuki Kodama* and Hideki Nakano

*Address all correspondence to: kodama-t@tachibana-u.ac.jp

Department of Physical Therapy, Faculty of Health Sciences, Kyoto Tachibana University, Kyoto, Japan

## References

[1] Cajal S, Ramon Y: Degeneration & Regeneration of the Nervous System. Trans. and edited by RM May ed. London: Oxford University Press; 1928.

[2] Merzenich MM, Nelson RJ, Stryker MP, Cynader MS, Schoppmann A, Zook JM: Somatosensory cortical map changes following digit amputation in adult monkeys. J Comp Neurol. 1984;224(4):591–605.

[3] Donoghue JP, Suner S, Sanes JN: Dynamic organization of primary motor cortex output to target muscles in adult rats. II. Rapid reorganization following motor nerve lesions. Exp Brain Res. 1990;79(3):492–503.

[4] Cohen LG, Bandinelli S, Findley TW, Hallett M: Motor reorganization after upper limb amputation in man. A study with focal magnetic stimulation. Brain. 1991;114(Pt 1B): 615–627.

[5] Sterr A, Müller MM, Elbert T, Rockstroh B, Pantev C, Taub E: Changed perceptions in Braille readers. Nature. 1998;391(6663):134–135.

[6] Elbert T, Pantev C, Wienbruch C, Rockstroh B, Taub E: Increased cortical representation of the fingers of the left hand in string players. Science. 1995;270(5234):305–307.

[7] Calautti C, Baron JC: Functional neuroimaging studies of motor recovery after stroke in adults: a review. Stroke. 2003;34(6):1553–1566.

[8] Nudo RJ, Milliken GW, Jenkins WM, Merzenich MM: Use-dependent alterations of movement representations in primary motor cortex of adult squirrel monkeys. J Neurosci. 1996;16(2):785–807.

[9] Hayward KS, Brauer SG: Dose of arm activity training during acute and subacute rehabilitation post stroke: a systematic review of the literature. Clin Rehabil. 2015;29(12):1234–1243.

[10] Döbrössy MD, Dunnett SB: The influence of environment and experience on neural grafts. Nat Rev Neurosci. 2001;2(12):871–879.

[11] Pollock A, Farmer SE, Brady MC, Langhorne P, Mead GE, Mehrholz J, van Wijck F: Interventions for improving upper limb function after stroke. Cochrane Database Syst Rev. 2014;11:CD010820.

[12] Guillot A, Di Rienzo F, Collet C: The neurofunctional architecture of motor imagery, in Advanced Brain Neuroimaging Topics in Health and Disease-Methods and Applications, Papageorgiou TD, Christopoulos GI, Smirnakis SM, editors. (Rijeka: InTech;) 2014: 433–456.

[13] Decety J: The neurophysiological basis of motor imagery. Behav Brain Res. 1996;77 (1–2):45–52.

[14] Molina-Luna K, Hertler B, Buitrago MM, Luft AR: Motor learning transiently changes cortical somatotopy. Neuroimage. 2008;40(4):1748–1754.

[15] Jenkinson PM, Haggard P, Ferreira NC, Fotopoulou A: Body ownership and attention in the mirror: insights from somatoparaphrenia and the rubber hand illusion. Neuropsychologia. 2013;51(8):1453–1462.

[16] Garbarini F, Fossataro C, Berti A, Gindri P, Romano D, Pia L, della Gatta F, Maravita A, Neppi-Modona M: When your arm becomes mine: pathological embodiment of alien

limbs using tools modulates own body representation. Neuropsychologia. 2015;70: 402–413.

[17] Lackner JR, Taublieb AB: Reciprocal interactions between the position sense representations of the two forearms. J Neurosci. 1983;3:2280–2285.

[18] Roll JP, Gilhodes JC: Proprioceptive sensory codes mediating movement trajectory perception: human hand vibration-induced drawing illusions. Can J Physiol Pharmacol. 1995;73(2):295–304.

[19] Naito E, Kochiyama T, Kitada R, Nakamura S, Matsumura M, Yonekura Y, Sadato N: Internally simulated movement sensations during motor imagery activate cortical motor areas and the cerebellum. J Neurosci. 2002;22(9):3683–3691.

[20] Kodama T, Nakano H, Ohsugi H, Murata S: Effects of vibratory stimulation-induced kinesthetic illusions on the neural activities of patients with stroke. J Phys Ther Sci. 2016;28(2):419–425.

[21] Eriksson PS, Perfilieva1 E, Björk-Eriksson T, Alborn AM, Nordborg C, Peterson DA, Gage FH: Neurogenesis in the adult human hippocampus. Nat Med. 1998;4:1313–1317.

[22] Murphy TH, Corbett D: Plasticity during stroke recovery: from synapse to behaviour. Nat Rev Neurosci. 2009;10(12):861–872.

[23] Toni N, Buchs PA, Nikonenko I, Bron CR, Muller D: LTP promotes formation of multiple spine synapses between a single axon terminal and a dendrite. Nature. 1999;402(6760):421–425.

[24] Hebb DO: The organization of behavior: a neuropsychological theory. New York: Wiley & Sons; 1949.

[25] Turrigiano GG, Leslie KR, Desai NS, Rutherford LC, Nelson SB: Activity-dependent scaling of quantal amplitude in neocortical neurons. Nature. 1998;391:892–896.

[26] Merzenich MM, Kaas JH, Wall J, Nelson RJ, Sur M, Felleman D: Topographic reorganization of somatosensory cortical areas 3b and 1 in adult monkeys following restricted deafferentation. Neuroscience. 1983;8(1):33–55.

[27] Ward NS, Brown MM, Thompson AJ, Frackowiak RS: Neural correlates of motor recovery after stroke: a longitudinal fMRI study. Brain. 2003;126:2476–2496.

[28] Grefkes C, Ward NS: Cortical reorganization after stroke: how much and how functional? Neuroscientist. 2014;20(1):56–70.

[29] Kantak SS, Stinear JW, Buch ER, Cohen LG: Rewiring the brain: potential role of the premotor cortex in motor control, learning, and recovery of function following brain injury. Neurorehabil Neural Repair. 2012;26(3):282–292.

[30] Gauthier LV, Taub E, Mark VW, Barghi A, Uswatte G: Atrophy of spared gray matter tissue predicts poorer motor recovery and rehabilitation response in chronic stroke. Stroke. 2012;43(2):453–457.

[31] Nudo RJ: Postinfarct cortical plasticity and behavioral recovery. Stroke. 2007;38(Suppl 2):840–845.

[32] Sharma N, Cohen LG: Recovery of motor function after stroke. Dev Psychobiol. 2012;54 (3):254–262.

[33] Geyer S, Ledberg A, Schleicher A, Kinomura S, Schormann T, Bürgel U, Klingberg T, Larsson J, Zilles K, Roland PE: Two different areas within the primary motor cortex of man. Nature. 1996;382:805–807.

[34] Rathelot JA, Strick PL: Subdivisions of primary motor cortex based on cortico-motoneuronal cells. Proc Natl Acad Sci USA. 2009;106(3):918–923.

[35] Strick PL, Preston JB: Sorting of somatosensory afferent information in primate motor cortex. Brain Res. 1978;156:364–368.

[36] Timmermans AA, Spooren AI, Kingma H, Seelen HA: Influence of task-oriented training content on skilled arm-hand performance in stroke: a systematic review. Neurorehabil Neural Repair. 2010;24(9):858–870.

[37] Plautz EJ, Milliken GW, Nudo RJ: Effects of repetitive motor training on movement representations in adult squirrel monkeys: role of use versus learning. Neurobiol Learn Mem. 2000;74(1):27–55.

[38] Dayan E, Cohen LG: Neuroplasticity subserving motor skill learning. Neuron. 2011;72 (3):443–454.

[39] Jeannerod M: The representing brain: neural correlates of motor intention and imagery. Behav Brain Sci. 1994;17(2):187–202.

[40] Bakker M, de Lange FP, Stevens JA, Toni I, Bloem BR: Motor imagery of gait: a quantitative approach. Exp Brain Res. 2007;179(3):497–504.

[41] McAvinue LP, Robertson IH: Relationship between visual and motor imagery. Percept Mot Skills. 2007;104(3 Pt 1):823–843.

[42] Hanakawa T, Immisch I, Toma K, Dimyan MA, Van Gelderen P, Hallett M: Functional properties of brain areas associated with motor execution and imagery. J Neurophysiol. 2003;89:989–1002.

[43] Erro R, Hirschbichler ST, Ricciardi L, Ryterska A, Antelmi E, Ganos C, Cordivari C, Tinazzi M, Edwards MJ, Bhatia KP: Mental rotation and working memory in musicians' dystonia. Brain Cogn. 2016;109:124–129.

[44] Farah MJ: The neural basis of mental imagery. Trends Neurosci. 1989;12(10):395–399.

[45] Hétu S, Grégoire M, Saimpont A, Coll MP, Eugène F, Michon PE, Jackson PL: The neural network of motor imagery: an ALE meta-analysis. Neurosci Biobehav Rev. 2013;37 (5):930–949.

[46] Deiber MP, Ibañez V, Sadato N, Hallett M: Cerebral structures participating in motor preparation in humans: a positron emission tomography study. J Neurophysiol. 1996;75 (1):233–247.

[47] Stephan KM, Fink GR, Passingham RE, Silbersweig D, Ceballos-Baumann AO, Frith CD, Frackowiak RS: Functional anatomy of the mental representation of upper extremity movements in healthy subjects. J Neurophysiol. 1995;73(1):373–386.

[48] Jeannerod M: Neural simulation of action: a unifying mechanism for motor cognition. Neuroimage. 2001;14(1 Pt 2):S103–S109.

[49] Szameitat AJ, Shen S, Conforto A, Sterr A: Cortical activation during executed, imagined, observed, and passive wrist movements in healthy volunteers and stroke patients. Neuroimage. 2012;62(1):266–280.

[50] Di Rienzo F, Collet C, Hoyek N, Guillot A: Impact of neurologic deficits on motor imagery: a systematic review of clinical evaluations. Neuropsychol Rev. 2014;24(2):116–147.

[51] Takemi M, Masakado Y, Liu M, Ushiba J: Event-related desynchronization reflects downregulation of intracortical inhibition in human primary motor cortex. J Neurophysiol. 2013;110(5):1158–1166.

[52] Sharma N, Jones PS, Carpenter TA, Baron JC: Mapping the involvement of BA 4a and 4p during motor imagery. Neuroimage. 2008;41(1):92–99.

[53] Ehrsson HH, Geyer S, Naito E: Imagery of voluntary movement of fingers, toes, and tongue activates corresponding body-part-specific motor representations. J Neurophysiol. 2003;90(5):3304–3316.

[54] Guillot A, Collet C, Nguyen VA, Malouin F, Richards C, Doyon J: Functional neuroanatomical networks associated with expertise in motor imagery. Neuroimage. 2008;41 (4):1471–1483.

[55] Solodkin A, Hlustik P, Chen EE, Small SL: Fine modulation in network activation during motor execution and motor imagery. Cereb Cortex. 2004;14(11):1246–1255.

[56] Kasess CH, Windischberger C, Cunnington R, Lanzenberger R, Pezawas L, Moser E: The suppressive influence of SMA on M1 in motor imagery revealed by fMRI and dynamic causal modeling. Neuroimage. 2008;40(2):828–837.

[57] Guillot A, Di Rienzo F, Macintyre T, Moran A, Collet C: Imagining is not doing but involves specific motor commands: a review of experimental data related to motor inhibition. Front Hum Neurosci. 2012;6:247.

[58] Lorey B, Pilgramm S, Bischoff M, Stark R, Vaitl D, Kindermann S, Munzert J, Zentgraf K: Activation of the parieto-premotor network is associated with vivid motor imagery-a parametric fMRI study. PLoS One. 2011;6(5):e20368.

[59] Daly JJ, Wolpaw JR: Brain-computer interfaces in neurological rehabilitation. Lancet Neurol. 2008;7(11):1032–1043.

[60] Ramos-Murguialday A, Broetz D, Rea M, Läer L, Yilmaz O, Brasil FL, Liberati G, Curado MR, Garcia-Cossio E, Vyziotis A, Cho W, Agostini M, Soares E, Soekadar S, Caria A, Cohen LG, Birbaumer N: Brain-machine interface in chronic stroke rehabilitation: a controlled study. Ann Neurol. 2013;74(1):100–108.

[61] Goodale MA, Westwood DA, Milner AD: Two distinct modes of control for object-directed action. Prog Brain Res. 2004;144:131–144.

[62] Blajenkova O, Kozhevnikov M, Motes MA: Object-spatial imagery: a new self-report imagery questionnaire. Appl Cogn Psychol. 2006;20(2);239–263.

[63] Macrae D, Troll E: The defect of function in visual agnosia. Brain. 1956;79:94–110.

[64] Ghez C, Gordon J, Ghilardi MF: Impairments of reaching movements in patients without proprioception. II. Effects of visual information on accuracy. J Neurophysiol. 1995;73 (1):361–372.

[65] Naito E, Morita T, Amemiya K: Body representations in the human brain revealed by kinesthetic illusions and their essential contributions to motor control and corporeal awareness. Neurosci Res. 2016;104:16–30.

[66] Head H, Holmes G: Sensory disturbances from cerebral lesions. Brain. 1911;34:102–254.

[67] Goodwin GM, McCloskey DI, Matthews PBC: The contribution of muscle afferents to kinaesthesia shown by vibration induced illusions of movement and by the effects of paralysing joint afferents. Brain. 1972;95:705–748.

[68] Naito E, Roland PE, Ehrsson HH: I feel my hand moving: a new role of the primary motor cortex in somatic perception of limb movement. Neuron. 2002;36:979–988.

[69] Harada T, Saito DN, Kashikura K, Sato T, Yonekura Y, Honda M, Sadato N: Asymmetrical neural substrates of tactile discrimination in humans: a functional magnetic resonance imaging study. J Neurosci. 2004;24:7524–7530.

[70] Pfurtscheller G, Neuper C: Motor imagery activates primary sensorimotor area in humans. Neurosci Lett. 1997;239:65–68.

[71] Muthukumaraswamy SD, Johnson BW, McNair NA: Mu rhythm modulation during observation of an object-directed grasp. Brain Res Cogn Brain Res. 2004;19:195–201.

[72] Naito E, Nakashima T, Kito T, Aramaki Y, Okada T, Sadato N: Human limb-specific and non-limb-specific brain representations during kinesthetic illusory movements of the upper and lower extremities. Eur Neurosci. 2007;25:3476–3487.

[73] Naito E, Ehrsson HH, Geyer S, Zilles K, Roland PE: Illusory arm movements activate cortical motor areas: a positron emission tomography study. J Neurosci. 1999;19: 6134–6144.

[74] Burke D, Hagbarth KE, Löfstedt L, Wallin BG: The responses of human muscle spindle endings to vibration during isometric contraction. J Physiol. 1976;261:695–711.

[75] Pascual-Marqui RD, Michel CM, Lehmann D: Low resolution brain electromagnetic tomography: a new method for localizing electrical activity in the brain. Int J Psychophysiol. 1994;18:49–65.

[76] Pascual-Marqui RD: Standardized low-resolution brain electromagnetic tomography (sLORETA): technical details. Methods Find Exp Clin Pharmacol. 2002;24:5–12.

[77] Collins DL, Holmes CJ, Peters TK, et al.: Automatic 3-D model-based neuroanatomical segmentation. Hum Brain Mapping. 1995;3:190–208.

[78] Pascual-Marqui RD: Instantaneous and lagged measurements of linear and nonlinear dependence between groups of multivariate time series: frequency decomposition. arXiv. 2007;0711:1455.

[79] Sadato N, Nakamura S, Oohashi T, et al.: Neural networks for generation and suppression of alpha rhythm: a PET study. Neuroreport. 1998;9:893–897.

[80] Tanji J, Okano K, Sato KC: Neuronal activity in cortical motor areas related to ipsilateral, contralateral, and bilateral digit movements of the monkey. J Neurophysiol. 1988;60:325–342.

[81] Naito E: Sensing limb movements in the motor cortex: how humans sense limb movement. Neuroscientist. 2004;10:73–82.

[82] Boussaoud D: Attention versus intention in the primate premotor cortex. Neuroimage. 2001;14:40–45.

[83] Van de Winckel A, Sunaert S, Wenderoth N, et al.: Passive somatosensory discrimination tasks in healthy volunteers: differential networks involved in familiar versus unfamiliar shape and length discrimination. Neuroimage. 2005;26:441–453.

[84] Chung GH, Han YM, Jeong SH, et al.: Functional heterogeneity of the supplementary motor area. AJNR Am J Neuroradiol. 2005;26:1819–1823.

[85] Rowland LM, Shadmehr R, Kravitz D, Holcomb HH: Sequential neural changes during motor learning in schizophrenia. Psychiatry Res. 2008;163(1):1–12.

[86] Pezawas L, Verchinski BA, Mattay VS, Callicott JH, Kolachana BS, Straub RE, Egan MF, Meyer-Lindenberg A, Weinberger DR: The brain-derived neurotrophic factor val 66 met polymorphism and variation in human cortical morphology. J Neurosci. 2004;24:10099–10102.

# 3

# Effects of Repetitive Finger Movements on the Short-Latency Somatosensory-Evoked Potentials

Yoshinori Yamamoto and Naoki Kado

**Abstract**

When performing a movement, many features of sensory information are used as inputs and integrated. Smooth movement is possible by selecting necessary information from all-sensory inputs. The somatosensory input of movement is adjusted at different levels such as at the level of the spinal cord, brainstem, and sensory cortex. However, sensory tests used by physical therapists provide only the sensory information that is perceivable through the parietal association fields. On the other hand, there is a somatosensory-evoked potentials (SEPs) in the tests of the somatic sensory function. An understanding of the SEPs enables the evaluation of the posterior track. Therefore, it is possible to determine if the adjustment of somatosensory inputs occurs at any stage. The SEP amplitude is decreased by passive and voluntary movement. Further, characteristic decrease in the SEP amplitude is noted with an increase in the speed and intensity of movement. Thus, it is important for us to understand the relationship between motor tasks and somatosensory inputs. In this chapter, we introduce our study on the relationship between physical movements and somatosensory inputs, and make recommendations for practicing physical therapy.

**Keywords:** somatosensory-evoked potentials, finger movements, somatosensory

## 1. Introduction

When performing a movement, all sensory information is not perceived at a conscious level, and the necessary sensory information is selected from all available information. For example, elaborate movements of the finger require conscious perception of somatosensory and optic information, but the sensory information associated with the trunk and lower limbs is not consciously perceived. In addition, the sensory information to execute finger movement changes according to the location of the body parts and direction of the motor task. In this manner, it is possible to perform smooth movements by extracting the necessary sensory information from the vast sensory information available. Somatosensory inputs are integrated by sensory receptors and through the somatosensory area and the parietal association fields. Mechanisms that adjust the sensory inputs to the sensory conducting pathway before and during movement exist. These mechanisms act at various stages, ranging from the spinal cord to the cerebral cortex. For example, the reflex is patterning the movement output from sensory input by spinal cord and brainstem. Walking and chewing are automatically generated movements based on sensory inputs delivered to the midbrain and the pons. The need for the cerebral cortex to act in order to execute these movements is optional. The initial stages of motor learning are associated with extensive sensory feedback. Advancement of motor learning requires adjustments of sensory inputs in advance by feed-forward mechanisms. It has been shown that the necessary sensory inputs and integration mechanisms vary depending on the exercise conditions. However, sensory tests used by physical therapists require subjects to recognize and judge movement based on sensory information from the sensory receptor. Therefore, it is difficult to evaluate the exact somatosensory pathway associated with movement.

The inspection of the sensory function has led to the observation if somatosensory-evoked potentials (SEPs). SEPs are able to evaluate the funiculus posterior. SEPs can be classified into short-latency, middle-latency, and long-latency, based on the latency of the SEP waveform. A 50 ms from stimulation electrical is a component of short-latency. In particular, the component within 20 ms is called short-latency SEPs. Short-latency SEPs are stable-evoked potentials generated in the cerebral cortex through inputs from peripheral nerves, and they are hardly affected by the level of consciousness. Potentials evoked with a latency of 50–100 ms are classified as middle-latency SEPs, while those evoked with a latency beyond 100 ms are called long-latency SEPs. Since middle-latency SEPs are generated in the cerebral cortex, they are susceptible to the attention level and can be modulated by the sleep state. Next is explaining of latency and components in short-latency SEP in upper limbs. SEPs can be defined by their polarity (positive/negative) and latency (short/middle/long). The N9 waveform is first recorded from the upper limbs upon electrical stimulation of the median nerve with the wrist joint. The N9 is a negative wave appearing at the latency of about 9 ms from electrical stimulation. The origin of N9 is believed to be the action potential derived from the brachial plexus. The N13 waveform is recorded next, and it is said to originate from the postsynaptic potential derived from the brachial plexus. The N20 and P25 waveforms are recorded following the N9 waveform. The origin of N20 is believed to be the 3b area while that of P25 is said to be postsynaptic potential derived from the one area [1].

On the topic of the influence of movement on SEPs, Giblin reported for the first time that the amplitude of cerebral cortex SEPs decreased during voluntary movement [2]. Numerous papers have reported the changes in SEPs during upper and lower limb movements. It is known that the SEP amplitude decreases during voluntary movement. In other words, sensory inputs are inhibited during voluntary movement [2]. This decrease in the SEP amplitude is called gating and can be mediated by two mechanisms, namely centripetal gating and centrifugal gating. In centripetal gating, the afferent impulse from the peripheral receptor due to voluntary movement and the afferent impulse from the peripheral nerve stimulation are input at the same time, resulting in interferences such as occlusion and lateral inhibition. In centrifugal gating, efferent impulses from exercise-related areas in response to voluntary movement suppress afferent impulses from peripheral nerve stimulation [3]. Voluntary movement affects both centripetal and centrifugal gating mechanisms. The SEP amplitude decreases with increases in movement speed [4] and load [5, 6]. This gating is thought to play a role in performing accurate movement by eliminating unnecessary somatosensory information [7]. We studied the effects of finger movement on short-latency SEPs. Previous studies have reported that the SEP amplitude varies with the type of motor task. Therefore, we will introduce our research on the influence of differences in motor tasks on SEPs and provide recommendations for physical therapy.

## 2. Effects of repetitive finger movements performed at different frequencies on the somatosensory-evoked potentials

When sensory inputs are facilitated, select the slow movement. It is important to understand the influence of movement frequency and speed on sensory function during physical therapy. Therefore, we examined the effects of repetitive finger movements performed at different frequencies on the sensory system of the ipsilateral upper arm [8]. The sample consisted of 13 healthy adult subjects. The SEPs were recorded by stimulating the right median nerve during movement of the right index finger and while at rest. The subjects were required to perform motor tasks involving repetitive flexion and extension of the metacarpophalangeal (MP) joint of the right index finger, and the movement frequencies used were 0.5, 1, and 3 Hz. The amplitude and latency of SEPs are shown in **Figures 1** and **2**. There was no significant difference in the N9 and N13 amplitudes between rest and task conditions. The amplitudes of the N20 and P25 waveforms were significantly lower at a movement frequency of 3 Hz than those at rest. The latencies of the N9, N13, N20, and P25 waveforms were not significantly different between rest and task conditions.

In this study, the SEPs recorded from the ipsilateral brachial plexus and nucleus cuneatus did not change even if the frequency of repetitive movements of the right index finger was increased. It was suggested that repetitive movements at 3 Hz suppress somatosensory inputs to areas higher in level than the 3b. This inhibition was likely due to an increase in the movement frequency. Sadato et al. reported that significant activation of the primary somatosensory cortex was not observed during flexion of the right index finger at movement frequencies of 0.25 and 0.5 Hz but reported that significant activation was observed as the frequency increased from 1 to 4 Hz [9]. Blinkenberg et al. reported that the contralateral primary motor cortex, primary somatosensory cortex, supplementary motor cortex, and cerebellum were activated at movement frequencies of 0.5–4 Hz during finger tapping movement of the right index finger [10]. In addition, they reported a significant positive correlation between the movement frequency and cerebral blood flow in the primary motor and primary somatosensory cortices. Similarly, this study also noted a possibility of increase in the exercise-related area or the extent of activation with an increase in movement frequency. In addition, it was possible that sensory inputs to proprioceptors and mechanoreceptors increase

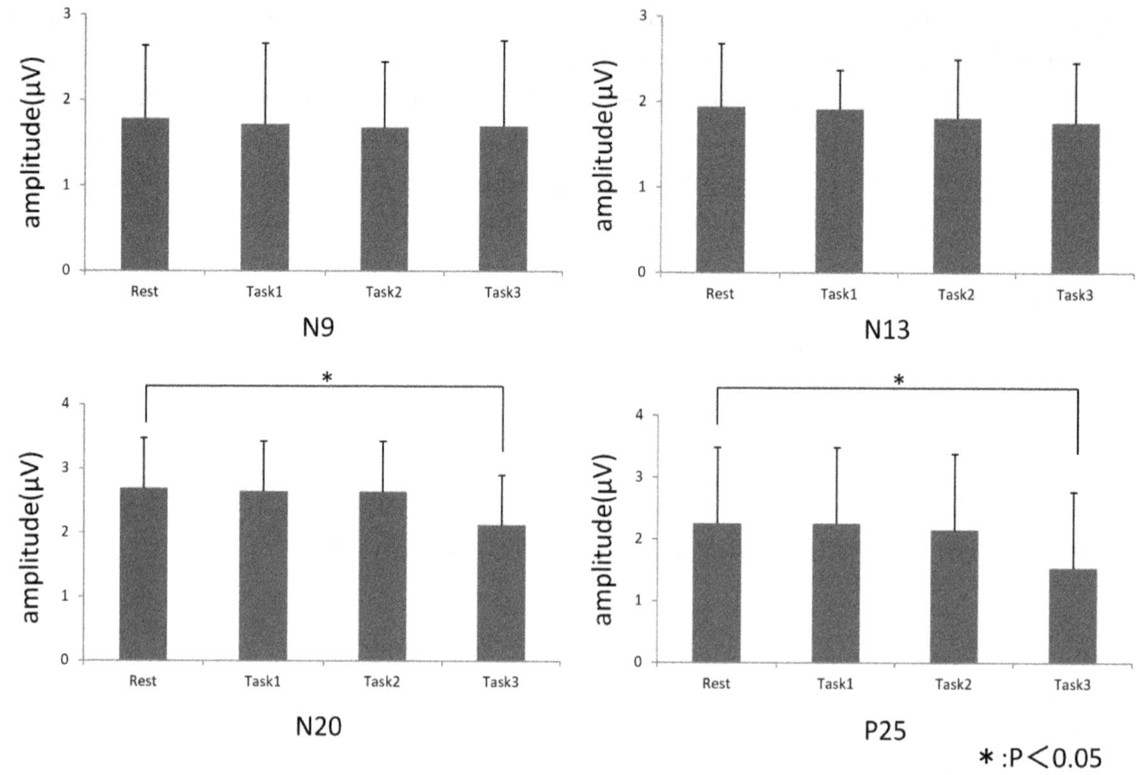


**Figure 1.** The change on the somatosensory-evoked potential amplitude when repetitive finger movements performed at different frequencies.

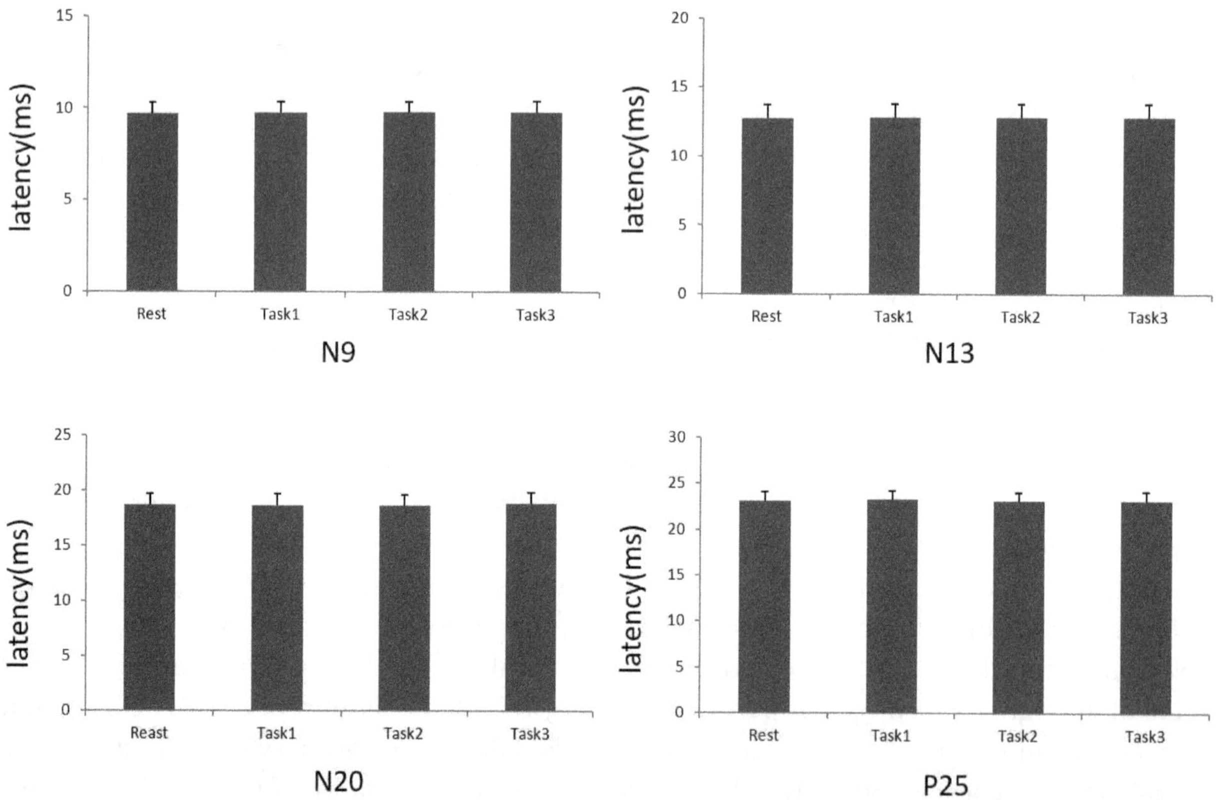


**Figure 2.** The change on the somatosensory-evoked potential latency when repetitive finger movements performed at different frequencies.

with movement. In precedence study of SEPs, it reported that the SEP amplitude decreased with an increase in the movement speed [4]. Both centripetal gating and centrifugal gating mechanisms might play a role in this effect. Similarly, this study also noted the possibility of suppression of the somatosensory input by the two gating mechanisms at a repetitive finger movement frequency of 3 Hz. Repetitive finger movements at low frequencies (such as in tasks 1 and 2) may elicit significant activation of exercise-related areas and decreases in the sensory input. Therefore, it was not affected by gating and no change in somatosensory inputs between rest and task conditions was expected. Cheron et al. reported that most gating arises in the cortex [11]. In this study too, it was considered that gating occurs at the cortical level, which may be the reason for why no change was observed in the nucleus cuneatus activation.

## 3. Effects of non-periodic repetitive finger movements on the short-latency somatosensory-evoked potentials

Periodic movements, such as walking, involve patterns of movement that mainly employ feed-forward neural mechanisms. On the other hand, non-periodic and unpredictable movements require sensory feedback for online modulation of movement. It is believed that the exercise programs employed for periodic and non-periodic movements are different. Therefore, we studied the effects of non-periodic repetitive finger movements on short-latency somatosensory evoked potentials (SEPs) [12]. A total of 11 healthy adult subjects were included in the study. The motor task involved flexion and extension of the right index finger MP joint in response to a specific auditory signal. Task 1 involved presenting a sound with a 1000-ms periodic interval, while task 2 involved randomly presenting sounds with 750-, 1000-, and 1250-ms periodic intervals. The number of movements performed during each task was the same. The amplitude and latency of SEPs are shown in **Figures 3** and **4**. The N9 and N13 amplitudes were not significantly different between rest and either of the tasks. The N20 and P25 amplitudes were significantly lower in task 2 than at rest. The N9, N13, N20, and P25 latencies were not significantly different between rest and either of the tasks.

This study suggests that non-periodic movement were decreased of the N20 and p25 amplitudes. In addition, it was guessed that non-periodic movement were suppress somatosensory inputs to areas higher in level than the 3b. Thaut reported that changes of 20% or more from the baseline interval due to sound was able to easily notice a change of time interval [13]. In this study, the time interval of non-periodic movement was set to 25% of that before and after 1000 ms. Laultz et al. reported that when comparing periodic and non-periodic movements, cerebral blood flow related to non-periodic movement was significantly higher in the ipsilateral cerebellar nuclei, contralateral thalamic dorsal lateral nucleus, and contralateral sensory motor area [14]. This report indicated that the activity in the cerebellum-thalamus-sensory motor pathway can control and correct the movement. Ivry et al. reported that the cerebellum lobus posterior pars lateralis participated in the regulation of exercise timing during non-periodic movements [15]. These reports show that non-periodic movement was influenced by the timing of exercise; this effect is mediated by the cerebellum lobus posterior pars lateralis and the online control of movement is achieved

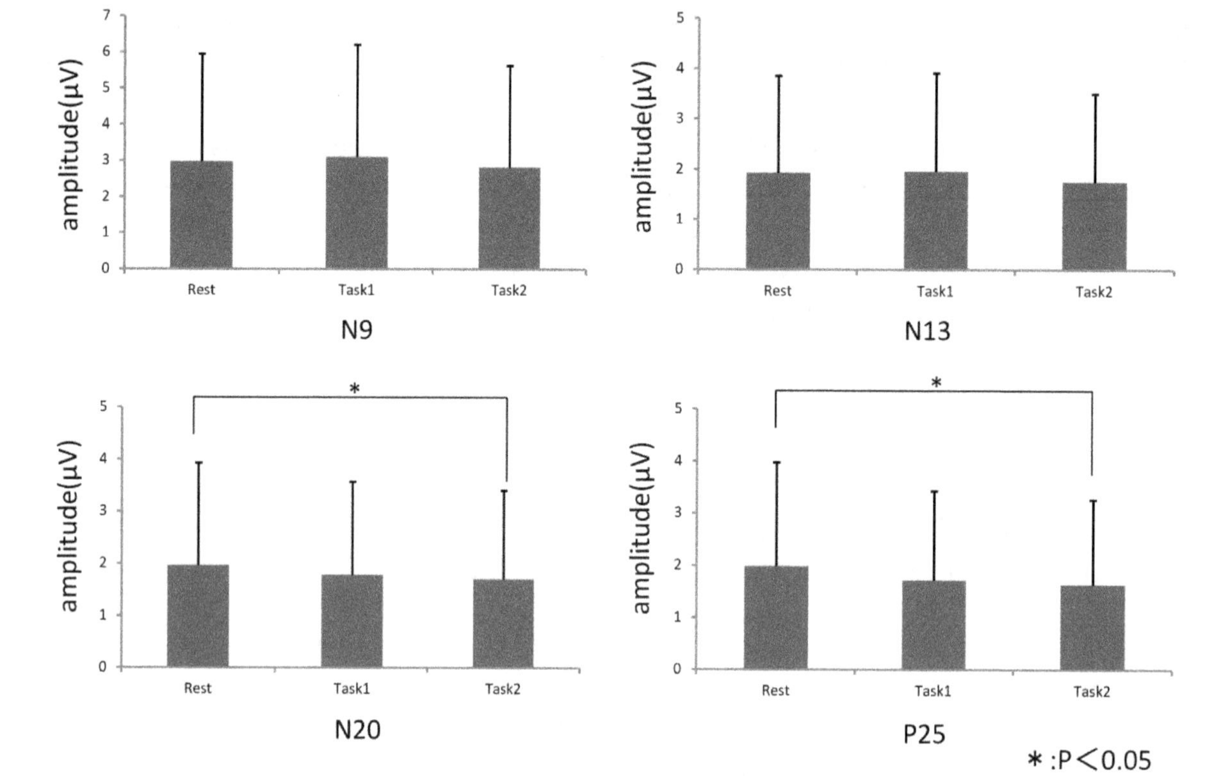


**Figure 3.** The change on the somatosensory-evoked potential amplitude when non-periodic repetitive finger movements.

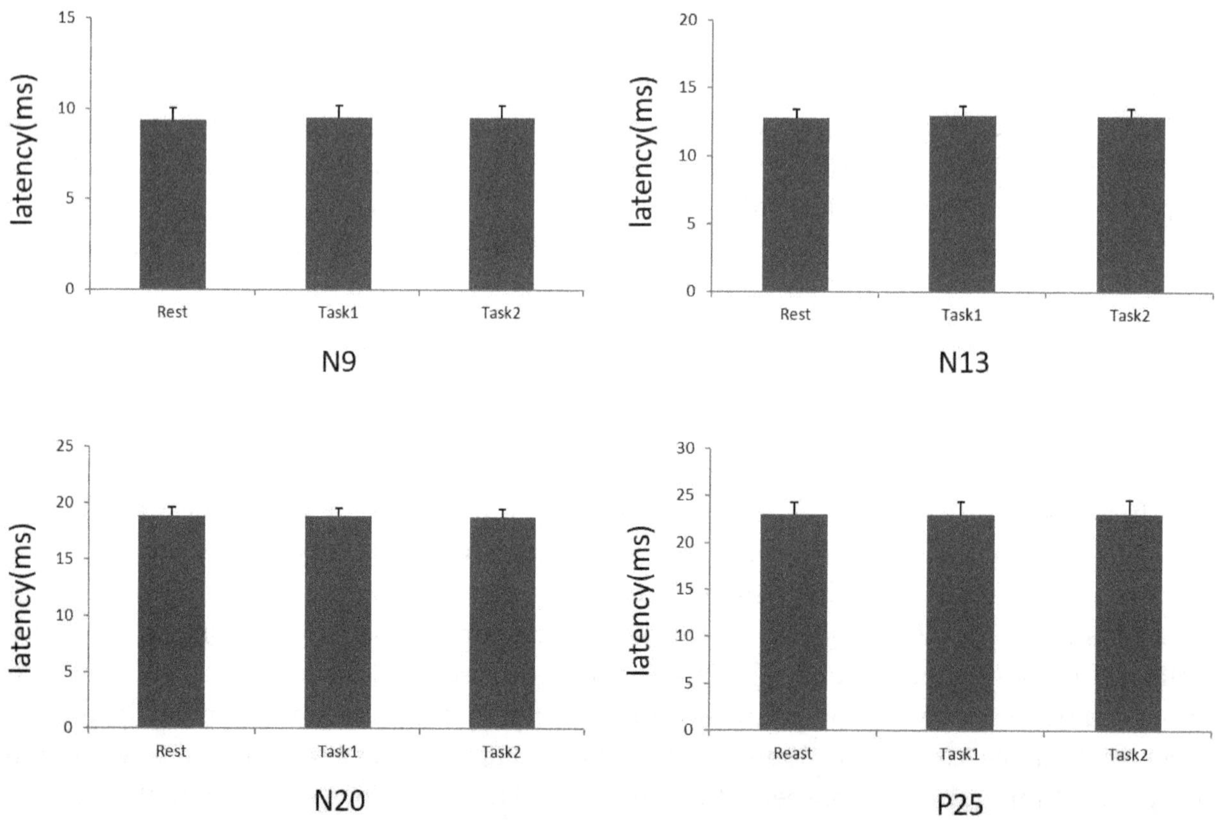


**Figure 4.** The change on the somatosensory-evoked potential latency when non-periodic repetitive finger movements.

through activity in the cerebellum-thalamus-sensory motor pathway. Furthermore, Ivry et al. reported that bilateral activities in the supplementary motor area, prefrontal cortex, gyrus cinguli, sensory motor cortex, and basal ganglia, and continuous attention paid to the time of non-periodic movement allowed for the prior preparation for the movement [15]. These reports showed that non-periodic movement was influenced by preparation and attention and timing and control. This study suggests that non-periodic movement was influenced to timing of exercise participating in the cerebellum lobus posterior pars lateralis and to controls exercise participating in the cerebellum-thalamus-sensory motor pathway. In addition, the results suggest that non-periodic movement is influenced by preparation, attention, timing, and control, and that this effect may be mediated by activity in the prefrontal cortex, gyrus cinguli, and supplementary motor area. However, it was reported that awakening (sleep/wake state) and attention influence long- and medium-latency SEPs, but not short-latency SEPs. In this study, decreases in the amplitudes of N20 and P25 SEPs were not influenced by the level of preparation or vigilance/awakening, and their amplitudes were influenced by exercise timing and control. The activity of motor-related areas was considered to have an inhibitory effect on the SEPs recorded from the somatosensory area, thalamus, and posterior nucleus. In addition, it was guessed that nerve cells possible to excited against somatosensory input by overlap of the motor-related area and electrical stimulation. Based on these findings, a mechanism underlying the effects of non-periodic repetitive finger movements on the SEPs was proposed: Activity of the cerebellum lobus posterior pars lateralis and cerebellum-thalamus-sensory motor cortex pathway inhibited activity in the thalamus and primary somatosensory cortex, which led to the inhibition of somatosensory inputs projecting from the primary motor cortex to the primary somatosensory cortex. And it was thought that refractory period occurred against stimulation of upper limb due to increase of activity of primary somatosensory cortex. Each amplitude of periodic movement showed no significant difference in each task compared with the rest. Sadato et al. reported that the activity of the primary somatosensory cortex in the flexion movement of the right index finger does not show a significant difference at the movement frequency of 4000 and 2000 ms [10]. However, it reported that a significant difference was recognized as increasing from 1000 to 250 ms. Del et al. reported that activity of the cerebellum was high with 500 ms than 2000 ms, 1000 ms in the tapping of the right index finger [16]. It was speculated that significant cerebellar activity was not recognized at an exercise frequency of about 1000 ms (such as that in task 1), and it was not affected by gating from exercise-related areas.

## 4. Clinical suggestion

In the early stages of motor learning, sensory feedback is required to identify and understand the expected movement. Movement using sensory feedback is slow, which allows for online correction of movement mediated by the cortex. Low-frequency movements (0.5 and 1 Hz) were not observed to be suppressed by sensory inputs, while high-frequency movements (3 Hz) were suppressed by sensory inputs. For performing smooth high-frequency movements, it is critical to suppress unnecessary sensory inputs. Moreover, it is necessary to suppress unnecessary sensory input while performing non-periodic movements for timing adjustment and motion control. Based on the results of this study, low frequency movement and periodic movement are considered beneficial while performing physical therapy aimed at stimulating sensory inputs. As motor learning progresses, it is necessary to introduce high-frequency and non-periodic movements in the therapy protocol. Thus, the frequency and style of movement and the stage of motor learning must be taken into account when determining the sensory inputs to be used in a physical therapy regimen.

## 5. Conclusion

It has been consistently reported that the SEP amplitude decreases during exercise. It was believed that this reduction in SEP amplitude suppresses the sensory input by gating and allows for smooth motion control by making use of only the necessary somatosensory information. Therefore, it is important to understand the relationship between sensory input and motor output when performing physical therapy.

## Author details

Yoshinori Yamamoto[1*] and Naoki Kado[2]

*Address all correspondence to: y.caluo@gmail.com

1 Department of Rehabilitation, Sakakibara Hakuho Hospital, Mie, Japan

2 Kobe College of Rehabilitation and Welfare, Hyogo, Japan

## References

[1] Allison T, McCarthy G, Wood CC, Darcey TM, Spencer DD, Williamson PD. Human cortical potentials evoked by stimulation of the median nerve. I. Cytoarchitectonic areas generating short-latency activity. J Neurophysiol. 1989;62(3):694–710.

[2] Gblin DR. Somatosensory evoked potentials in healthy subjects and in patients with lesions of the nervous system. Ann N Y Acad Sci. 1964;112(8):93–142.

[3] Jones SJ, Halonen JP, Shawkat F. Centrifugal and centripetal mechanisms involved in the 'gating' of cortical SEPs during movement. Elecyroencephalogr Clin Neurophysiol. 1989;74(1):36–45.

[4] Rushton DM, Rothwell JC, Craggs MD. Gating of somatosensory evoked potentials during different kinds of movement in man. Brain. 1981;104(3):465–491.

[5] Angel RW, Boylls CC, Weinrich M. Cerebral evoked potential and somatosensory perception. Neurology. 1984;34(1):123–126.

[6] Cohen LG, Starr A. Vibration and muscle contraction affect somatosensory evoked potentials. Neurology. 1985;35(5):691–698.

[7] Cohen LG, Starr A. Localization, timing and specificity of gating of somatosensory evoked potentials during active movement in man. Brain. 1987;110(2):451–467.

[8] Yamamoto Y, Kado N, Suzuki T. Effects of repetitive finger movements performed at different frequencies on the somatosensory evoked potentials (in Japanese). J Phys Therapy Sci. 2013;28(2):257–260.

[9] Sadato N, Ibanez V, Campell G, Deiber MP, Le Bihan D, Hallett M. Frequency-dependent changes of regional blood flow during finger movements: functional MRI compared to PET. J Cereb Blood Metab. 1997;17(6):670–679.

[10] Blinkenberg M, Borde C, Holm S, Svarer C, Andersen J, Paulson OB, Law I. Rate dependence of regional cerebral activation during performance of a repetitive motor task: A PET study. J Cereb Blood Flow Metab. 1996;16(5):794–803.

[11] Cheron G, Borenstein S. Specific gating of the early somatosensory evoked potentials during active movement. Electroencephalogr Clin Neurophysiol. 1987;67(6):537–548.

[12] Yamamoto Y, Kado N, Suzuki T. Effects of non-periodic repetitive finger movements on the short-latency somatosensory evoked potentials (in Japanese). Jpn J Clin Neurophysiol. 2015(2);43:65–69.

[13] Thaut MH, editor. Rhythm, music, and the brain: Scientific foundations and clinical applications. New York: Routledge; 2008, pp. 4–45.

[14] Lautz K, Specht K, Shah NJ, Jancke L. Tapping movement according to regular and irregular visual timing signals investigated with fMRI. Neuro Rep. 2000;11(6):1301–1306.

[15] Ivry RB, Keele SW, Diener HC. Dissociation of the lateral and medial cerebellum in movement timing and movement execution. Exp Brain Res. 1988;73(1):167–180.

[16] Del Olmo MF, Cheeran B, Koch G, Rothwell JC. Role of the cerebellum in externally paced rhythmic finger movements. J Neurophysiol. 2007;98(1):145–152.

4

# The Effect of Motor Imagery on Spinal Motor Neuron Excitability and its Clinical use in Physical Therapy

Yoshibumi Bunno, Yuki Fukumoto,

Todo Marina and Chieko Onigata

**Abstract**

We investigated the influence of the imagined muscle contraction strengths on spinal motor neuron excitability in healthy volunteers. F-wave was used for assessing spinal motor excitability. The F-waves during motor imagery (MI) under 10, 30, 50, 70, and 100% maximal voluntary contractions (MVCs) were compared. Furthermore, we investigated changes of the F-waves during motor imagery for 5 min. Motor imagery under 10, 30, 50, 70, and 100% maximal voluntary contractions can increase spinal motor neuron excitability. However, the imagined muscle contraction strengths were not involved in changes of spinal motor neuron excitability. Additionally, spinal motor neuron excitability after 5 min from onset of motor imagery returned to the rest level. Thus, in clinical use of motor imagery, slightly imagined muscle contraction strength is enough for facilitating spinal motor neuron excitability. Also, duration of motor imagery needs to be considered.

**Keywords:** motor imagery, F-wave, imagined muscle contraction strength, duration, physical therapy

## 1. Introduction

Motor imagery (MI) is defined as a cognitive process in which the subjects imagine that they perform movements without actually performing movements and muscle contractions [1].

MI has been shown to improve various motor functions in healthy subjects. Specifically, Yue and Cole [2] suggested that MI of little finger abduction under maximal voluntary contraction (MVC) for 4weeks could increase muscle strength. Additionally, MI of ankle dorsiflexion under MVC for 4weeks could increase muscle strength [3]. Also, Guillot et al. [4] suggested that muscle flexibility was improved after MI of stretching for 5weeks. Furthermore, in clinical settings, MI can be applied in physical therapy for patients with damage to the central nervous system, such as stroke, Parkinson's disease, and spinal cord injury.

The effects of MI have been discussed in numerous neurophysiological studies. Various brain activities, including primary motor area, supplementary motor area, premotor area, somatosensory area, prefrontal cortex, parietal lobule, cingulate area, cerebellum, and basal ganglia, were activated during MI by using positron emission tomography (PET), functional magnetic resonance imaging (fMRI), and near infrared spectroscopy (NIRS) [5–8]. These regions were also activated in motor execution. Thus, MI and motor execution are considered to share common neural networks. Furthermore, enhanced corticospinal excitability may explain the increase in motor evoked potentials (MEPs) amplitude by applying transcranial magnetic stimulation (TMS) over the primary motor area during MI [9]. These previous studies suggested that MI can facilitate the central nervous system.

However, other studies could not show the certain results in spinal motor neuron excitability during MI by using the F-wave, H-reflex, and T-reflex. The F-wave, H-reflex, and T-reflex are considered as indices of spinal motor neuron excitability. We previously studied spinal motor neuron excitability during MI of isometric thenar muscle activity. The persistence and F/M amplitude ratio during MI of thenar muscle activity under 50% MVC were significantly increased compared to that at rest [10]. Taniguchi et al. [11] reported that the F/M amplitude ratio after volitional relaxation for 3h was significantly decreased. When subjects did volitional relaxation and MI of thumb abduction simultaneously, the F/M amplitude ratio was maintained at that before volitional relaxation level. This indicated that MI can increase spinal motor neuron excitability. Whereas Kasai et al. [9] reported that the H-reflex amplitude was not changed during MI of wrist flexion movement, Oishi et al. [12] reported that there are various results in the H-reflex amplitude during MI in speed skaters. Thus, it might be suggested that spinal motor neuron excitability was not always increased during MI, although MI can increase the central nervous system.

Our final goal is to find the way that MI obtained the most beneficial effect. To assess spinal motor neuron excitability is as important as the central nervous system, because we think that facilitation of spinal motor neuron excitability is required for improvement of motor function. Thus, in this chapter, we would like to introduce our previous work about spinal motor neuron excitability during MI under various MI conditions. First, we described spinal motor neuron excitability during MI under various imagined muscle contraction strengths. Next, we described the influence of duration of MI on spinal motor neuron excitability. Additionally, at the end of the chapter, we discuss how to apply MI to physical therapy.

## 2. Spinal motor neuron excitability of MI under various imagined muscle contractions

### 2.1. Spinal motor neuron excitability of MI under 10, 30, 50, and 70% MVC

#### *2.1.1. Purpose*

We previously reported that spinal motor neuron excitability during MI of isometric thenar muscle activity under 50% MVC was significantly increased in comparison with that at rest [10]. In actual motion, Suzuki et al. [15] compared spinal motor neuron excitability during actual isometric thenar muscle activity under 25, 50, 75, and 100% MVC. The persistence and F/M amplitude ratio increased linearly with the muscle contraction strength. Spinal motor neuron excitability during MI increases linearly with the imagined muscle contraction strength if MI and motor execution share common neural networks. However, it was unclear whether the imagined muscle contraction strength affects the changes of spinal motor neuron excitability. Then, we investigated changes of spinal motor neuron excitability during MI of isometric thenar muscle activity under various imagined muscle contraction strengths. Specifically, we used 10, 30, 50, and 70% MVC for the imagined muscle contraction strength. In addition, we assessed spinal motor neuron excitability by using F-wave.

#### *2.1.2. Materials*

We included 10 healthy volunteers (5 males and 5 females; mean age, 28.7±4.5years. All subjects provided informed consent prior to the study's commencement. This study was approved by the Research Ethics Committee at Kansai University of Health Sciences. The experiments were conducted in accordance with the Declaration of Helsinki.

#### *2.1.3. Methods*

Subjects were in a supine position with muscles relaxed and instructed to fix one eye on a pinch meter monitor [digital indicator F304A (unipulse)] throughout the test (**Figure 1**). Abrasive gel was applied to keep the skin impedance below 5kΩ. The temperature was maintained at 25°C. A Viking Quest electromyography (EMG) machine (Natus Medical Inc., Pleasanton, USA) was used for F-wave recording (**Figure 1**). We recorded F-waves from the left thenar muscles after stimulating the left median nerve. A pair of disks was attached with collodion to the skin over the belly and the bones of the metacarpophalangeal joint of the thumb. The stimulating electrodes comprised the cathode placed over the left median nerve 3cm proximal to the palmar crease, and the anode was placed 2cm more proximally (**Figure 2**). The maximal stimulus was determined by delivering 0.2-ms square-wave pulses of increasing intensity to elicit the largest compound muscle action potential (M-wave). The supramaximal stimuli (adjusted up to 20% higher than the maximum stimulus intensity) were delivered at 0.5Hz. The bandwidth filter ranged from 2Hz to 3kHz.

We showed the typical F-wave forms from thenar muscle after applying 30 electrical stimuli on the median nerve (**Figure 3**).

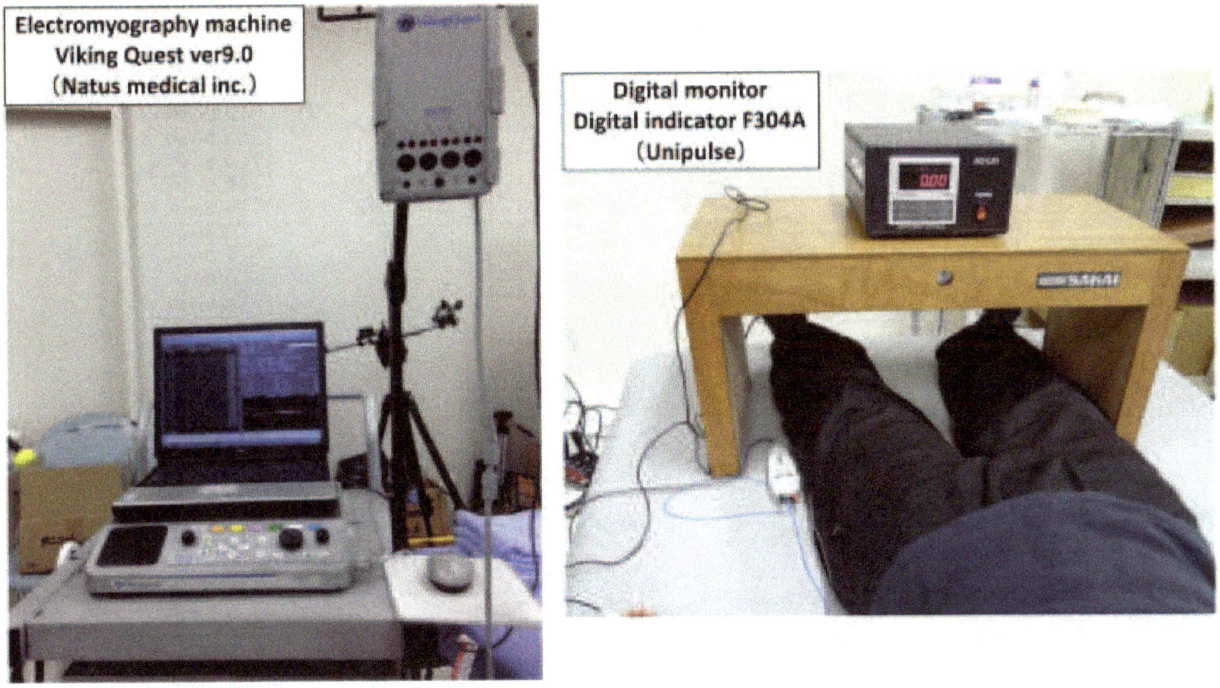


**Figure 1.** The F-wave recording instruments.

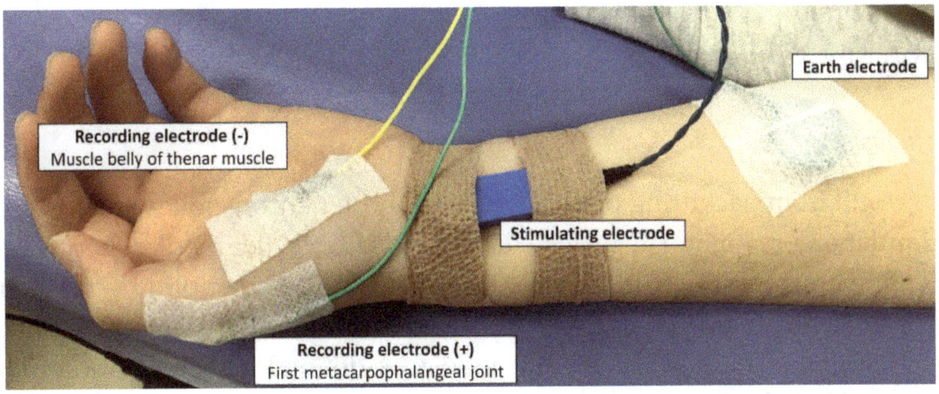


**Figure 2.** The F-wave recording condition.

In the resting trial (rest), the F-waves were recorded during relaxation. Next, we measured MVC by asking the subjects to apply maximum pressure to the pinch meter sensor between left thumb and index finger for 10s. Subsequently, the subjects were required to learn isometric thenar muscle activity under 10% MVC for 1min. The subjects were instructed to keep the 10% MVC value, which was displayed on the digital pinch meter monitor. For MI trial, the subjects were instructed to imagine 10% MVC thenar muscle activity while holding the sensor between their thumb and index finger without exerting any muscle contractions. F-waves were measured both during (10% MI) and immediately after 10% MI (post). The above process was defined as the MI using a 10% MVC condition (10% MI condition). This training process was repeated for MI of 30, 50, and 70% of MVC, and F-waves were recorded as described. Trials under these conditions were performed randomly on different days.

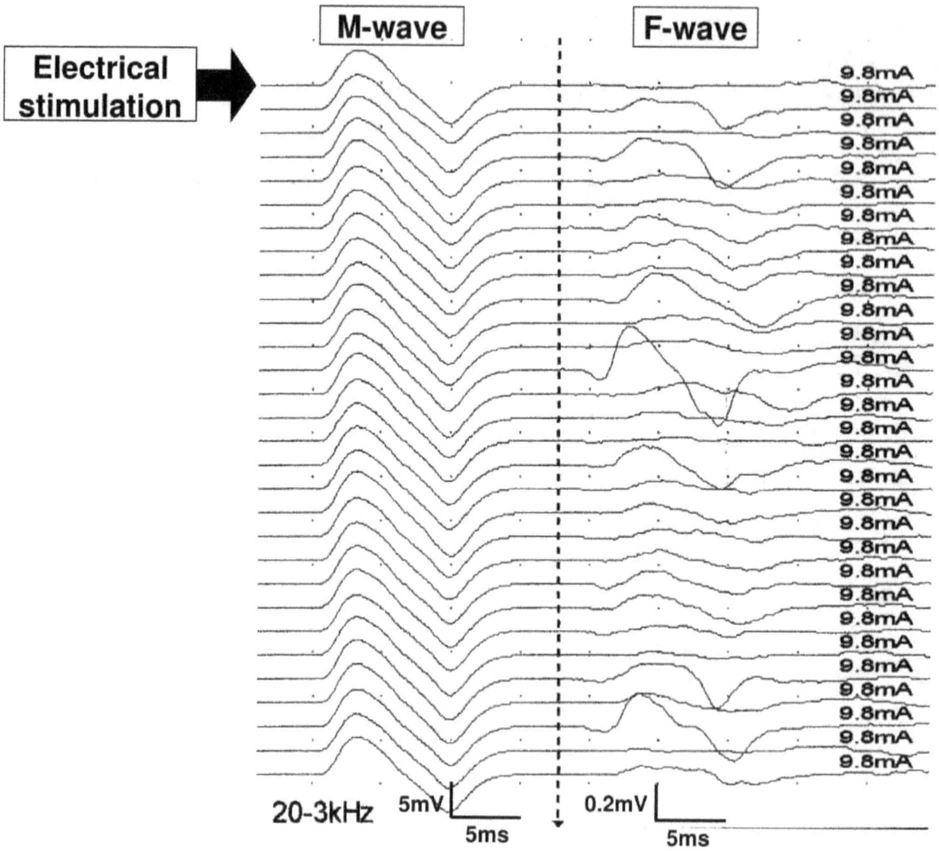


**Figure 3.** The typical F-wave forms.

### *2.1.4. Date analysis*

The F-waves result from backfiring of spinal anterior horn neurons following distal antidromic electrical stimulation of $\alpha$-motor neurons [16–18], in this case the median nerve. The F-waves from 30 stimuli were analyzed with respect to persistence, F/M amplitude ratio, and latency. Persistence was defined as the number of measurable F-wave responses divided by 30 supramaximal stimuli. The F/M amplitude ratio was defined as the mean amplitude of all responses divided by M-wave amplitude. Latency was defined as the mean latency from the time of stimulation to onset of measurable F-waves. Persistence reflects the number of backfiring anterior horn cells [17, 18]. The F/M amplitude ratio reflects the number of backfiring anterior horn cells and the excitability of individual cells [17, 18]. Therefore, these parameters are considered to be the indexes of spinal motor neuron excitability.

### *2.1.5. Statistical analysis*

The normality of F-wave data was confirmed using the Kolmogorov-Smirnov and Shapiro-Wilk tests. The persistence, F/M amplitude ratio, and latency among three trials (rest, MI, post) under each MI condition (10% MI, 30% MI, 50% MI, and 70% MI conditions) were compared using the Friedman test and Scheffe's post hoc test. The relative values among the four MI conditions were compared using the Friedman test. We used IBM SPSS statistics ver.19 for all statistical analysis.

### 2.1.6. Results

Persistence during MI under the four MI conditions was significantly increased compared to that at rest (Scheffe's test; 10% MI vs rest, 70% MI vs rest, $^{**}p<0.01$; 30% MI vs rest, 50% MI vs rest, $^{*}p<0.05$; **Figures 4–7**). Persistence immediately after MI was significantly decreased compared with that at MI (Scheffe's test; 10% MI vs post, 30% MI vs post, 70% MI vs post, $^{*}p<0.05$; **Figures 4, 5,** and **7**). Persistence at post tended to be decreased compared with that at 50% MI (Scheffe's test; $p=0.067$; **Figure 6**).

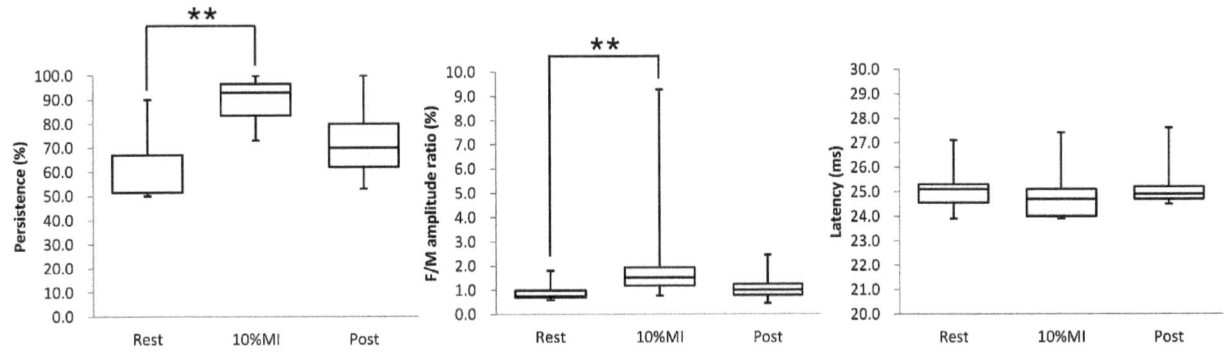


**Figure 4.** The F-waves at rest, MI, and post trials under the 10% MI condition.

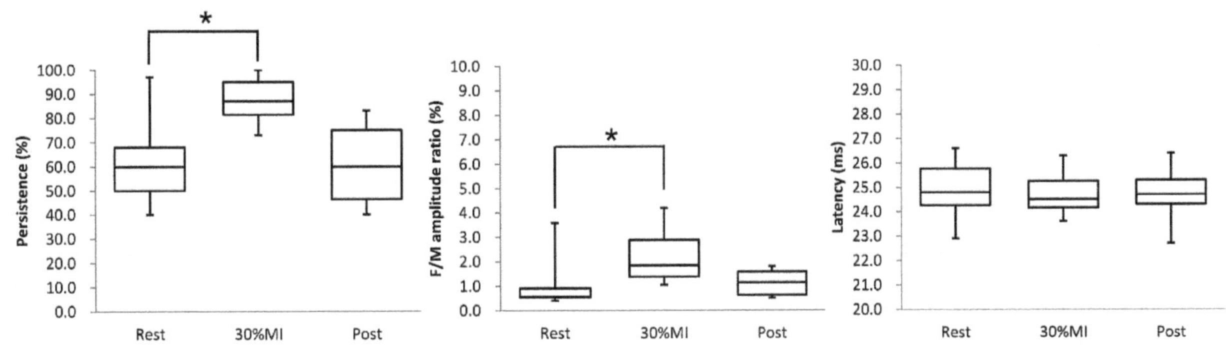


**Figure 5.** The F-waves at rest, MI, and post trials under the 30% MI condition.

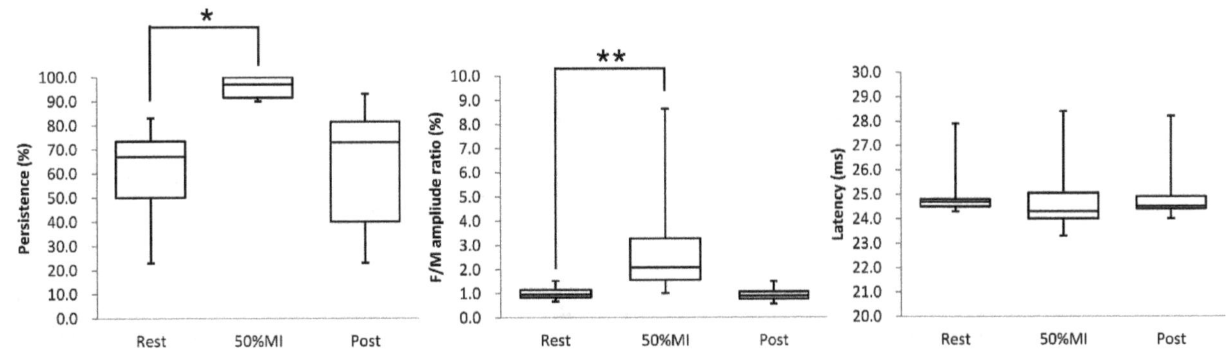


**Figure 6.** The F-waves at rest, MI, and post trials under 50% MI condition.

The F/M amplitude ratio during MI under the three MI conditions was significantly increased compared to that at rest (Scheffe's test; 10% MI vs rest, 50% MI vs rest, **$p<0.01$; 30% MI vs rest, *$p<0.05$; **Figures 4–6**). The F/M amplitude ratio during 70% MI tended to be increased compared to that at rest (Scheffe's test; $p=0.082$; **Figure 7**). The F/M amplitude ratio immediately after 50% MI was significantly decreased compared to that at 50% MI (Scheffe's test; *$p<0.05$; **Figure 6**).

Alternatively, no significant differences in latency were observed among three trials (rest, MI, and post) under the four MI conditions (**Figures 4–7**).

The relative values of persistence, F/M amplitude ratio, and latency did not exhibit significant differences among the four MI conditions (**Figures 8–10**).

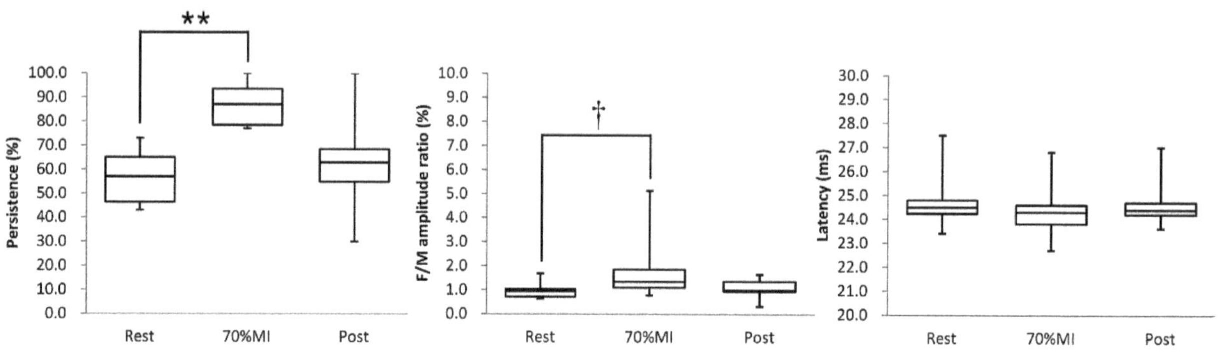


**Figure 7.** The F-waves at rest, MI, and post trials under 70% MI condition.

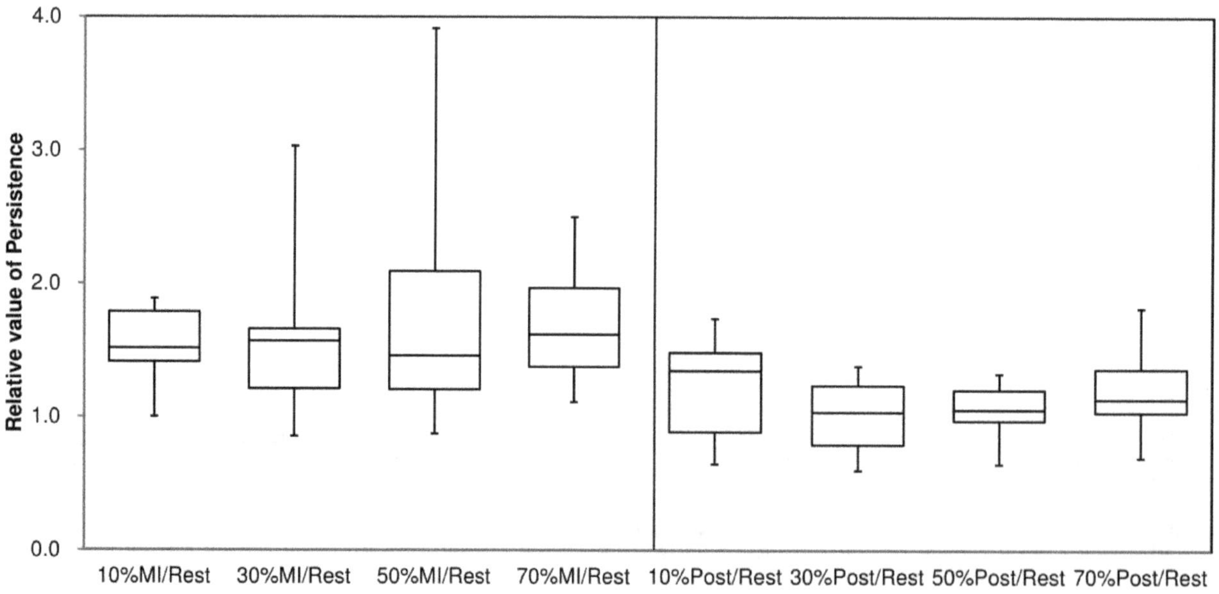


**Figure 8.** Comparison of relative values of persistence among the four MI conditions.

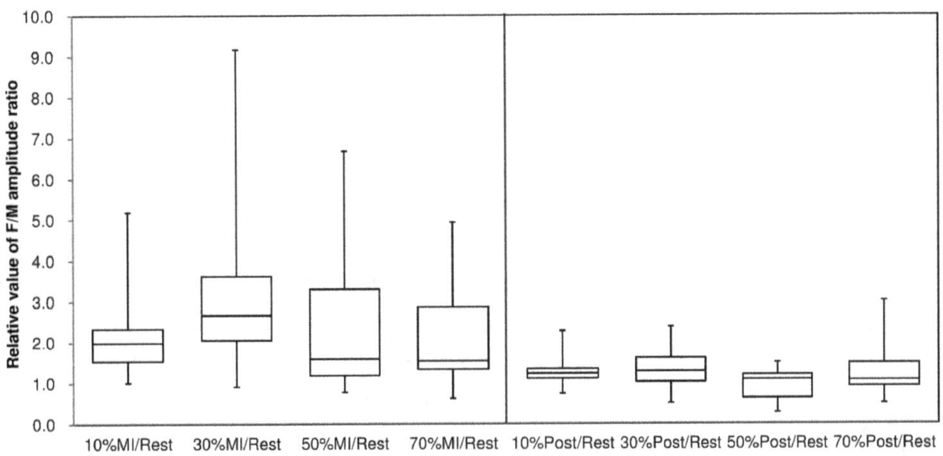


**Figure 9.** Comparison of relative values of F/M amplitude ratio among the four MI conditions.

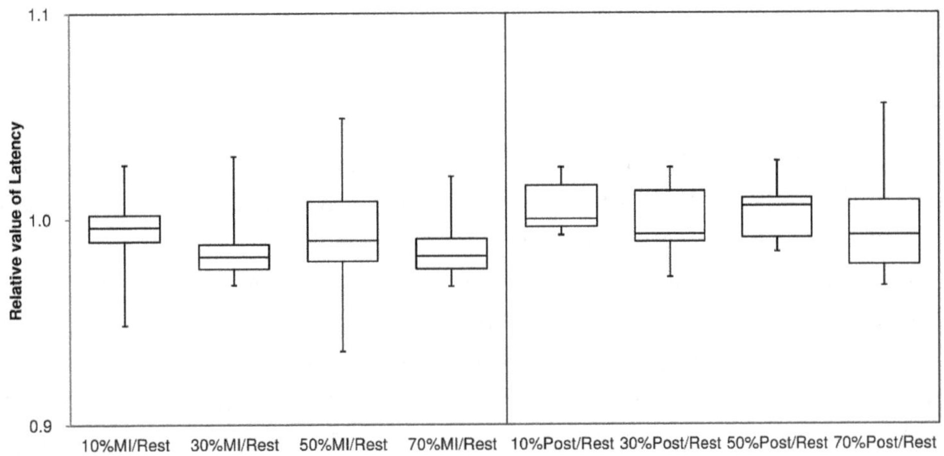


**Figure 10.** Comparison of relative values of latency among the four MI conditions.

## 2.2. Spinal motor neuron excitability during MI under 50 and 100% MVC

### *2.2.1. Purpose*

In previous work, MI under 10, 30, 50, and 70% MVC was shown to increase spinal motor neuron excitability [13, 14]. The imagined muscle contraction strengths did not influence the facilitation amount of spinal motor neuron excitability [13, 14]. However, Cowley et al. [20] suggested that the H-reflex amplitude during MI of plantar flexion under 100% MVC was significantly higher than that under 50% MVC. Therefore, we hypothesized that the MI of thenar muscle activity under 100% MVC will be higher than that under 50% MVC. In this study, we investigated spinal motor neuron excitability during MI under 50 and 100% MVC.

### *2.2.2. Materials*

We included 15 healthy subjects (13 males; 2 females; mean age, 25.3±5.04years). All subjects provided informed consent prior to the study's commencement. This study was approved by the Research Ethics Committee at Graduate School of Kansai University of Health Sciences. The experiments were conducted in accordance with the Declaration of Helsinki.

### 2.2.3. Methods

The environment and conditions of the F-wave recording are the same as in previous work. The protocol of this study is as follows. In the resting trial (rest), the F-waves were recorded during relaxation. Next, we measured 100% MVC; that is, the subjects held the sensor of the pinch meter while exerting their maximum effort for 10s. Subsequently, the subjects were instructed to learn the isometric thenar muscle activity under 100% MVC for 1min as a motor task. They performed the activity using visual feedback while watching the digital monitor of the pinch meter. They were then instructed to perform MI of learned thenar muscle activity under 100% MVC by holding the sensor between the thumb and index finger. F-waves were recorded during the MI (100% MI). F-waves were recorded immediately after 100% MI trial (post). We defined the above process as the MI using the 100% MVC condition (100% MI condition). With regard to the MI using the 50% MVC condition (50% MI condition), F-waves were recorded using the same process. These conditions were randomly performed on different days.

### 2.2.4. Statistical analysis

For statistical analysis, the normality of F-wave data was confirmed using the Kolmogorov-Smirnov and Shapiro-Wilk tests. Persistence, F/M amplitude ratio, and latency among three trials (rest, MI, and post) under each MVC MI condition were compared using the Friedman test and Scheffe's post hoc test. We also evaluated the relative values obtained under the two MI conditions by dividing the values of persistence, F/M amplitude ratio, and latency at rest with those obtained during MI at post. The relative values between the two MI conditions were compared using the Wilcoxon signed rank test. The significance level was set at $p<0.05$. We used IBM SPSS statistics ver.19 for statistical analysis.

### 2.2.5. Results

Persistence during MI under the two MI conditions was significantly increased compared with that at rest (Scheffe's test; $^{**}p<0.01$; **Figures 11** and **12**). Persistence immediately after MI (at post) under the two MI conditions did not show significant differences compared with that at rest (**Figures 11** and **12**). No significant differences were observed between the relative values of persistence obtained under the two MI conditions (**Figure 13**).

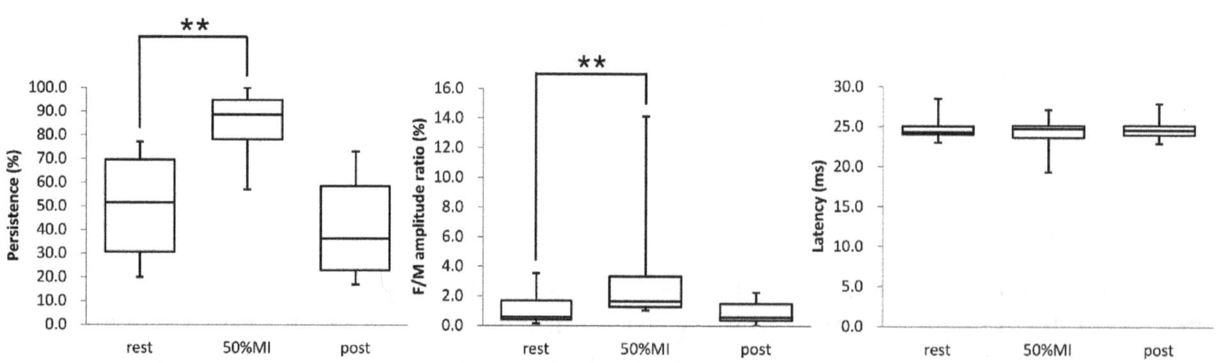


**Figure 11.** Changes in the F-wave under 50% MI condition.

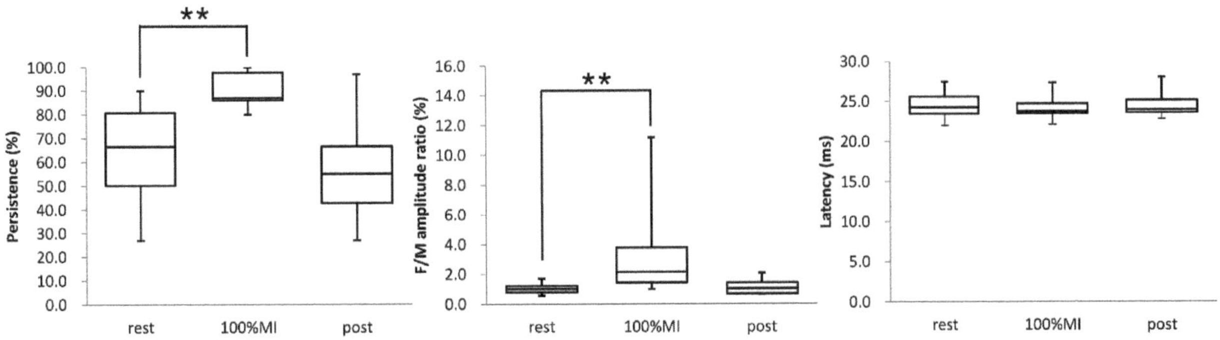


**Figure 12.** Changes in the F-wave under 100% MI condition.

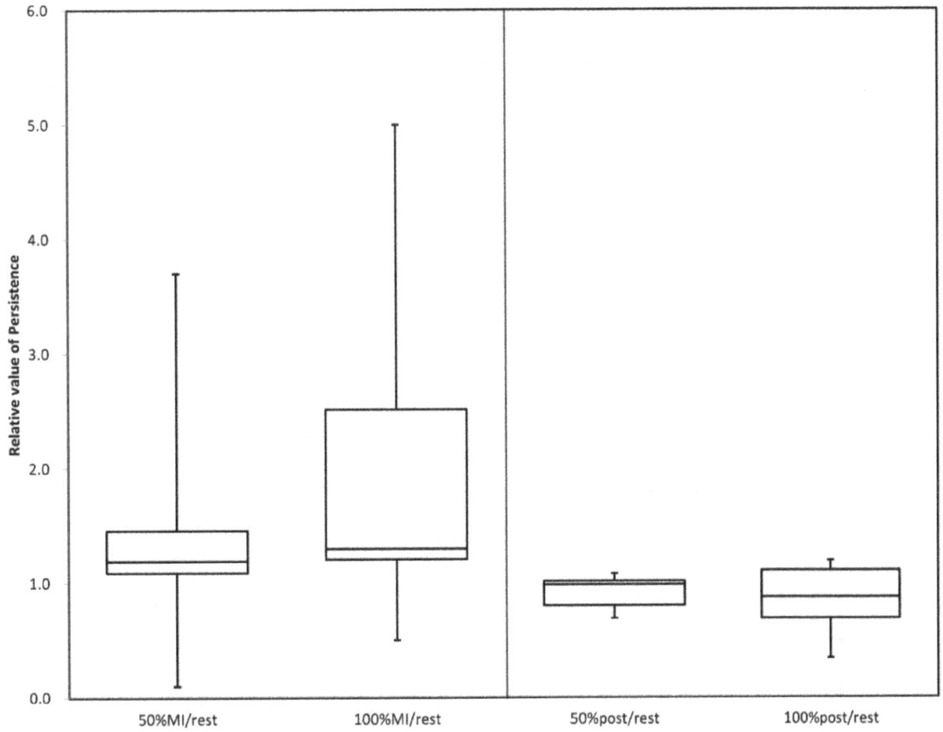


**Figure 13.** Comparison of relative values of persistence between 50 and 100% MI condition.

The F/M amplitude ratio during MI under the two MI conditions was significantly increased compared with that at rest (Scheffe's test; $^{**}p<0.01$; **Figures 11** and **12**). The F/M amplitude ratio immediately after MI (at post) under the two MI conditions did not show a significant difference compared with that at rest (**Figures 11** and **12**). No significant differences were observed between the relative values of F/M amplitude ratio obtained under the two MI conditions (**Figure 14**).

There were no significant differences in latency among three trials (rest, MI, post) under the two conditions (**Figures 11** and **12**). No significant differences were observed between the relative values of latency obtained under the two MI conditions (**Figure 15**).

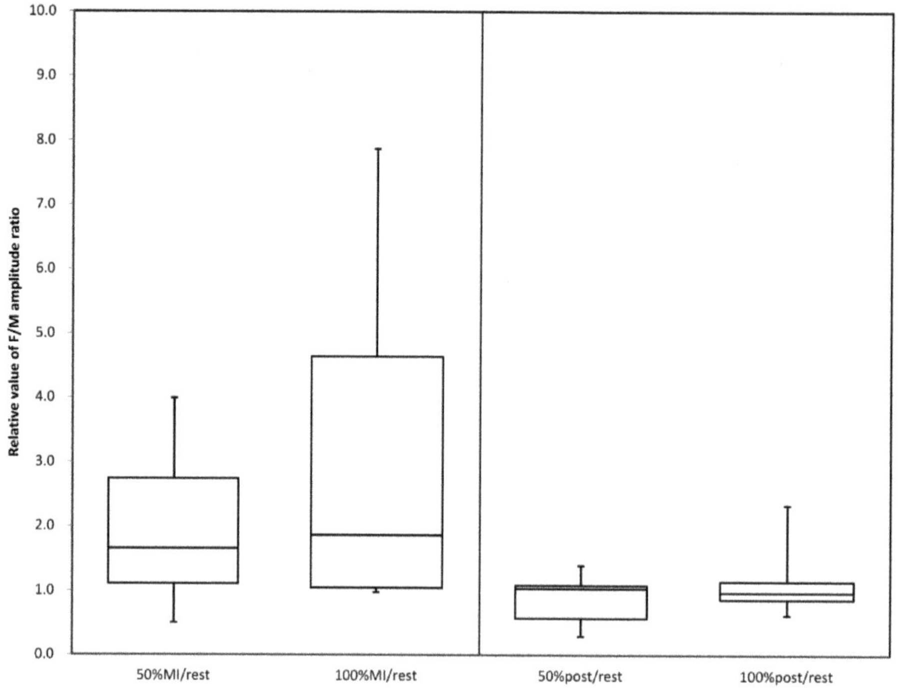


**Figure 14.** Comparison of relative values of F/M amplitude ratio between 50 and 100% MI condition.

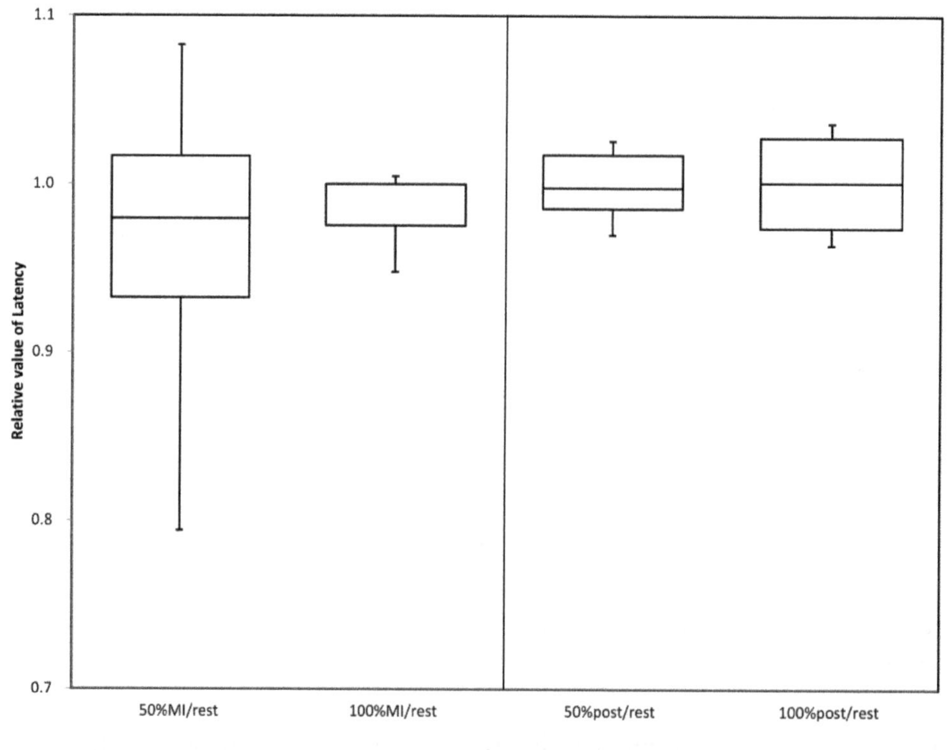


**Figure 15.** Comparison of relative values of latency between 50 and 100% MI condition.

## 2.3. Discussion

### 2.3.1. *Spinal motor neuron excitability during MI of thenar muscle activity*

Summarizing the previous work, MI of isometric thenar muscle activity under 10, 30, 50, 70, and 100% MVC can increase spinal motor neuron excitability. However, excitability does not vary with the imagined muscle contraction strengths.

Concerning the increase of spinal motor neuron excitability during MI, it was considered to influence the descending pathways corresponding to the thenar muscle. The previous studies have demonstrated that the activation of multiple cortical and subcortical regions contributes to motor preparation and planning during MI [5–8]. The activities of multiple brain regions as motor preparation and planning plausibly increased spinal motor neuron excitability via the corticospinal and/or extrapyramidal tract. Furthermore, MI is the mental rehearsal of a movement without any overt movement and muscle contraction [1]. Therefore, it is considered that motor inhibiting function was participated in simultaneously with motor preparation and planning. The supplementary motor area and premotor area are known to have functions of motor planning and inhibition in the GO/NO-GO task [21, 22]. Thus, spinal motor neuron excitability during MI may be generated by various functions (i.e., motor planning, preparation, and inhibition). In summary, it is plausible that the activation of multiple brain regions contributes to motor planning, preparation, and inhibition during MI increased spinal motor neuron excitability via the corticospinal and/or extrapyramidal tract.

Additionally, participants in all previous studies were instructed to perform MI while holding the sensor of a pinch meter. Therefore, the influence of haptic and proprioceptive perceptions during MI while holding the sensor on spinal motor neuron excitability should be considered. Mizuguchi et al. [23] reported that the MEP amplitude during MI was larger when a ball was squeezed than when no ball was held. Suzuki et al. [10] analyzed the changes in spinal motor neuron excitability between with and without holding the sensor MI tasks. The F-waves during MI while holding the sensor were greatly facilitated than without holding the sensor. The haptic and proprioceptive perceptions also contribute to the increase in spinal motor neuron excitability together with MI-activated pathways.

### 2.3.2. *The changes of spinal motor neuron excitability during MI under different imagined muscle contraction strengths*

Our previous results suggested that the facilitation amount of spinal motor neuron excitability during MI under various imagined muscle contraction strengths (i.e., 10, 30, 50, 70, and 100% MVC) was similar. There are several previous studies investigating the changes of spinal motor neuron excitability of MI under different imagined muscle contraction strengths. Hale et al. [24] reported that the soleus H-reflex amplitude was significantly increased during MI of ankle plantar flexion under 20, 40, 60, 80, and 100% MVC than that at rest. However, no significant differences were observed in changes of the soleus H-reflex amplitude among five MI conditions. Bonnet et al. [25] reported that the soleus H-reflex amplitude was significantly increased during MI of ankle plantar flexion under 2 and 10% than that at rest. Additionally, there were no significant differences in changes of the soleus H-reflex amplitude between 2 and 10% MI condition. Similarly, Aoyama and Kaneko [26] reported that there were no differences in changes of the soleus H-reflex amplitude ratio between 50 and 100% MVC MI condition, although the H-reflex amplitude was increased during MI under two imagined muscle contraction strengths. In actual movement, spinal motor neuron excitability was increased linearly with muscle contraction strengths [15]. However, higher imagined muscle contraction strengths did not progressively enhance spinal motor neuron excitability. Concerning these results, also, one possibility is the contribution of a neural mechanism that inhibits actual movement and muscle contraction during MI. Park and Li [27] reported that the MEPs amplitude during MI of finger flexion or extension under 10, 20, 30, 40, 50, and 60% MVC was significantly higher than that at rest. However, there were no significant differences in changes of the MEPs amplitude among all MI conditions. Similarly, an event-related potential study found that the magnitude of primary motor cortex activity during MI did not correlate with the imagined contraction strengths but supplementary motor area and premotor area activities during MI did [28]. As mentioned above, supplementary motor area and premotor area have crucial roles in larger force generation [29], motor planning, preparation, and motor inhibition [21, 22]. Therefore, the supplementary motor area and premotor area may inhibit the actual muscle activity depending on the muscle contraction strength. These inputs from the supplementary motor area and premotor area may suppress any additional excitability conferred by MI with high imagined contraction strength. Furthermore, spinal motor neuron excitability during MI is thought to be affected by the central nervous system via the corticospinal and extrapyramidal tract. Thus, the degree of the changes of spinal motor neuron excitability during MI under different imagined muscle contraction strengths may be modulated by both excitatory and inhibitory inputs from the central nervous system.

MI ability is a factor that affects spinal motor neuron excitability. Lorey et al. [30] studied the relationship between activation of the cerebral cortex during MI and the vividness of MI by fMRI. The primary motor cortex, premotor area, primary somatosensory area, inferior parietal lobe and superior parietal lobe, putamen, and cerebellum showed activation during MI. In particular, activation of the premotor area, parietal lobule, and cerebellum was associated with increased vividness of MI, suggesting a correlation between the activation of the cerebral cortex and vividness of the MI. Therefore, MI ability may be a possible factor that affects spinal motor neuron excitability.

However, Bonnet et al. [25] reported that the T-reflex amplitude during MI under 10% MVC was significantly higher than that under 2% MVC. Additionally, Cowley et al. [20] reported that the soleus H-reflex amplitude ratio during MI under 100% MVC was significantly higher than that under 50% MVC. To clarify the reason why these results differed from our previous results, further research will be required.

### 2.4. Conclusion

We investigated spinal motor neuron excitability during MI of isometric thenar muscle activity under 10, 30, 50, 70, and 100% MVC [13, 14, 19]. As a result, MI of isometric thenar muscle activity can facilitate spinal motor neuron excitability. However, the imagined muscle contraction strengths were not involved in the changes of spinal motor neuron excitability.

# 3. Whether duration of MI affects spinal motor neuron excitability?

## 3.1. Purpose

Our previous work suggested that MI can increase spinal motor neuron excitability, and differences in the imagined muscle contraction strengths are not involved in changes of spinal motor neuron excitability. Therefore, the previous results implied that MI of isometric thenar muscle activity under slight MVC (i.e., 10% MVC) can substantially facilitate spinal motor neuron excitability. Described in the introduction, one of our final goals is to find the way that MI obtained the most beneficial effect. Hale et al. [24] suggested that spinal motor neuron excitability was gradually increased with the number of MI trials. Gentili et al. [31] proposed that a number of MI trials are necessary to improve motor performance. To obtain a more beneficial effect of MI, the number of MI practices is considered to be important. On the other hand, in the optimal duration of MI that can facilitate motor performance, the most is unclear. Previous research used various durations of MI session, which ranged from a few seconds to approximately 200min (for review, see Driskell et al. [32]). A meta-analysis by Driskell et al. [32] suggested that a longer MI session does not always provide a beneficial effect on sports performance. Furthermore, they recommended approximately 20min to achieve a more beneficial effect. Hinshaw [33] also suggested that MI for 10–15min was considered to elicit the largest effect on performance, and Twining [34] indicated that 5min is the temporal limitation when we can concentrate and perform MI. Alternatively, the influence of duration of MI on the changes of spinal motor neuron excitability is not apparent. In our previous work [10, 13, 14, 19], participants were asked to perform MI for 1min. Thus, this research aimed to investigate the influence of MI for 5min on spinal motor neuron excitability by analyzing F-waves.

## 3.2. Materials

We included 10 healthy volunteers (8 males; 2 females; mean age, 25.3±5.0years). All participants gave their written informed consent prior to the study's commencement. This study was approved by the Research Ethics Committee at Graduate School of Kansai University of Health Sciences. The experiment was conducted in accordance with the Declaration of Helsinki.

## 3.3. Methods

The environment and conditions of the F-wave recording are the same as those for previous work. The protocol of this study is as follows. For the resting trial (rest), the F-waves were recorded while the muscle was relaxed. For the MI trial, participants first learned how to perform isometric thenar muscle activity under 50% MVC as a motor task for 1min. They were then instructed to imagine the isometric thenar muscle activity under 50% MVC by holding the sensor between the thumb and index finger for 5min. The F-waves were recorded at 1, 3, and 5 min after the onset of motor imagery (1min MI, 3min MI, and 5min MI, respectively). Immediately after MI, the F-waves were recorded (post).

## 3.4. Statistical analysis

For statistical analysis, first, the normality of F-wave data was confirmed using the Shapiro-Wilk tests. Persistence, F/M amplitude ratio, and latency among five trials (rest, 1min MI, 3min

MI, 5min MI, and post, respectively) were compared using the Friedman test and Scheffe's post hoc test. The significance level was set at $p<0.05$. We used IBM SPSS statistics ver.19 for statistical analysis.

### 3.5. Results

Persistence at 1 and 5min MI was significantly greater than that at rest (Scheffe's test, $^{**}p<0.01$; **Figure 16**). Also, persistence at 3min MI was significantly greater than that at rest (Scheffe's test, $^{*}p<0.05$; **Figure 16**). Additionally, persistence at 1, 3, and 5min MI had similar results (**Figure 16**).

The F/M amplitude ratios at 1 and 3min MI were significantly greater than those at rest, at 1 min MI (Scheffe's test, $^{**}p<0.01$), and at 3min MI (Scheffe's test, $^{*}p<0.05$; **Figure 16**). However, the F/M amplitude ratio at 5min MI was similar compared with that at rest (**Figure 16**). Additionally, the F/M amplitude ratio at 5min MI was significantly smaller than that at 1 and 3min MI (Scheffe's test, $^{*}p<0.05$; **Figure 16**).

Immediately after MI, persistence and the F/M amplitude ratio recovered to the rest level (**Figure 16**).

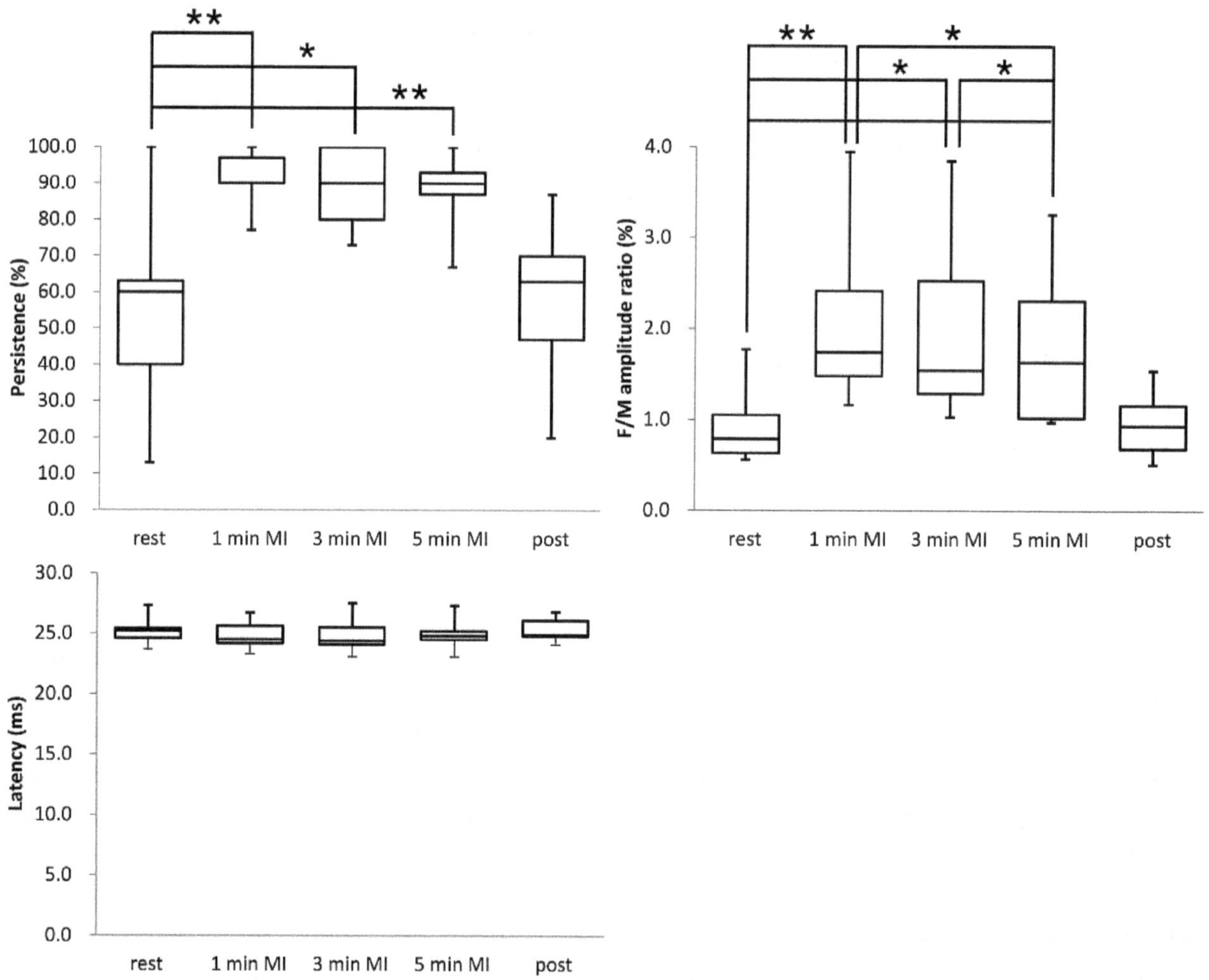


**Figure 16.** Changes of the F-waves during MI for 5min.

There were no significant differences in latency among all five trials (**Figure 16**).

### 3.6. Discussion

In our previous study, it is plausibly possible that participants did MI for 5 min because the persistence and F/M amplitude ratio were increased compared with those at rest. Specifically, persistence during MI for 5 min was kept significantly higher compared with that at rest. The F/M amplitude ratios at 1 and 3 min MI were significantly higher compared with those at rest. However, the F/M amplitude ratio at 5 min MI was significantly smaller compared with that at 1 and 3 min MI. Therefore, the facilitation effect of spinal motor neuron excitability by MI may be decreased between 3 and 5 min after the initial MI.

In regard to the F/M amplitude ratio at 5 min MI being significantly decreased compared to that at 1 and 3 min MI, there are several considerable factors. The first possible factor is the habituation of MI. MI is closely related to attentional processing [35]. Brain activation was decreased by habituation after the cognitive motor task required sustained attention (e.g., continuous performance test: CPT) for 10 min. Furthermore, corticospinal excitability was diminished by habituation [36]. Also, at the spinal level, T-reflex amplitude was significantly decreased by habituation after sustained mental work load (e.g., a paced two-choice serial reaction task) for 20 min [37]. Hence, it is considered that the further activation of the central nervous system and spinal level during MI might not be required by habituation.

The second possible factor is mental fatigue. Mental fatigue alters motor performance. Specifically, high-load mental cognitive tasks (e.g., incongruent Stroop task) for about 20 min altered maximal force production of elbow flexor [38], and task-induced mental fatigue altered the speed accuracy of actual performance and MI [39]. Furthermore, repetitive MI led to participants having difficulties in maintaining focused attention on imagined movement. Repetitive MI of pointing tasks did significantly extend the duration of actual performance [40]. Also, in regard to influence of repetitive MI on the central nervous system excitability, repetitive MI of handgrip movements significantly decreased the MEPs amplitude compared with that at rest [41]. Considering the previous results, it is possible that mental fatigue evoked by sustained mental exertion induced significant reduction in the F/M amplitude ratio to the rest level.

In our previous study, despite reduction of the facilitation effect of the F/M amplitude ratio 5 min after MI, persistence during MI for 5 min was kept at a higher level compared with that at rest. In previous research using electromyography (EMG), muscle fatigue reduced the maximal force production and mean power frequency, and it conversely increased the EMG amplitude [42]. Previous researchers interpreted these phenomena to additional recruitment of motor units, an increased firing rate, and synchronization of motor units' recruitment [43]. Furthermore, Levenez et al. [44] demonstrated that sustained dorsiflexion under 50% MVC induced decline of soleus H-reflex amplitude. Rossi et al. [45] demonstrated that sustained MVC of abductor digiti minimi induced decline of the F-wave amplitude, although the F-wave persistence was unchanged. Therefore, depression of the facilitation effect of the F/M amplitude after 5 min from the onset of MI implicated decline of the individual anterior cell excitability. Further, regarding the result that persistence was kept at a higher level during MI for 5 min compared with that at rest, it is considered that there was additional recruitment and/or increasing firing rate of the anterior horn cells to compensate for the decrease of individual anterior horn cell excitability evoked by mental fatigue.

Finally, we considered the practice time and vividness of MI as a possible factor. Using MI in physical practice for learning motor skills, Twining [34] indicated that 5min is the temporal limitation when we can concentrate and perform MI. In mental chronometry, the time required for actual performance and executing it mentally was similar [46]. In other words, it was difficult for participants to perform MI accurately for more than 1min. In the present research, participants practiced isometric thenar muscle activity under 50% MVC as a motor task for only 1min. Hence, practice time for 1min might be insufficient to learn entirely the thenar muscle activity under 50% MVC. Indeed, introspective comments recorded from subjects after MI for 5min indicated that they felt difficulty in performing MI vividly with time. From the viewpoint that the time required to execute and imagine the movement is similar [46], it may be necessary to match the time of task practice and MI. However, we did not study the time-dependent change of the vividness of MI precisely in the present research, and further research will be required.

### 3.7. Conclusion

We investigated the change of spinal motor neuron excitability during MI for 5min. Persistence was significantly increased during MI for 5min. However, the F/M amplitude ratio at 5min returned to the rest level. As a result, MI for 5min may affect spinal motor neuron excitability. Thus, the duration of MI needs to be considered.

## 4. The use of MI in clinical settings

From the results of our previous work [13, 14, 19], MI of isometric thenar muscle activity under 10, 30, 50, 70, and 100% MVC can facilitate spinal motor neuron excitability. Furthermore, the imagined muscle contraction strength is not involved in changes of spinal motor neuron excitability. In other words, MI under slight MVC (10% MVC) can sufficiently increase spinal motor neuron excitability. In the study about duration of MI, the F/M amplitude ratio returned to rest level between 3 and 5min after initial MI. It is considered that the adequate duration of MI might be 1 or 3min.

Finally, we discuss the application of MI to patients in clinical settings. Functional reorganization of the central nervous system may be elicited after brain and spinal cord injury. After brain and spinal cord injury, motor cortex excitability decreased due to various factors, including the damage of neural substrates, loss of sensory inputs, and disuse of the affected limb [47]. The corticospinal excitability would be decreased following the significant decrease of both size and number of the corticospinal neurons [48]. Therefore, we considered that facilitating the excitability of the central and spinal neural level could be necessary for improvement of motor function. MI can increase the MEPs amplitude in patients with post-stroke [49] and spinal cord injury [50], and the F-waves post-stroke [51]. From these previous results, we believe that MI is the effective method for improvement of motor function after damage to the central nervous system.

## Author details

Yoshibumi Bunno[1*], Yuki Fukumoto[1], Todo Marina[2] and Chieko Onigata[2]

*Address all correspondence to: yoshibumi_b@yahoo.co.jp

1 Graduate School of Health Sciences, Graduate School of Kansai University of Health Sciences and Clinical Physical Therapy Laboratory, Faculty of Health Sciences, Kansai University of Health Sciences, Wakaba, Kumatori, Sennan, Osaka, Japan

2 Clinical Physical Therapy Laboratory, Faculty of Health Sciences, Kansai University of Health Sciences, Osaka, Japan

## References

[1] Guillot A, Rienzo FD, Maclntyre T, et al. Imagining is not doing but involves specific motor commands: a review of experimental data related to motor inhibition. Front Hum Neurosci. 2012;6:247.

[2] Yue G, Cole KJ. Strength increases from of motor program: comparison of training with maximal voluntary and imagined muscle contractions. J Neurophysiol. 1992;67:1114–1123.

[3] Ranganathan VK, Siemionow V, Liu JZ et al. From mental power to muscle power-gaining strength by using mind. Neuropsychologia. 2004;42:944–956.

[4] Guillot A, Tolleron C, Collet C. Does motor imagery enhance stretching and flexibility? J Sports Sci. 2010;28:291–298.

[5] Luft AR, Skalej M, Stefanou A, et al. Comparing motion- and imagery-related activation in the human cerebellum: a functional MRI study. Hum Brain Mapp. 1998;6:105–113.

[6] Lotze M, Montoya P, Erb M, et al. Activation of cortical and cerebellar motor areas during executed and imagined hand movements: an fMRI study. J Cogn Neurosci. 1999;11:491–501.

[7] Matsuda T, Watanabe S, Kuruma H, et al. Neural correlates of chopsticks exercise for the non-dominant hand: comparison among the movement, images and imitations—a functional MRI study. Rigakuryoho Kagaku. 2011;26:117–122 (in Japanese).

[8] Stephan KM, Fink GR, Passingham RE, et al. Functional anatomy of the mental representation of upper extremity movements in healthy subjects. J Neurophysiol. 1995;73:373–386.

[9] Kasai T, Kawai S, Kawanishi M, et al. Evidence for facilitation of motor evoked potentials (MEPs) induced by motor imagery. Brain Res. 1997;744:147–150.

[10] Suzuki T, Bunno Y, Onigata C, et al. Excitability of spinal neural function during several motor imagery tasks involving isometric opponens pollicis activity. NeuroRehabilitation. 2013;33:171–176.

[11] Taniguchi S, Kimura J, Yamada T, et al. Effect of motion imagery to counter rest-induced suppression of F-wave as a measure of anterior horn cell excitability. Clin Neurophysiol. 2008;119:1346–1352.

[12] Oishi K, Kimura M, Yasukawa M, et al. Amplitude reduction of H-reflex during mental movement simulation in elite athletes. Behav Brain Res. 1994;62:55–61.

[13] Bunno Y, Yurugi Y, Onigata C, et al. Influence of motor imagery of isometric opponens pollicis activity on the excitability of spinal motor neurons: a comparison using different muscle contraction strengths. J Phys Ther Sci. 2014;26:1069–1073.

[14] Bunno Y, Onigata C, Suzuki T. The imagined muscle contraction strengths did not affect the changes of spinal motor neurons excitability. J Nov Physiother. 2016;S3:008.

[15] Suzuki T, Fujiwara T, Takeda I. Excitability of the spinal motor neuron pool and F-waves during isometric ipsilateral and contralateral contraction. Physiother Theory Pract. 1993;9:19–24.

[16] Suzuki T, Saitoh E. Recommendations for the practice of the evoked EMG; H-reflex and F-wave. Guidelines of the International Federation of Clinical Neurophysiology. Rigakuryoho Kagaku. 2000;15:187–192 (in Japanese).

[17] Mesrati F, Vecchierini MF. F-waves neurophysiology and clinical value. Clin Neurophysiol. 2004;34:217–243.

[18] Fisher MA. F-waves—physiology and clinical uses. Sci World J. 2007;7:144–160.

[19] Bunno Y, Onigata C, Suzuki T. Excitability of spinal motor neuron excitability during motor imagery of thenar muscle activity under maximal voluntary contractions of 50% and 100%. J Phys Ther Sci. 2015;27:2775–2778.

[20] Cowley PM, Clark BC, Ploutz-Snyder LL. Kinesthetic motor imagery and spinal excitability: the effect of contraction intensity and spatial localization. Clin Neurophysiol. 2008;119:1849–1856.

[21] Nakata H, Sakamoto K, Ferretti A, et al. Somato-motor inhibitory processing in humans: an event-related functional MRI study. Neuroimage. 2008;39:1858–1866.

[22] Watanabe J, Sugiura M, Sato K, et al. The human prefrontal and parietal association cortices are involved in NO-GO performances: an event-related fMRI study. Neuroimage. 2002;17:1207–1216.

[23] Mizuguchi N, Sakamoto M, Muraoka T, et al. The modulation of corticospinal excitability during motor imagery of action with objects. PLoS One. 2011;6:e26006.

[24] Hale BS, Raglin JS, Koceja DM. Kinesthetic motor imagery and spinal excitability: the effect of contraction intensity and spatial localization. Behav Brain Res. 2003;142: 81–87.

[25] Bonnet M, Decety J, Jeannerod M, et al. Mental simulation of an action modulates the excitability of spinal reflex pathways in man. Cogn Brain Res. 1997;5:221–228.

[26] Aoyama T, Kaneko F. The effect of motor imagery on gain modulation of the spinal reflex. Brain Res. 2011;1372:41–48.

[27] Park WH, Li S. No graded responses of finger muscles to TMS during motor imagery of isometric finger force. Neurosci Lett. 2011;494:255–259.

[28] Romero DH, Lacourse MG, Lawrence KE, et al. Event-related potentials as a function of movement parameter variations during motor imagery and isometric action. Behav Brain Res. 2000;117:83–96.

[29] Oda S, Shibata M, Moritani T. Force-dependent changes in movement-related cortical potentials. J Electromyogr Kinesiol. 1996;6:247–252.

[30] Lorey B, Pilgramm S, Bischoff M, et al. Activation of the parieto-premotor network is associated with vivid motor imagery—a parametric fMRI study. PLoS One. 2011;6: e20368.

[31] Gentili R, Han CE, Schwelghofer N, et al. Motor learning without doing: Trial-by-Trial improvement in motor performance during mental training. J Neurophysiol. 2010;104:774–783.

[32] Driskell J, Copper C, Moran A. Does mental practice enhance performance? J Appl Phychol. 1994;79:481–492.

[33] Hinshaw KE. The effects of mental practice on motor skill performance: critical evaluation and meta-analysis. Imagin Cogn Pers. 1991;11:3–35.

[34] Twining WE. Mental practice and physical practice in learning a motor skill. Res Q. 1949;20:432–435.

[35] Decety J. The neurophysiological basis of motor imagery. Behav Brain Res. 1996;77:45–52.

[36] Tana MG, Montin E, Cerutti S, et al. Exploring cortical attentional system by using fMRI during a continuous perfomance test. Comput Intell Neurosci. 2010;2010:329213.

[37] Brunia CH, Zwaga HJ, van Boxtel A. Tendon reflex amplitude with increasing task difficulty. Ergonomics. 1973;16:495–499.

[38] Bray SR, Graham JD, Martin Ginis KA, et al. Cognitive task performance causes impaired maximum force production in human hand flexor muscles. Biol Psychol. 2012;89:195–200.

[39] Guillot A, Haguenauer M, Dittmar A, et al. Effect of a fatiguing protocol on motor imagery accuracy. Eur J Appl Physiol. 2005;95:186–190.

[40] Rozand V, Lebon F, Stapley PJ, et al. A prolonged motor imagery session alter imagined and actual movement durations: potential implications for neurorehabilitation. Behav Brain Res. 2016;297:67–75.

[41] Kluger BM, Palmer C, Shattuck JT, et al. Motor evoked potential depression following repetitive central motor initiation. Exp Brain Res. 2012;216:585–590.

[42] De Luca CJ. The use of surface electromyography in biomechanics. J Appl Biomechanics. 1997;13:135–163.

[43] Moritani T, Muro M, Nagata A. Intramuscular and surface electromyogram changes during muscle fatigue. J Appl Physiol. 1986;60:402–411.

[44] Levenez M, Kotzamanidis C, Carpentler A, et al. Spinal reflexes and coactivation of ankle muscles during a submaximal fatiguing contraction. J Appl Physiol. 2005;99:1182–1188.

[45] Rossi A, Rossi S, Ginanneschi F. Activity-dependent changes in intrinsic excitability of human spinal motoneurones produced by natural activity. J Neurophysiol. 2012;108:2473–2480.

[46] Guillot A, Collet C. Duration of mentally simulated movement: a review. J Motor Behav. 2005;37:10–20.

[47] Liepert J, Bauder H, Miltner WHR, et al. Treatment-induced cortical reorganization after stroke in humans. Stroke. 2000;31:1210–1216.

[48] Wrigley PJ, Gustin SM, Macey PM, et al. Anatomical changes in human motor cortex and motor pathways following complete thoracic spinal cord injury. Cereb Cortex. 2009;19: 224–232.

[49] Cicinelli P, Marconi B, Zaccagnini M, et al. Imagery-induced cortical excitability changes in stroke: a transcranial magnetic stimulation study. Cereb Cortex. 2006;16:247–253.

[50] Cramer SC, Nelles G, Benson RR, et al. A functional MRI study of subjects recovered from hemiparetic stroke. Stroke. 1997;28:2518–2527.

[51] Naseri M, Petramfar P, Ashraf A. Effect of motor imagery on the F-wave parameters in hemiparetic stroke survivors. Ann Rehabil Med. 2015;39:401–408.

5

# The Study of Action Observation Therapy in Neurological Diseases: A Few Technical Considerations

Julio Plata-Bello

**Abstract**

Action observation therapy (AOT) is a developing neurorehabilitative tool, which is based on the existence of the mirror neuron system (MNS). This neural network involves motor regions, and its main feature is that it is activated not only during the execution of an action, but also during the observation of the same action. Bearing in mind this "dual" activation, the AOT proposes that motor symptoms of different neurological disorders can improve with the observation and imitation of different actions. While several studies have shown the benefits of this therapy, others have been less favorable indicating a lack of clarity in the field. The present study focuses on previously undiscussed aspects regarding this therapy: from the kind of actions used in the therapy to the scales that should be used to measure the results of AOT. Differences and similarities between virtual reality-based therapies and AOT are also discussed. The considerations made here about all such aspects may be useful for future studies and possible applications of AOT.

**Keywords:** mirror neurons, neurological rehabilitation, rehabilitation interventions, action observation, motor recovery

## 1. Introduction

Action observation therapy (AOT) is based on the well-known "mirror mechanism." AOT alludes to the activation of motor-related areas not only when an action is performed, but also when the action is observed [1]. This mechanism was first described in the premotor cortex of the macaque [2], and over the last two decades, several studies have focused on the identification, description and characterization of the human brain regions that present this mechanism [3–5]. Nowadays, there is much agreement about the existence of a neural network formed by regions that present the "mirror mechanism." The most consistent regions are located in the frontal lobe [mainly in the inferior frontal gyrus (IFG)] and in the posterior parietal lobe [mainly in the inferior parietal lobule (IPL)] [1, 4], though there are other regions that may also be involved [6, 7]. This brain network is the so-called mirror neuron system (MNS) (**Figure 1**).

The dual activation of the MNS has been associated with the ability to understand the actions performed by others [3, 8]. Bearing this in mind, it is easy to deduce that the MNS is essential for imitation and, eventually, for action learning [9–11]. Several experiments have provided some evidence in this respect and have led to the suggestion of the possible role of action observation (i.e., MNS activation) in motor rehabilitation. Effectively, the activation of motor regions during the simple observation of an action may result in an improvement of motor impairment; this is the AOT hypothesis. However, the MNS is associated not only with motor functions, but also with social cognition. Many authors agree in considering the involvement of the MNS in social interaction and in the relationship between people and the environment [4, 12]. This consideration makes the AOT not only a motor rehabilitation program, but also a functional recovery program.

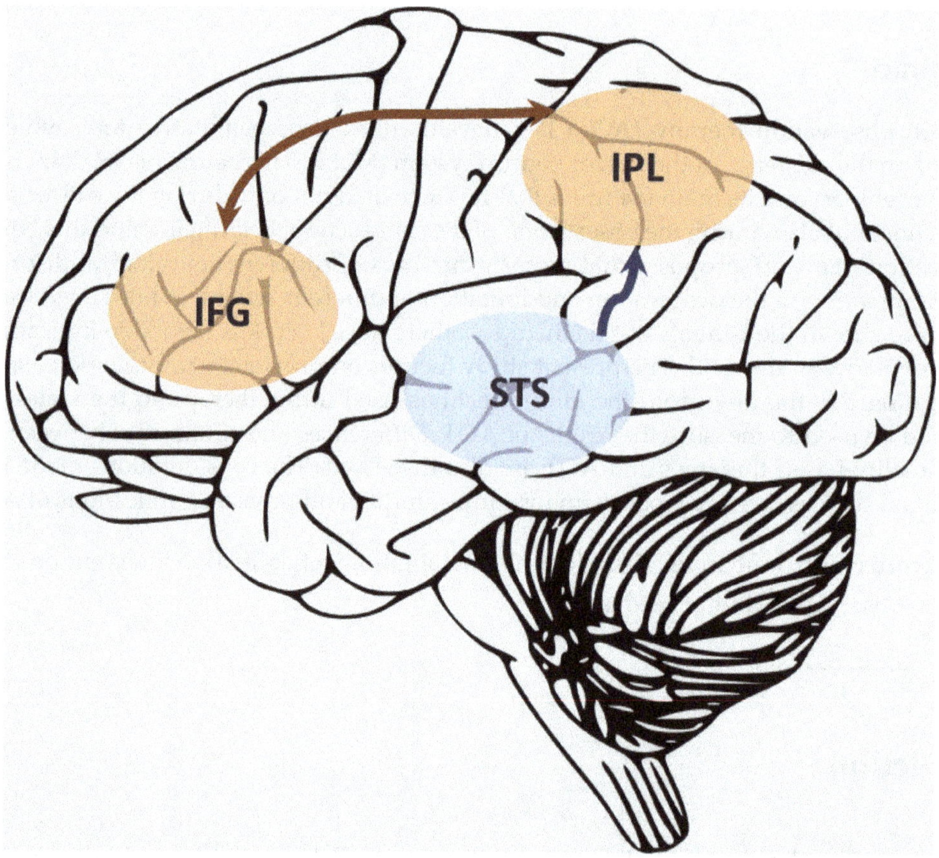


**Figure 1.** The MNS in humans. Many functional studies have shown that many brain regions present mirror properties. Apart from premotor cortex (PMC), parietal and temporal regions are also activated when an action is executed or observed and this is clearly related with the important role that mirror neurons seem to play in many aspects of social cognition (language, empathy, learning process, etc.). Because of this, it has been suggested that developmental MNS dysfunction leads to disordered social cognition in humans, including autism spectrum disorders. Anyway, the most studied areas that present mirror properties in humans are the inferior frontal gyrus (IFG) corresponding to BA 44 and inferior parietal lobule (IPL), corresponding to BA 40. Both form the core of the known parietal-frontal mirror neuron system (MNS). The superior temporal sulcus (STS) is consistently activated during the observation of human movements and seems to play a prominent role in the flux of information to the MNS.

Bearing in mind only neurological diseases, stroke is, unmistakably, the most common neurological disease where AOT has been tested. Motor impairment and aphasia were the most common features of the stroke patients included in trials and prospective observational studies [13–20]. For both clinical conditions, the majority of the studies reported a clear benefit of AOT, with a maintained improvement in the motor condition and the functional status. In fact, the benefit of this therapy has been remarked on in a recent evidenced-based review of the literature concerning the effect of AOT in upper limb dysfunction after stroke [21].

AOT has also been used in other movement disorders such as Parkinson's disease and cerebral palsy, though the number of studies that have focused on these diseases is much lower than those focused on stroke. In any case, the application of AOT leads to an improvement in gait and bradykinesia in Parkinsonian patients [22–24] and in the functional status in cerebral palsy's infants [25]. Finally, cognitive benefits have been reported after the application of AOT in Alzheimer's disease [26].

New and different studies about AOT need to be performed in order to properly identify the role of this therapy in the rehabilitation of neurological disorders. Some weaknesses in the current literature about AOT can be identified. For example, most of the previously cited studies included patients with a chronic evolution of their diseases (more than 6 months after the onset) and not in the acute or subacute phase of the disease, where the therapy might also show efficacy (or even more). Furthermore, the number of patients is highly variable between the different studies and the differences in the period where patients were exposed between the different studies are large. However, these methodological aspects are not the only ones that must be considered when AOT is going to be applied. In the present work, we stress the importance of adequately selecting the actions to be used during therapy as well as the correct scale for evaluating the results of AOT. The consideration of these aspects in future studies may help to provide a better understanding of the MNS and to know the real impact of the therapy in patient's recovery. This study also discusses the differences and similarities that exist between virtual reality-based therapies, an innovative approach that is being increasingly applied in rehabilitation centers. Finally, future perspectives about AOT research are proposed.

## 2. Which actions should be used in AOT?

One major issue about AOT is the kind of action that should be used in order to get the maximum benefit. Most of the actions that have been employed in AOT studies consist of upper limb transitive actions (i.e., actions with object interaction, e.g., using a pencil). These are usually daily actions that have been selected on the basis of their ecological value [27]. This kind of action has been shown to have increased MNS activity in neuroimaging studies [15, 28] and corticospinal facilitation in transcranial magnetic stimulation (TMS) [29, 30].

Although the benefits of AOT have been demonstrated with the use of transitive actions, the use of intransitive ones (i.e., actions without object interaction, e.g., the opposition of the index finger and the thumb as the pantomime of a precision grasping) may also be considered for use in this therapy. Intransitive actions lead to an activation of the human MNS (there is new evidence of this activation in primates too) in a more restrictive way than transitive actions do [31, 32]. In fact, the activity of the MNS when intransitive actions are observed tends to predominantly activate posterior parietal regions more than premotor areas [31, 33]. Minor activation of the MNS does not have to mean that an AOT based on these actions had less benefit than using transitive ones. It is known that part of the brain activity obtained with the use of transitive actions is due to the presence of an object and a more complex scenario where the action takes part [34]. In this respect, many patients with neurological disorders may have attention deficits or less capacity to follow the action continuously, because there are many factors that catch the observer's attention (e.g., the object features) and they may become cognitively overloaded. Furthermore, when patients are asked to imitate the motor actions, the imitation of simple and intransitive actions would be effortless than the performance of complex and transitive ones. Consequently, future studies should incorporate intransitive actions to those which patients must observe to evaluate the efficacy of the AOT using these actions. Although they will lead to less brain activity, the patient can be more focused on the effector as well as on the kinematics of the action, and neither on the object which the effector interacts with nor on the context where the action takes place.

On the other hand, another factor that must be considered in AOT is the visual perspective from which the motor acts of others are observed. It has been demonstrated that the majority of mirror neurons in the monkey premotor cortex are view-dependent (i.e., they are only activated when the action is presented in a specific visual perspective) [35, 36] and, depending on the point of view, action observation leads to different activations of the MNS [37]. In this sense, certain evidence exists that an egocentric view (i.e., first-person perspective) of an action leads to higher brain activity than a third-person view [30] (**Figure 2**). Moreover, studies in monkeys have revealed the existence of some subcategories of mirror neurons that are selective for specific space positions, right or left hand, and for specific directions [2, 38]. Although these

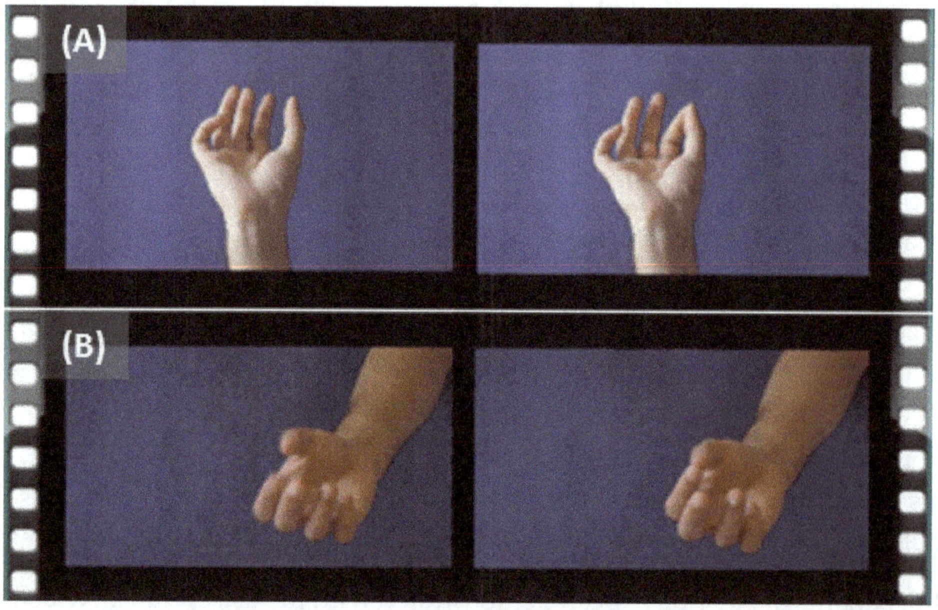


**Figure 2.** Different visual perspectives. First-person perspective (A) and third-person perspective (B) of an intransitive motor action (index to thumb opposition task). First-person perspective seems to conduct to higher MNS activity than a third-person view.

properties have been less studied in the human MNS, its presence in non-human primates makes it easy to assume the existence of this diversity among the mirror neurons of human beings. Thus, the MNS is important for visuospatial and visuoperceptive abilities. Bearing this in mind, patients who are candidates for AOT should be previously tested in these functions with proper neuropsychological assessment. This evaluation may allow the adaption of the kind of actions that are shown to the patient in order to achieve better and faster results.

## 3. Measuring AOT results: what matters?

One of the most important aspects when considering AOT is to adequately evaluate the results. The use of an appropriate scale or index is a basic requisite to analyze the efficacy of any rehabilitative therapy. Previous studies have reported the efficacy of the AOT in terms of changes in scales that measured specific clinical aspects of each neurological disease. For instance, some stroke-based studies expressed the efficacy of AOT with changes in Upper Extremity Fugl-Meyer Motor Assessment (FMA) and Functional Test of the Hemiparetic Upper Extremity (FTHUE) [20]; similarly, the application of AOT in Parkinson's disease patients was measured with a 39-item Parkinson Disease Questionnaire (PDQ-39) [24]. Although the specific scales are vital for understanding the effect of MNS therapy in the clinical symptoms of each neurological disease, the broad implications of AOT (considering its effect on the MNS with motor and cognitive implications) mean that these scales are restricted. Moreover, these scales should also be versatile enough to be applied to the majority of the spectrum of neurological diseases where AOT may be applied. Thus, it seems reasonable to propose a more general scale or index to evaluate the results of AOT in terms of functional recovery.

Functioning is a generic term defined by the World Health Organization (WHO), which includes the positive aspects of the interaction between an individual (with a certain health condition) and the contextual factors (personal and environmental factors). This leads to a definition of disability as the restriction of a person's functioning. Neurorehabilitative approaches must converge in a recovery in the functioning that may have been lost as a result of the disease. Therefore, the efficacy of this kind of therapy has to be measured by functional scales.

There are several functional scales described in the literature. Bearing in mind its extensive applicability in neurological diseases, broad extended use and adaptability, the Barthel Index (BI) can be considered as a trustworthy scale for evaluating AOT results. The BI was designed in 1965 by Mohoney and Barthel [39] and has been subsequently modified by many others. The modification made by Granger et al. [40] should be mentioned as it is probably the most used version of the BI nowadays. The BI modified (BIm) consists of the evaluation of the independency degree when a patient performs 15 basic daily life activities (BDLA). Granger et al. grouped the activities into two subscales: one measuring the capacity to take care of themselves and the other determining the degree of mobility (**Table 1**). The BIm is a highly sensitive, valid and feasible, which is able to detect progress or impairment during the evolution of a rehabilitation program [41]. Furthermore, it is an inexpensive tool, which does not take up much of the examiner's time.

| | Independent | Assistance | Dependent |
|---|---|---|---|
| **Personal care** | | | |
| Drinking using a glass | 4 | 0 | 0 |
| Eating | 6 | 0 | 0 |
| Dressing the upper part of the body | 5 | 3 | 0 |
| Dressing the lower part of the body | 7 | 4 | 0 |
| Putting on prosthesis | 0 | −2 | 0 |
| Tidying up | 5 | 0 | 0 |
| Bathing | 6 | 0 | 0 |
| Urine control | 10 | 5 | 0 |
| Fecal control | 10 | 5 | 0 |
| **Mobility** | | | |
| Sitting/getting up from a chair/bed | 15 | 7 | 0 |
| Use of the toilet | 6 | 3 | 0 |
| Getting in/out to the shower1 | 1 | 0 | 0 |
| Walking 50 m | 15 | 10 | 0 |
| Going down/upstairs | 10 | 5 | 0 |
| Propelling a wheelchair | 5 | 0 | 0 |
| **Score** | | | |
| 0–20 | Complete disabled | | |
| 21–60 | Severe disabled | | |
| 61–90 | Moderate disabled | | |
| 91–99 | Slight disabled | | |
| 100 | Independent | | |

**Table 1.** Barthel Index modified by Granger et al. Adapted from Granger et al. [40].

However, the evaluation of the capacity to perform the BDLA may not be enough to appropriately measure the impact of the AOT. "Instrumental daily life activities" (IDLA) and "advanced daily life activities" (ADLA) have been defined as activities that allow a person to be independent in the community (IDLA) (e.g., going to the supermarket, cooking) and to develop a social role (ADLA) (e.g., working, practicing sports, religion). The measurement of the capacity to develop these activities would provide a more holistic picture of the patient's situation before and after the application of AOT. It would be interesting to evaluate the results of AOT using specific scales for IDLA and ADLA, because the MNS is clearly involved in the normal development of these activities.

One of the scales for IDLA assessment is the Lawton and Brody scale, which consists of eight items related to daily activities (e.g., use of transport) which are asked directly to the patient or the caregiver [42]. It is a highly sensitive scale and has a high inter- and intra-observer correlation coefficient. However, the main disadvantage of this scale is that it was conceived for the elderly population, and thus, its application might be restricted.

Furthermore, it should be recognized that the evaluation of IDLA and ADLA is more complex than other evaluations and such activities are influenced by the culture and the geographical environment of the patient. Therefore, some effort needs to be made for testing new scales to approach the evaluation of IDLA and ADLA and apply them (with BDLA scales) to the measurement of AOT impact.

## 4. AOT and virtual reality: two heads of the same coin

AOT is not the only rehabilitative tool that has been investigated in the last decade to improve the functional status of patients with neurological disorders. The application of virtual reality (VR) approaches in the field of rehabilitation is extensively reported, and it has been shown to have certain benefits, not only in the recovery of motor dysfunctions [43], but also in improving cognitive impairment [44, 45]. VR therapies are based on the generation of a real-time three-dimensional environment that makes the patients feels as if they are in a real situation [46]. Normally, the patient is situated in front of a monitor and is required to perform actions with the impaired limb (or with the non-impaired limb when the deficit is notable). These actions are recognized by a movement sensor, and the patient receives the feedback by means of the monitor, observing different movements or consequences of the performed actions. The feedback will depend on which VR program has been initiated. For instance, a VR program may consist of a box moving from one side to the other; the patient performs an action and observes the displacement of the boxes on the screen). These VR approaches have demonstrated their usefulness in several neurological disorders [43, 47–49], with stroke being the subject of the largest number of studies. In fact, a recent Cochrane meta-analysis concluded that VR leads to an improvement in upper limb function and recommended its use as a complementary therapy to the usual therapy for improving the activity of daily living function [50].

VR therapy has some aspects in common with AOT. The feedback in both therapies consists of an observation task (although the feedback of VR is usually over dimensioned); moreover, patients can be requested to interact with the elements they observe, with an imitation (AOT) or by trying to modify a condition in the virtual environment. Thus, VR and AOT modulate the MNS to achieve an improvement in the functional condition of patients. In this respect, some studies have shown the presence of an intense MNS activity during VR tasks [51, 52].

However, although these therapies share common features in the conditions they use, as well as the neural substrates they take advantage of, there are important feasibility and applicability differences. On the one hand, VR therapy requires a more sophisticated informatics structure than AOT; thus, it may be less efficient and makes this therapy less practical for use at home. On the other hand, the instructions and the tasks of VR therapies are more complex than those applied in AOT (i.e., simply observing or imitating a movement). Therefore, although VR and AOT may be complementary rehabilitation tools, AOT may be more widely used than VR in different socioeconomic environments.

## 5. Future perspectives

The road that AOT has to travel until it can be considered a standard therapy in neurorehabilitation is still long. Although some randomized trials have been published reporting the efficacy of this therapy in stroke, Parkinson's disease and cerebral palsy patients, new studies are necessary (considering the heterogeneity in the scales used for measuring the efficacy and in the period of treatment). Furthermore, other neuropathological conditions should be considered in such trials. For example, multiple sclerosis or traumatic brain injury patients could also benefit from AOT, but no randomized trials with this kind of patients have been performed to date.

On the other hand, apart from the aspects that have been discussed above, it would also be interesting if new studies reported the results of neurofunctional studies (i.e., neuroimaging and/or other functional tests). It would provide much information about the functioning of the MNS in different pathological conditions as well as the plastic changes in the brain that may be associated with the use of AOT.

Further study of AOT may generate a new weapon in the armory against the functional and social limitations produced by neurological disorders. The decrease of such limitations is clearly associated with an improvement in the quality of life and survival periods of the patients, thanks to the reduction of complication rates (associated with the aforementioned limitations). Therefore, new and appropriate research is needed to convert the AOT in a standard therapy in our hospitals and rehabilitative centers.

## Acknowledgements

We would like to thank all members of the research group "Neurochemistry and Neuroimaging" of the University of La Laguna for their ideas and contributions to the preparation of this chapter.

## Author details

Julio Plata-Bello[1,2]

Address all correspondence to: jplata5@hotmail.com

1 Department of Neurosurgery, Hospital Universitario de Canarias, Spain

2 Magnetic Resonance Imaging Service for Biomedical Research, University of La Laguna, Spain

## References

[1] Rizzolatti G, Craighero L. The mirror-neuron system. Annu Rev Neurosci 2004;27:169–92. doi:10.1146/annurev.neuro.27.070203.144230

[2] Gallese V, Fadiga L, Fogassi L, et al. Action recognition in the premotor cortex. Brain 1996;119(Pt 2):593–609.

[3] Hari R, Forss N, Avikainen S, et al. Activation of human primary motor cortex during action observation: a neuromagnetic study. Proc Natl Acad Sci USA 1998;95:15061–5. http://www.pubmedcentral.nih.gov/articlerender.fcgi?artid=24575&tool=pmcentrez&rendertype=abstract

[4] Rizzolatti G, Sinigaglia C. The functional role of the parieto-frontal mirror circuit: interpretations and misinterpretations. Nat Rev Neurosci 2010;11:264–74. doi:10.1038/nrn2805

[5] Glenberg AM. Introduction to the mirror neuron forum. Perspect Psychol Sci 2011;6:363–8. doi:10.1177/1745691611412386

[6] Overwalle F Van. Social cognition and the brain : a meta-analysis. Hum Brain Mapp 2009;858:829–58. doi:10.1002/hbm.20547

[7] Molenberghs P, Cunnington R, Mattingley JB. Brain regions with mirror properties: a meta-analysis of 125 human fMRI studies. Neurosci Biobehav Rev 2012;36:341–9. doi:10.1016/j.neubiorev.2011.07.004

[8] Schmidt RC, Fitzpatrick P, Caron R, et al. Understanding social motor coordination. Hum Mov Sci 2011;30:834–45. doi:10.1016/j.humov.2010.05.014

[9] Buccino G, Vogt S, Ritzl A, et al. Neural circuits underlying imitation learning of hand actions: an event-related fMRI study. Neuron 2004;42:323–34.

[10] Catmur C, Walsh V, Heyes C. Sensorimotor learning configures the human mirror system. Curr Biol 2007;17:1527–31. doi:10.1016/j.cub.2007.08.006

[11] Vogt S, Thomaschke R. From visuo-motor interactions to imitation learning: behavioural and brain imaging studies. J Sports Sci 2007;25:497–517. doi:10.1080/02640410600946779

[12] Gallese V, Keysers C, Rizzolatti G. A unifying view of the basis of social cognition. Trends Cogn Sci 2004;8:396–403. doi:10.1016/j.tics.2004.07.002

[13] Celnik P, Webster B, Glasser DM, et al. Effects of action observation on physical training after stroke. Stroke 2008;39:1814–20. doi:10.1161/STROKEAHA.107.508184

[14] Bhasin A, Padma Srivastava M V, Kumaran SS, et al. Neural interface of mirror therapy in chronic stroke patients: a functional magnetic resonance imaging study. Neurol India 2012;60:570–6. doi:10.4103/0028-3886.105188

[15] Ertelt D, Small S, Solodkin A, et al. Action observation has a positive impact on rehabilitation of motor deficits after stroke. Neuroimage 2007;36 Suppl 2:T164–73. doi:10.1016/j.neuroimage.2007.03.043

[16] Franceschini M, Agosti M, Cantagallo A, et al. Mirror neurons: action observation treatment as a tool in stroke rehabilitation. Eur J Phys Rehabil Med 2010;46:517–23.

[17] Franceschini M, Ceravolo MG, Agosti M, et al. Clinical relevance of action observation in upper-limb stroke rehabilitation: a possible role in recovery of functional dexterity. A randomized clinical trial. Neurorehabil Neural Repair 2012;26:456–62. doi:10.1177/1545968311427406

[18] Michielsen ME, Selles RW, van der Geest JN, et al. Motor recovery and cortical reorganization after mirror therapy in chronic stroke patients: a phase II randomized controlled trial. Neurorehabil Neural Repair 2011;25:223–33. doi:10.1177/1545968310385127

[19] Sampson M, Shau Y-W, King MJ. Bilateral upper limb trainer with virtual reality for post-stroke rehabilitation: case series report. Disabil Rehabil Assist Technol 2012;7:55–62. doi:10.3109/17483107.2011.562959

[20] Sugg K, Müller S, Winstein C, et al. Does action observation training with immediate physical practice improve hemiparetic upper-limb function in chronic stroke? Neurorehabil Neural Repair 2015;29:807–17. doi:10.1177/1545968314565512

[21] Kim K. Action observation for upper limb function after stroke: evidence-based review of randomized controlled trials. J Phys Ther Sci 2015;27:3315–7. doi:10.1589/jpts.27.3315

[22] Pelosin E, Avanzino L, Bove M, et al. Action observation improves freezing of gait in patients with Parkinson's disease. Neurorehabil Neural Repair 2010;24:746–52. doi:10.1177/1545968310368685

[23] Pelosin E, Bove M, Ruggeri P, et al. Reduction of bradykinesia of finger movements by a single session of action observation in Parkinson disease. Neurorehabil Neural Repair 2013;27:552–60. doi:10.1177/1545968312471905

[24] Jaywant A, Ellis TD, Roy S, et al. Randomized controlled trial of a home-based action observation intervention to improve walking in Parkinson disease. Arch Phys Med Rehabil 2016;97:665–73. doi:10.1016/j.apmr.2015.12.029

[25] Buccino G, Arisi D, Gough P, et al. Improving upper limb motor functions through action observation treatment: a pilot study in children with cerebral palsy. Dev Med Child Neurol 2012;54:822–8. doi:10.1111/j.1469-8749.2012.04334.x

[26] Eggermont LHP, Swaab DF, Hol EM, et al. Observation of hand movements by older persons with dementia: effects on cognition: a pilot study. Dement Geriatr Cogn Disord 2009;27:366–74. doi:10.1159/000209311

[27] Buccino G. Action observation treatment: a novel tool in neurorehabilitation. Philos Trans R Soc Lond B Biol Sci 2014;369:20130185. doi:10.1098/rstb.2013.0185

[28] Filimon F, Nelson JD, Hagler DJ, et al. Human cortical representations for reaching: mirror neurons for execution, observation, and imagery. Neuroimage 2007;37:1315–28. doi:10.1016/j.neuroimage.2007.06.008

[29] Enticott PG, Kennedy H a, Bradshaw JL, et al. Understanding mirror neurons: evidence for enhanced corticospinal excitability during the observation of transitive but not intransitive hand gestures. Neuropsychologia 2010;48:2675–80. doi:10.1016/j.neuropsychologia.2010.05.014

[30] Fitzgibbon BM, Fitzgerald PB, Enticott PG. An examination of the influence of visuomotor associations on interpersonal motor resonance. Neuropsychologia 2014;56:439–46. doi:10.1016/j.neuropsychologia.2014.02.018

[31] Plata-Bello J, Modroño C, Marcano F, et al. The mirror neuron system and motor dexterity: what happens? Neuroscience 2014;275:285–95.

[32] Jonas M, Siebner HR, Biermann-Ruben K, et al. Do simple intransitive finger movements consistently activate frontoparietal mirror neuron areas in humans? Neuroimage 2007;36 Suppl 2:T44–53.

[33] Plata-Bello J, Modroño C, Marcano F, et al. Observation of simple intransitive actions: the effect of familiarity. PLoS One 2013;8:e74485.

[34] Molnar-Szakacs I, Kaplan J, Greenfield PM, et al. Observing complex action sequences: the role of the fronto-parietal mirror neuron system. Neuroimage 2006;33:923–35.

[35] Caggiano V, Fogassi L, Rizzolatti G, et al. View-based encoding of actions in mirror neurons of area f5 in macaque premotor cortex. Curr Biol 2011;21:144–8. doi:10.1016/j.cub.2010.12.022

[36] Rizzolatti G, Fogassi L. The mirror mechanism: recent findings and perspectives. Philos Trans R Soc Lond B Biol Sci 2014;369:20130420. doi:10.1098/rstb.2013.0420

[37] Caggiano V, Giese M, Thier P, et al. Encoding of point of view during action observation in the local field potentials of macaque area F5. Eur J Neurosci 2015;41:466–76. doi:10.1111/ejn.12793

[38] Caggiano V, Fogassi L, Rizzolatti G, et al. Mirror neurons differentially encode the peripersonal and extrapersonal space of monkeys. Science 2009;324:403–6. doi:10.1126/science.1166818

[39] Mahoney FI, Barthel DW. Functional evaluation: the Barthel Index. MD State Med J 1965;14:61–5.

[40] Granger CV, Dewis LS, Peters NC, et al. Stroke rehabilitation: analysis of repeated Barthel index measures. Arch Phys Med Rehabil 1979;60:14–7.

[41] Cid-Ruzafa J, Damián-Moreno J. Disability evaluation: Barthel's index. Rev española salud pública 1996;71:127–37.

[42] Lawton MP, Brody EM. Assessment of older people: self-maintaining and instrumental activities of daily living. Gerontologist 1969;9:179–86.

[43] Yoon J, Chun MH, Lee SJ, et al. Effect of virtual reality-based rehabilitation on upper-extremity function in patients with brain tumor: controlled trial. Am J Phys Med Rehabil 2015;94:449–59. doi:10.1097/PHM.0000000000000192

[44] García-Betances RI, Jiménez-Mixco V, Arredondo MT, et al. Using virtual reality for cognitive training of the elderly. Am J Alzheimers Dis Other Demen 2015;30:49–54. doi:10.1177/1533317514545866

[45] Yang S, Chun MH, Son YR. Effect of virtual reality on cognitive dysfunction in patients with brain tumor. Ann Rehabil Med 2014;38:726–33. doi:10.5535/arm.2014.38.6.726

[46] Holden MK. Virtual environments for motor rehabilitation: review. Cyberpsychol Behav 2005;8:187–211; discussion 212–9. doi:10.1089/cpb.2005.8.187

[47] Liao Y-Y, Yang Y-R, Cheng S-J, et al. Virtual reality-based training to improve obstacle-crossing performance and dynamic balance in patients with Parkinson's disease. Neurorehabil Neural Repair 2015;29:658–67. doi:10.1177/1545968314562111

[48] Eftekharsadat B, Babaei-Ghazani A, Mohammadzadeh M, et al. Effect of virtual reality-based balance training in multiple sclerosis. Neurol Res 2015;37:539–44. doi:10.1179/1743132815Y.0000000013

[49] Lloréns R, Gil-Gómez J-A, Alcañiz M, et al. Improvement in balance using a virtual reality-based stepping exercise: a randomized controlled trial involving individuals with chronic stroke. Clin Rehabil 2015;29:261–8. doi:10.1177/0269215514543333

[50] Laver KE, George S, Thomas S, et al. Virtual reality for stroke rehabilitation. Cochrane database Syst Rev 2015;2:CD008349.

[51] Prochnow D, Bermúdez i Badia S, Schmidt J, et al. A functional magnetic resonance imaging study of visuomotor processing in a virtual reality-based paradigm: rehabilitation gaming system. Eur J Neurosci 2013;37:1441–7. doi:10.1111/ejn.12157

[52] Modroño C, Plata-Bello J, Zelaya F, et al. Enhancing sensorimotor activity by controlling virtual objects with gaze. PLoS One 2015;10:e0121562. doi:10.1371/journal.pone.0121562

# 6

# Physical Therapy for Cerebellar Ataxia

Akiyoshi Matsugi

**Abstract**

Ataxia, the incoordination and balance dysfunction in movements without muscle weakness, causes gait and postural disturbance in patients with stroke, multiple sclerosis, and degeneration in the cerebellum. The aim of this article was to provide a narrative review of the previous reports on physical therapy for mainly cerebellar ataxia offering various opinions. Some systematic reviews and randomized control trial studies, which were searched in the electronic databases using terms "ataxia" and "physical therapy," enable a strategy for physical therapy for cerebellar ataxia. Intensive physical therapy more than 1 hour per day for at least 4 weeks, focused on balance, gait, and strength training in hospital and home for patients with degenerative cerebellar ataxia can improve ataxia, gait ability, and activity of daily living. Furthermore, the weighting on the torso, using treadmill, noninvasive brain stimulation over the cerebellum for neuromodulation to facilitate motor learning, and neurophysiological assessment have a potential to improve the effect of physical therapy on cerebellar ataxia. Previous findings indicated that physical therapy is time restricted; therefore, its long-term effect and the effect of new optional neurophysiological methods should be studied.

**Keywords:** ataxia, cerebellum, physical therapy, balance training, noninvasive brain stimulation, stroke, degenerative ataxia, multiple sclerosis

## 1. Introduction

Incoordination and balance dysfunction in movements without muscle weakness are the most accepted definition of ataxia, which has three subcategories: sensory, vestibular [1], and cerebellar ataxia [2, 3]. When the cerebellum is damaged, activity of daily living (ADL) is disturbed in patients with the ataxia owing to diseases, such as spinocerebellar degeneration [4–8], multiple sclerosis (MS) [2, 3, 9–13], and stroke [14–17]. In contrast, these can have several causes in children, such as infection and tumor [18].

The cerebellum contributes to sensory motor control [3, 19–25], gait [11, 21, 26–31], and balance [5] for maintenance of upright posture. Furthermore, the cerebellum has an important role in motor learning [32] and adaptation [33]. Therefore, if the cerebellum is damaged, then these functions are disturbed, and dysmetria, tremor, rebound phenomenon, dysdiadochokinesia, dyssynergia, and hypotonia [24, 34].

Intervention is provided to patients with cerebellar ataxia to recover motor function and ADL. The intervention for rehabilitation includes medication [35, 36], surgery, and physical therapy [6, 9]. The effect of medication and surgery depends on the cause of ataxia and extent of neuronal damage [37, 38]; however, there is no radical treatment for these diseases yet.

Patients with cerebellar damage have impaired motor learning [15, 39–46], but their ataxia, gait, and ADL can be improved. Studies with high methodological quality and scientific evidence regarding the intervention using physical therapy for cerebellar ataxia occur as systematic reviews, randomized control trials (RCT), and guidelines. Systematic reviews can particularly provide important information on physical therapy use for cerebellar ataxia. The systematic reviews offer various viewpoints to solve various clinical questions. The aim of this article was to review the important points for physical therapy to improve the motor function and ADL in patients with cerebellar ataxia and to search for the point which we should study in the future to establish the evidence of the effect of physical therapy for cerebellar ataxia. Based on these previous findings and opinions in this search, I will mention about recommended and possible physical therapy which includes the measure and intervention for cerebellar ataxia and ADL in the patients with cerebellar damage.

## 2. Method of search

A search for articles written in English, using the word "ataxia," was performed by the author in electronic databases of the Physiotherapy Evidence Database (PEDro), which is provided by the George Institute for Global Health for Physical Therapy. The searched systematic reviews were scrutinized based on the aim of the articles, including RCTs for physical therapy, and the year of publication of the target articles. Subsequently, article search was conducted using the words "ataxia" and "physical therapy" or "physiotherapy" in PubMed [1970–2016]. The effective methods of measurement and intervention for ataxia were mainly assessed transversely in systematic reviews and RCT studies. Furthermore, other than these reports, we also considered the possible method of measure and intervention for cerebellar ataxia.

## 3. Review

Six systematic reviews [6, 9, 10, 36, 47, 48] written in English regarding physical therapy were searched in these databases. Six RCTs [2, 49–54] were included in these systematic reviews that were published before October 2016. In addition, another RCT [55] was found in PubMed, upon searching for all systematic reviews and RCT reports regarding physical therapy that were published from 1980 to 2016. An article regarding intensive physical therapy for spinocerebellar degeneration (SCD) written by Miyai et al. [50] was referred in three review articles [10, 47, 48], which were all systematic reviews published after 2012, as the most influential study with high methodological quality and scientific evidence on physical therapy for patients with degenerative cerebellar ataxia. These RCTs regarding MS or SCD were included in these reviews and that regarding stroke was not included. No RCT report on the long-term effect of physical therapy for cerebellar ataxia was found. In addition, no study regarding the meta-analysis on physical therapy for cerebellar ataxia was found.

### 3.1. Outcome measure for physical therapy

#### *3.1.1. Evaluation for ataxia, balance, gait ability, and ADL*

The definition of function and ADL should be measured before and after physical therapy [10, 34] because clients and therapists must judge the effectiveness of the intervention. Clinical scales are often used for investigating the effect of physical therapy. In cerebellar ataxia, the most often used specific scales for the severity of cerebellar ataxia in previous studies were the scale for the assessment and rating of ataxia (SARA) [5, 10, 16, 56–59] and international cooperative ataxia rating scale (ICARS) [55, 57, 60–64]. These scales include the measurement of not only incoordination movement of the upper and lower extremities but also balance in sitting, standing, and gait [10, 56, 62]. The Berg balance scale (BBS) was most often used in previous studies to measure balance ability comprehensively [5, 16, 26, 28, 51, 54, 62, 65–70]. Timed up and go test [54, 64, 69], 10-m walk test [5, 66], 2-min walking test [62], and 6-min walking test [10] were used to measure the gait ability in previous studies. Furthermore, the functional independence measure (FIM) was often used to measure the ADL in patients with cerebellar ataxia [4, 50]. These scales are recommended and should be used to measure for severity of cerebellar ataxia and ability of balance and gait before and after physical therapy for cerebellar ataxia.

In previous studies regarding stroke rehabilitation, the parameter, which measures severity of impairment and disability, is often used to predict for functional outcome and destination from hospital [71–83]. A report indicated that continued recovery is possible in cerebellar ataxia by trauma [84], but no report on the prediction of the rehabilitation outcome in patients with degenerative cerebellar ataxic was found. Therefore, the method of prediction of rehabilitation outcome using these measures in patients with cerebellar ataxia should be studied.

#### *3.1.2. Possible scales for ataxia and postural disorder*

Another possible test has been reported in a previous study regarding ataxia and postural disorder. Force control test was conducted to test the ability of force control by muscle contraction in the extremity by using a dynamometer in the isometric testing mode with Biodex (Medical Inc., Shirley, NY) [30]. The inadequacy of force control by muscle contraction can cause posture and gait disturbances [30]. The repetitive and alternate movement with both legs is acquired in locomotion, such as gait and pedaling. Therefore, we may measure the amplitude and speed in these motions because the amplitude and speed of repetitive motion, which involve pedaling movement with both legs, are disturbed in patients with cerebellar ataxia [85]. The performance of leg placement task has a strong relationship with gait disturbance in patients with cerebellar ataxia [86]. Subjective visual vertical (SVV) is often measured in stroke patients [87, 88] because SVV deviated to one side laterally and the bias causes dysfunction of postural control in stroke patients not only with palsy [88] but also with cerebellar ataxia [89, 90]. The reason why SVV bias occurs in cerebellar patients is the estimated contamination of vestibular disorder, but it is unclear, so further study is needed.

#### *3.1.3. Evaluation with neuroimaging*

A functional magnetic resonance imaging (MRI) study revealed that cerebellar somatotopic maps are associated with voluntary limb movement in lobules and sublobules in the rostral and caudal spinocerebellar cortex [91]. Voluntary limb movement is disturbed in patients with the atrophy in intermediate and lateral cerebellum, which can be evaluated with MRI [92–94]. Furthermore, a voxel-based lesion-symptom mapping study using MRI revealed that limb ataxia was significantly correlated with lesions of the interposed and part of the dentate nuclei and ataxia of posture and gait was significantly correlated with lesions of the fastigial nuclei, including interposed nuclei [63]. Subsequently, MRI is useful to estimate location causing incoordination movement.

#### *3.1.4. Neurophysiological evaluation*

The motor-evoked potential induced by transcranial magnetic stimulation (TMS) over the primary motor cortex is inhibited by TMS over the contralateral cerebellum [95, 96]. This cerebellar brain inhibition (CBI) [95, 97–103] is modulated in patients with cerebellar ataxia [99, 103] and in healthy adults after motor learning [32], indicating that CBI reflects excitability of the cerebellum and the function of connectivity of the cerebellum and other tissues associated with motor control and learning [104]. Therefore, CBI may be useful for estimation whether ataxia may be due to the disturbance of the input, output, or cerebellum itself and the effect of physical therapy in cerebellar plastic change [61].

The cerebellum has output to the vestibular nuclei, red nuclei, reticular formation, and functional corroboration with the brainstem [105]. The vestibulospinal, rubrospinal, and reticulospinal tracts play an important role in postural control [106]. A previous study reported the possibility that cerebellar TMS facilitates spinal reflex [107] mediated with these extrapyramidal tracts [108]. This cerebellar spinal facilitation (CSpF) [107, 108] is modulated by motor tasks [107], which require cerebellar excitation [109]. In contrast, cerebellar TMS induces long latency electromyographic response (C-LER) in the hand muscles [110–112] particularly during visually guided manual tracking tasks and in the lower muscles [113–115], which can be mediated by the vestibulospinal and reticulospinal tracts because C-LER is affected by the task-modulated excitability of these tracts [114, 115]. Therefore, CSpF and C-LER may be useful to detect the function of cerebellar output and that of the cerebellum itself.

## 3.2. Intervention

### 3.2.1. *Intensive physical therapy*

Three systematic reviews [10, 47, 48] and two narrative review articles [37, 116] introduced and recommended intensive physical therapy for cerebellar ataxia in patient with SCD within 1 year from diagnosis [50]. Physical and occupational therapies, which were 2 hours × 5 days + 1 hour × 2 days per week for 4 weeks, were applied to patient in the hospital. This intensive physical therapy, which focused on balance, gait, and muscle strengthening, can improve SARA score and gait speed in the hospital, but the effect was carried over only until 12 weeks after the training, but not 24 weeks [50]. In another study including the patient with a diagnosis of SCD for more than 1 year, intensive physical therapy, which was 1 hour × 3 days per week for 4 weeks, including coordinative training, improves SARA and gait ability, and the period of effect was 8 weeks post-rehabilitation [52, 53]. Therefore, intensive physical therapy that is focused on balance, gait, and muscle strengthening can be recommended for patients with SCD with cerebellar ataxia to improve their severity of ataxia and gait ability. However, these effects can be restrictive in time; hence, continuing therapy intermittently and further studies acquiring more long-term effects are necessary.

In patients with cerebellar stroke, intensive training for the upper limb with cerebellar ataxia can improve the upper function [17]. In this study, the modified constraint-induced movement therapy was conducted for patients with subacute stroke, resulting in the improvement of the upper limb function. However, whether the effect harbors for more than 1 week is not known.

The study was conducted regarding the intensive physical therapy to chronic MS patient who does not have sufficient walking ability. The patients received physiotherapy for two sessions of 45-min each week on different days for 8 weeks. The result suggests that the intensive intervention can mildly improve the upper function and mobility in chronic MS patients [49].

### 3.2.2. *Balance training*

Balance training is an important intervention for patients with cerebellar ataxia [50, 52, 53, 117]. A previous RCT study revealed that balance training with placement on the torso with less than 1.5% of patient's body weight improves gait ability in patients with cerebellar ataxia with MS [10, 54]. Small weights were applied to the torso on a specially constructed vestlike garment that allowed Velcro application of weights to the front, back, or sides of the torso between the shoulders and waist to maintain the balance of the upright posture [54]. This balance-based torso weighting (BBTW) can be useful for treatment of cerebellar ataxic gait.

In another report that is not RCT, balance training without weighting can improve gait function in patients with SCD using the PhysioTools™ General Exercises First Edition software (PhysioTools; Tampere, Finland) in own home [64]. The home-based exercise program was modified by physical therapist based on severity of ataxia, and the tools, which were chair, exercise ball, or balance disk, were applied [64]. The improvement of gait function was maintained 4 weeks after the final training [64]. This balance training can be effective at home after rehabilitation in hospital.

A rehabilitation program including foot sensory stimulation, balance, and gait training with limited vision was adapted to patients with ataxic neuropathy. The results suggest that there is a possibility that the intervention improves the motor function in patient with ataxic neuropathies [69].

Trunk stabilization and locomotor training in cerebellar ataxia can improve the balance score [66]. Furthermore, core stability exercise increases trunk stability to facilitate skilled motor behavior of the upper extremities [118].

### 3.2.3. *Gait training*

The gait in patients with degenerative cerebellar ataxia is disturbed [28, 29]; however, no RCT report focused on especially gait training for patients with cerebellar ataxia. Human locomotor adaptive learning is proportional to the depression of cerebellar excitability [33], and patients with ataxia with cerebellar damage have partially impaired in motor learning [14, 41, 45, 46], but some previous studies reported that gait training can improve the function of gait. The locomotive training on the ground is applied [84], and the treadmill training is applied to cerebellar ataxic gait in adults [5, 66, 119–121] and children [120], resulting to the intervention that contributes gait function improvement in this report. Furthermore, body-weight support on a treadmill can improve balance and gait function with severe cerebellar ataxia [66].

Task-oriented (disability-focused) or facilitation (impairment-based) approach was conducted to cerebellar ataxia in MS to improve gait ability [51]. Both approaches improved gait function, but no significant difference was found on the effect in both approaches. Another possible gait function improvement on cerebellar ataxia was reported; auditory feedback control therapy can improve ataxic gait in MS [122], and orthopedic shoes were used to improve gait in Friedreich's ataxia in a single case report [123].

### 3.2.4. *Noninvasive brain stimulation (NIBS)*

NIBS, which is repetitive TMS (rTMS) [96, 98] and transcranial direct current stimulation (tDCS) [124], over the primary motor cortex can modulate the excitability of the motor cortex [125] and is often used as an effective tool for enhancing behavioral training after stroke with hemiplegia [125–128]. Furthermore, the NIBS to the cerebellum modulates cerebellar excitability [98, 129–131], motor function [132, 133], and motor learning [32, 134–138] in healthy population. In patients with cerebellar ataxia, some previous studies reported about the effect of tDCS to the cerebellum on motor function [131, 139–141]. A double-blind, randomized and sham-controlled study revealed that cerebellar tDCS improved SARA, ICARS, nine-hole peg test, and gait speed [141]. But it is not clear whether the effect remains for a long term. In another report, tDCS over the cerebellum and contralateral motor cortex reduced postural and action tremor due to the degenerative cerebellum in patients [140]. rTMS over the cerebellum in patients with cerebellar stroke and cerebellar ataxia improves ICARS subscore on gait and posture with improvement in neurophysiological parameters, such as CBI [61]. Therefore, some recent report revealed that NIBS over the cerebellum transiently improve ataxia and gait disturbance; however, there are no report on the long-term effect in any RCT.

## 4. Conclusion

Gait, balance, and ADL are disturbed in patients with cerebellar ataxia owing to diseases, such as stroke, SCD, and MS. Severity of cerebellar ataxia depends on the disease. The interventions for cerebellar ataxia are medication, surgery, and physical therapy to improve and maintain their function of gait, balance, and ADL due to cerebellar ataxia. However, very few reports, which are systematic reviews, RCT studies, and meta-analysis studies, on physical therapy for cerebellar ataxia with high methodological quality and scientific evidence, were found compared with rehabilitation for hemiplegia due to stroke.

Some systematic reviews introduced and recommended intensive physical therapy more than 1 hour per day for at least 4 weeks, which focused on balance, gait, and strengthening training for degenerative cerebellar ataxia in hospital and own home. However, these effects can be restrictive in time; therefore, the therapy should be applied intermittently. To facilitate the effect, the intervention program should be modified by physical therapist based on results of evaluation using SARA, ICARS, BBS, walking test, FIM, neuroimaging, and neurophysiological assessments. The weighting on the torso, treadmill, balance ball, balance disk, and the software to instruct the exercise can improve the effect of physical therapy in hospital and own home. NIBS over the cerebellum for neuromodulation to facilitate motor learning has potential to improve the effect of physical therapy for cerebellar ataxia. Previous findings indicated that physical therapy for cerebellar ataxia is time restricted; therefore, the long-term effect and the effect of new optional neurophysiological methods should be studied in patient with stroke, SCD, and MS.

## Acknowledgements

This work was supported by Shijonawate Gakuen University and JSPS KAKENHI (Grant Number 15K16422).

## Author details

Akiyoshi Matsugi

Address all correspondence to: a-matsugi@reha.shijonawate-gakuen.ac.jp

Faculty of Rehabilitation, Shijonawate Gakuen University, Osaka, Japan

## References

[1] Strupp M, Brandt T. Current treatment of vestibular, ocular motor disorders and nystagmus. Ther Adv Neurol Disord. 2009;2(4):223–239.

[2] Armutlu K, Karabudak R, Nurlu G. Physiotherapy approaches in the treatment of ataxic multiple sclerosis: a pilot study. Neurorehabil Neural Repair. 2001;15(3):203–211.

[3] Manto M, Bower JM, Conforto AB, Delgado-Garcia JM, da Guarda SN, Gerwig M, et al. Consensus paper: roles of the cerebellum in motor control—the diversity of ideas on cerebellar involvement in movement. Cerebellum. 2012;11(2):457–487.

[4] Miyai I. Challenge of neurorehabilitation for cerebellar degenerative diseases. Cerebellum. 2012;11(2):436–437.

[5] Fonteyn EM, Heeren A, Engels JJ, Boer JJ, van de Warrenburg BP, Weerdesteyn V. Gait adaptability training improves obstacle avoidance and dynamic stability in patients with cerebellar degeneration. Gait Posture. 2014;40(1):247–251.

[6] Trujillo-Martín MM, Serrano-Aguilar P, Monton-Alvarez F, Carrillo-Fumero R. Effectiveness and safety of treatments for degenerative ataxias: a systematic review. Mov Disord. 2009;24(8):1111–1124.

[7] Zhuchenko O, Bailey J, Bonnen P, Ashizawa T, Stockton DW, Amos C, et al. Autosomal dominant cerebellar ataxia (SCA6) associated with small polyglutamine expansions in the alpha 1A-voltage-dependent calcium channel. Nat Genet. 1997;15(1):62–69.

[8] Nagaoka U, Takashima M, Ishikawa K, Yoshizawa K, Yoshizawa T, Ishikawa M, et al. A gene on SCA4 locus causes dominantly inherited pure cerebellar ataxia. Neurology. 2000;54(10):1971–1975.

[9] Mills RJ, Yap L, Young CA. Treatment for ataxia in multiple sclerosis. Cochrane Database Syst Rev. 2007;24(1):CD005029.

[10] Marquer A, Barbieri G, Pérennou D. The assessment and treatment of postural disorders in cerebellar ataxia: a systematic review. Ann Phys Rehabil Med. 2014;57(2):67–78.

[11] Stevens V, Goodman K, Rough K, Kraft GH. Gait impairment and optimizing mobility in multiple sclerosis. Phys Med Rehabil Clin N Am. 2013;24(4):573–592.

[12] Marsden J, Harris C. Cerebellar ataxia: pathophysiology and rehabilitation. Clin Rehabil. 2011;25(3):195–216.

[13] Peterson EW, Cho CC, von Koch L, Finlayson ML. Injurious falls among middle aged and older adults with multiple sclerosis. Arch Phys Med Rehabil. 2008;89(6):1031–1037.

[14] Hatakenaka M, Miyai I, Mihara M, Yagura H, Hattori N. Impaired motor learning by a pursuit rotor test reduces functional outcomes during rehabilitation of poststroke ataxia. Neurorehabil Neural Repair. 2012;26(3):293–300.

[15] Boyd LA, Winstein CJ. Cerebellar stroke impairs temporal but not spatial accuracy during implicit motor learning. Neurorehabil Neural Repair. 2004;18(3):134–143.

[16] Kim BR, Lim JH, Lee SA, Park S, Koh SE, Lee IS, et al. Usefulness of the scale for the assessment and rating of ataxia (SARA) in ataxic stroke patients. Ann Rehabil Med. 2011;35(6):772–780.

[17] Richards L, Senesac C, McGuirk T, Woodbury M, Howland D, Davis S, et al. Response to intensive upper extremity therapy by individuals with ataxia from stroke. Top Stroke Rehabil. 2008;15(3):262–271.

[18] Musselman KE, Stoyanov CT, Marasigan R, Jenkins ME, Konczak J, Morton SM, et al. Prevalence of ataxia in children: a systematic review. Neurology. 2014;82(1):80–89.

[19] Bastian AJ. Learning to predict the future: the cerebellum adapts feedforward movement control. Curr Opin Neurobiol. 2006;16(6):645–649.

[20] Scott SH. Optimal feedback control and the neural basis of volitional motor control. Nat Rev Neurosci. 2004;5(7):532–546.

[21] Jankovic J. Gait disorders. Neurol Clin. 2015;33(1):249–268.

[22] Manto M, Oulad Ben Taib N. The contributions of the cerebellum in sensorimotor control: what are the prevailing opinions which will guide forthcoming studies?. Cerebellum. 2013;12(3):313–315.

[23] Bastian AJ, Zackowski KM, Thach WT. Cerebellar ataxia: torque deficiency or torque mismatch between joints?. J Neurophysiol. 2000;83(5):3019–3030.

[24] Bastian AJ. Mechanisms of ataxia. Phys Ther. 1997;77(6):672–675.

[25] Stoodley CJ, Schmahmann JD. Evidence for topographic organization in the cerebellum of motor control versus cognitive and affective processing. Cortex. 2010;46(7):831–844.

[26] Ustinova KI, Chernikova LA, Dull A, Perkins J. Physical therapy for correcting postural and coordination deficits in patients with mild-to-moderate traumatic brain injury. Physiother Theory Pract. 2015;31(1):1–7.

[27] Goodworth AD, Paquette C, Jones GM, Block EW, Fletcher WA, Hu B, et al. Linear and angular control of circular walking in healthy older adults and subjects with cerebellar ataxia. Exp Brain Res. 2012;219(1):151–161.

[28] Jahn K, Zwergal A. Imaging supraspinal locomotor control in balance disorders. Restor Neurol Neurosci. 2010;28(1):105–114.

[29] Morton SM, Bastian AJ. Mechanisms of cerebellar gait ataxia. Cerebellum. 2007;6(1):79–86.

[30] Harris-Love MO, Siegel KL, Paul SM, Benson K. Rehabilitation management of Friedreich ataxia: lower extremity force-control variability and gait performance. Neurorehabil Neural Repair. 2004;18(2):117–124.

[31] Bodranghien F, Bastian A, Casali C, Hallett M, Louis ED, Manto M, et al. Consensus paper: revisiting the symptoms and signs of cerebellar syndrome. Cerebellum. 2016;15(3):369–391.

[32] Celnik P. Understanding and modulating motor learning with cerebellar stimulation. Cerebellum. 2015;14(2):171–174.

[33] Jayaram G, Galea JM, Bastian AJ, Celnik P. Human locomotor adaptive learning is proportional to depression of cerebellar excitability. Cereb Cortex. 2011;21(8):1901–1909.

[34] Tyson S, Watson A, Moss S, Troop H, Dean-Lofthouse G, Jorritsma S, et al. Development of a framework for the evidence-based choice of outcome measures in neurological physiotherapy. Disabil Rehabil. 2008;30(2):142–149.

[35] Revuelta GJ, Wilmot GR. Therapeutic interventions in the primary hereditary ataxias. Curr Treat Options Neurol. 2010;12(4):257–273.

[36] Vogel AP, Keage MJ, Johansson K, Schalling E. Treatment for dysphagia (swallowing difficulties) in hereditary ataxia. Cochrane Database Syst Rev. 2015;13(11):CD010169.

[37] Pandolfo M, Manto M. Cerebellar and afferent ataxias. Continuum (Minneap Minn). 2013;19(5 Movement Disorders):1312–1343.

[38] Ilg W, Bastian AJ, Boesch S, Burciu RG, Celnik P, Claassen J, et al. Consensus paper: management of degenerative cerebellar disorders. Cerebellum. 2014;13(2):248–268.

[39] Martin TA, Keating JG, Goodkin HP, Bastian AJ, Thach WT. Throwing while looking through prisms. I. Focal olivocerebellar lesions impair adaptation. Brain. 1996;119 (Pt 4):1183–1198.

[40] Maschke M, Gomez CM, Ebner TJ, Konczak J. Hereditary cerebellar ataxia progressively impairs force adaptation during goal-directed arm movements. J Neurophysiol. 2004;91(1):230–238.

[41] Morton SM, Bastian AJ. Prism adaptation during walking generalizes to reaching and requires the cerebellum. J Neurophysiol. 2004;92(4):2497–2509.

[42] Fernandez-Ruiz J, Velásquez-Perez L, Díaz R, Drucker-Colín R, Pérez-González R, Canales N, et al. Prism adaptation in spinocerebellar ataxia type 2. Neuropsychologia. 2007;45(12):2692–2698.

[43] Rabe K, Livne O, Gizewski ER, Aurich V, Beck A, Timmann D, et al. Adaptation to visuomotor rotation and force field perturbation is correlated to different brain areas in patients with cerebellar degeneration. J Neurophysiol. 2009;101(4):1961–1971.

[44] Molinari M, Leggio MG, Solida A, Ciorra R, Misciagna S, Silveri MC, et al. Cerebellum and procedural learning: evidence from focal cerebellar lesions. Brain. 1997;120 (Pt 10):1753–1762.

[45] Smiley-Oyen AL, Worringham CJ, Cross CL. Motor learning processes in a movement-scaling task in olivopontocerebellar atrophy and Parkinson's disease. Exp Brain Res. 2003;152(4):453–465.

[46] Spencer RM, Ivry RB. Sequence learning is preserved in individuals with cerebellar degeneration when the movements are directly cued. J Cogn Neurosci. 2009;21(7):1302–1310.

[47] Fonteyn EM, Keus SH, Verstappen CC, Schöls L, de Groot IJ, van de Warrenburg BP. The effectiveness of allied health care in patients with ataxia: a systematic review. J Neurol. 2014;261(2):251–258.

[48] Synofzik M, Ilg W. Motor training in degenerative spinocerebellar disease: ataxia-specific improvements by intensive physiotherapy and exergames. Biomed Res Int. 2014;2014:583507.

[49] Wiles CM, Newcombe RG, Fuller KJ, Shaw S, Furnival-Doran J, Pickersgill TP, et al. Controlled randomised crossover trial of the effects of physiotherapy on mobility in chronic multiple sclerosis. J Neurol Neurosurg Psychiatry. 2001;70(2):174–179.

[50] Miyai I, Ito M, Hattori N, Mihara M, Hatakenaka M, Yagura H, et al. Cerebellar ataxia rehabilitation trial in degenerative cerebellar diseases. Neurorehabil Neural Repair. 2012;26(5):515–522.

[51] Lord SE, Wade DT, Halligan PW. A comparison of two physiotherapy treatment approaches to improve walking in multiple sclerosis: a pilot randomized controlled study. Clin Rehabil. 1998;12(6):477–486.

[52] Ilg W, Synofzik M, Brotz D, Burkard S, Giese MA, Schols L. Intensive coordinative training improves motor performance in degenerative cerebellar disease. Neurology. 2009;73(22):1823–1830.

[53] Ilg W, Brotz D, Burkard S, Giese MA, Schols L, Synofzik M. Long-term effects of coordinative training in degenerative cerebellar disease. Mov Disord. 2010;25(13):2239–2246.

[54] Widener GL, Allen DD, Gibson-Horn C. Randomized clinical trial of balance-based torso weighting for improving upright mobility in people with multiple sclerosis. Neurorehabil Neural Repair. 2009;23(8):784–791.

[55] Chang YJ, Chou CC, Huang WT, Lu CS, Wong AM, Hsu MJ. Cycling regimen induces spinal circuitry plasticity and improves leg muscle coordination in individuals with spinocerebellar ataxia. Arch Phys Med Rehabil. 2015;96(6):1006–1013.

[56] Schmitz-Hübsch T, du Montcel ST, Baliko L, Berciano J, Boesch S, Depondt C, et al. Scale for the assessment and rating of ataxia: development of a new clinical scale. Neurology. 2006;66(11):1717–1720.

[57] Yabe I, Matsushima M, Soma H, Basri R, Sasaki H. Usefulness of the scale for assessment and rating of ataxia (SARA). J Neurol Sci. 2008;266(1–2):164–166.

[58] Kaut O, Jacobi H, Coch C, Prochnicki A, Minnerop M, Klockgether T, et al. A randomized pilot study of stochastic vibration therapy in spinocerebellar ataxia. Cerebellum. 2014;13(2):237–242.

[59] Pozzi NG, Minafra B, Zangaglia R, De Marzi R, Sandrini G, Priori A, et al. Transcranial direct current stimulation (tDCS) of the cortical motor areas in three cases of cerebellar ataxia. Cerebellum. 2014;13(1):109–112.

[60] Morton SM, Tseng YW, Zackowski KM, Daline JR, Bastian AJ. Longitudinal tracking of gait and balance impairments in cerebellar disease. Mov Disord. 2010;25(12):1944–1952.

[61] Bonnì S, Ponzo V, Caltagirone C, Koch G. Cerebellar theta burst stimulation in stroke patients with ataxia. Funct Neurol. 2014;29(1):41–45.

[62] Salci Y, Fil A, Armutlu K, Yildiz FG, Kurne A, Aksoy S, et al. Effects of different exercise modalities on ataxia in multiple sclerosis patients: a randomized controlled study. Disabil Rehabil. 2016;29:1-7.

[63] Schoch B, Dimitrova A, Gizewski ER, Timmann D. Functional localization in the human cerebellum based on voxelwise statistical analysis: a study of 90 patients. Neuroimage. 2006;30(1):36–51.

[64] Keller JL, Bastian AJ. A home balance exercise program improves walking in people with cerebellar ataxia. Neurorehabil Neural Repair. 2014;28(8):770–778.

[65] Blum L, Korner-Bitensky N. Usefulness of the berg balance scale in stroke rehabilitation: a systematic review. Phys Ther. 2008;88(5):559–566.

[66] Freund JE, Stetts DM. Use of trunk stabilization and locomotor training in an adult with cerebellar ataxia: a single system design. Physiother Theory Pract. 2010;26(7):447–458.

[67] Fujimoto C, Murofushi T, Chihara Y, Ushio M, Sugasawa K, Yamaguchi T, et al. Assessment of diagnostic accuracy of foam posturography for peripheral vestibular disorders: analysis of parameters related to visual and somatosensory dependence. Clin Neurophysiol. 2009;120(7):1408–1414.

[68] Matsuzaki S, Hashimoto M, Yuki S, Koyama A, Hirata Y, Ikeda M. The relationship between post-stroke depression and physical recovery. J Affect Disord. 2015;176:56–60.

[69] Missaoui B, Thoumie P. Balance training in ataxic neuropathies. Effects on balance and gait parameters. Gait Posture. 2013;38(3):471–476.

[70] Qiang W, Sonoda S, Suzuki M, Okamoto S, Saitoh E. Reliability and validity of a wheelchair collision test for screening behavioral assessment of unilateral neglect after stroke. Am J Phys Med Rehabil. 2005;84(3):161–166.

[71] Matsugi A, Tani K, Mitani Y, Oku K, Tamaru Y, Nagano K. Revision of the predictive method improves precision in the prediction of stroke outcomes for patients admitted to rehabilitation hospitals. J Phys Ther Sci. 2014;26(9):1429–1431.

[72] Matsugi A, Tani K, Tamaru Y, Yoshioka N, Yamashita A, Mori N, et al. Prediction of advisability of returning home using the home care score. Rehabil Res Pract. 2015;2015:501042.

[73] Matsugi A, Tani K, Yoshioka N, Yamashita A, Mori N, Oku K, et al. Prediction of destination at discharge from a comprehensive rehabilitation hospital using the home care score. J Phys Ther Sci. 2016;28(10):2737–2741.

[74] Sonoda S, Saitoh E, Nagai S, Okuyama Y, Suzuki T, Suzuki M. Stroke outcome prediction using reciprocal number of initial activities of daily living status. J Stroke Cerebrovasc Dis. 2005;14(1):8–11.

[75] Koyama T, Matsumoto K, Okuno T, Domen K. A new method for predicting functional recovery of stroke patients with hemiplegia: logarithmic modelling. Clin Rehabil. 2005;19(7):779–789.

[76] Koyama T, Matsumoto K, Okuno T, Domen K. Relationships between independence level of single motor-FIM items and FIM-motor scores in patients with hemiplegia after stroke: an ordinal logistic modelling study. J Rehabil Med. 2006;38(5):280–286.

[77] Inouye M. Predicting outcomes of patients in Japan after first acute stroke using a simple model. Am J Phys Med Rehabil. 2001;80(9):645–649.

[78] Inouye M, Kishi K, Ikeda Y, Takada M, Katoh J, Iwahashi M, et al. Prediction of functional outcome after stroke rehabilitation. Am J Phys Med Rehabil. 2000;79(6):513–518.

[79] Nguyen TA, Page A, Aggarwal A, Henke P. Social determinants of discharge destination for patients after stroke with low admission FIM instrument scores. Arch Phys Med Rehabil. 2007;88(6):740–744.

[80] Saji N, Kimura K, Ohsaka G, Higashi Y, Teramoto Y, Usui M, et al. Functional independence measure scores predict level of long-term care required by patients after stroke: a multicenter retrospective cohort study. Disabil Rehabil. 2015;37(4):331–337.

[81] Veerbeek JM, Kwakkel G, van Wegen EE, Ket JC, Heymans MW. Early prediction of outcome of activities of daily living after stroke: a systematic review. Stroke. 2011;42(5):1482–1488.

[82] Ween JE, Mernoff ST, Alexander MP. Recovery rates after stroke and their impact on outcome prediction. Neurorehabil Neural Repair. 2000;14(3):229–235.

[83] Matsugi A, Tani K, Tamara Y, Yoshioka N, Yamashita A, Mori N, et al. Home care score predicts the advisability of home care when it is difficult to predict it using the functional independence measure score. J Allied Health Sci. 2016;7(2):30–36.

[84] Freund JE, Stetts DM. Continued recovery in an adult with cerebellar ataxia. Physiother Theory Pract. 2013;29(2):150–158.

[85] Matsuo Y, Asai Y, Nomura T, Sato S, Inoue S, Mizukura I, et al. Intralimb incoordination in patients with ataxia. Neuroreport. 2003;14(16):2057–2059.

[86] Morton SM, Bastian AJ. Relative contributions of balance and voluntary leg-coordination deficits to cerebellar gait ataxia. J Neurophysiol. 2003;89(4):1844–1856.

[87] Tani K, Matsugi A, Uehara S, Kimura D. Abnormal bias in subjective vertical perception in a post-stroke astasia patient. J Phys Ther Sci. 2016;28(10):2979–2983.

[88] Reinhart S, Schaadt AK, Keller I, Hildebrandt H, Kerkhoff G, Utz K. Rotational coherent dot movement normalizes spatial disorientation of the subjective visual vertical in patients with rightsided stroke. Neuropsychologia. 2016;92:174–180.

[89] Baier B, Bense S, Dieterich M. Are signs of ocular tilt reaction in patients with cerebellar lesions mediated by the dentate nucleus?. Brain. 2008;131(Pt 6):1445–1454.

[90] Baier B, Dieterich M. Pusher syndrome in patients with cerebellar infarctions? J Neurol. 2012;259(7):1468–1469.

[91] Grodd W, Hülsmann E, Lotze M, Wildgruber D, Erb M. Sensorimotor mapping of the human cerebellum: fMRI evidence of somatotopic organization. Hum Brain Mapp. 2001;13(2):55–73.

[92] Timmann D, Brandauer B, Hermsdörfer J, Ilg W, Konczak J, Gerwig M, et al. Lesion-symptom mapping of the human cerebellum. Cerebellum. 2008;7(4):602–606.

[93] Timmann D, Konczak J, Ilg W, Donchin O, Hermsdörfer J, Gizewski ER, et al. Current advances in lesion-symptom mapping of the human cerebellum. Neuroscience. 2009;162(3):836–851.

[94] Burciu RG, Reinold J, Rabe K, Wondzinski E, Siebler M, Müller O, et al. Structural correlates of motor adaptation deficits in patients with acute focal lesions of the cerebellum. Exp Brain Res. 2014;232(9):2847–2857.

[95] Daskalakis ZJ, Paradiso GO, Christensen BK, Fitzgerald PB, Gunraj C, Chen R. Exploring the connectivity between the cerebellum and motor cortex in humans. J Physiol. 2004;557(Pt 2):689–700.

[96] Grimaldi G, Argyropoulos GP, Boehringer A, Celnik P, Edwards MJ, Ferrucci R, et al. Non-invasive cerebellar stimulation—a consensus paper. Cerebellum. 2014;13(1):121–138.

[97] Pinto AD, Chen R. Suppression of the motor cortex by magnetic stimulation of the cerebellum. Exp Brain Res. 2001;140(4):505–510.

[98] Popa T, Russo M, Meunier S. Long-lasting inhibition of cerebellar output. Brain Stimul. 2010;3(3):161–169.

[99] Groiss SJ, Ugawa Y. Cerebellar stimulation in ataxia. Cerebellum. 2012;11(2):440–442.

[100] Hamada M, Strigaro G, Murase N, Sadnicka A, Galea JM, Edwards MJ, et al. Cerebellar modulation of human associative plasticity. J Physiol. 2012;590(Pt 10):2365–2374.

[101] Hardwick RM, Lesage E, Miall RC. Cerebellar Transcranial Magnetic Stimulation: The Role of Coil Geometry and Tissue Depth. Brain Stimul. 2014;7:643-649.

[102] Iwata NK, Ugawa Y. The effects of cerebellar stimulation on the motor cortical excitability in neurological disorders: a review. Cerebellum. 2005;4(4):218–223.

[103] Ugawa Y, Uesaka Y, Terao Y, Hanajima R, Kanazawa I. Magnetic stimulation over the cerebellum in humans. Ann Neurol. 1995;37(6):703–713.

[104] Schmahmann JD, Pandya DN. The cerebrocerebellar system. Int Rev Neurobiol. 1997;41:31–60.

[105] Shinoda Y, Futami T, Kano M. Synaptic organization of the cerebello-thalamo-cerebral pathway in the cat. II. Input-output organization of single thalamocortical neurons in the ventrolateral thalamus. Neurosci Res. 1985;2(3):157–180.

[106] Takakusaki K. Neurophysiology of gait: from the spinal cord to the frontal lobe. Mov Disord. 2013;28(11):1483–1491.

[107] Matsugi A, Mori N, Uehara S, Kamata N, Oku K, Mukai K, et al. Task dependency of the long-latency facilitatory effect on the soleus H-reflex by cerebellar transcranial magnetic stimulation. Neuroreport. 2014;25(17):1375–1380.

[108] Matsugi A, Mori N, Uehara S, Kamata N, Oku K, Okada Y, et al. Effect of cerebellar transcranial magnetic stimulation on soleus Ia presynaptic and reciprocal inhibition. Neuroreport. 2015;26(3):139–143.

[109] Witt ST, Laird AR, Meyerand ME. Functional neuroimaging correlates of finger-tapping task variations: an ALE meta-analysis. Neuroimage. 2008;42(1):343–356.

[110] Matsugi A, Kamata N, Tanaka T, Hiraoka K. Long latency fluctuation of the finger movement evoked by cerebellar TMS during visually guided manual tracking task. Indian J Physiol Pharmacol. 2012;56(3):193–200.

[111] Matsugi A, Iwata Y, Mori N, Horino H, Hiraoka K. Long latency electromyographic response induced by transcranial magnetic stimulation over the cerebellum preferentially appears during continuous visually guided manual tracking task. Cerebellum. 2013;12(2):147–154.

[112] Hiraoka K, Horino K, Yagura A, Matsugi A. Cerebellar TMS evokes a long latency motor response in the hand during a visually guided manual tracking task. Cerebellum. 2010;9(3):454–460.

[113] Sakihara K, Yorifuji S, Ihara A, Izumi H, Kono K, Takahashi Y, et al. Transcranial magnetic stimulation over the cerebellum evokes late potential in the soleus muscle. Neurosci Res. 2003;46(2):257–262.

[114] Sakihara K, Hirata M, Nakagawa S, Fujiwara N, Sekino M, Ueno S, et al. Late response evoked by cerebellar stimuli: effect of optokinetic stimulation. Neuroreport. 2007;18(9):891–894.

[115] Hosokawa S, Hirata M, Goto T, Yanagisawa T, Sugata H, Araki T, et al. Cerebellar-related long latency motor response in upper limb musculature by transcranial magnetic stimulation of the cerebellum. Neuroreport. 2014;25(6):353–357.

[116] Maring JR, Croarkin E. Presentation and progression of Friedreich ataxia and implications for physical therapist examination. Phys Ther. 2007;87(12):1687–1696.

[117] Ilg W, Schatton C, Schicks J, Giese MA, Schöls L, Synofzik M. Video game-based coordinative training improves ataxia in children with degenerative ataxia. Neurology. 2012;79(20):2056–2060.

[118] Miyake Y, Kobayashi R, Kelepecz D, Nakajima M. Core exercises elevate trunk stability to facilitate skilled motor behavior of the upper extremities. J Bodyw Mov Ther. 2013;17(2):259–265.

[119] Bultmann U, Pierscianek D, Gizewski ER, Schoch B, Fritsche N, Timmann D, et al. Functional recovery and rehabilitation of postural impairment and gait ataxia in patients with acute cerebellar stroke. Gait Posture. 2014;39(1):563–569.

[120] Cernak K, Stevens V, Price R, Shumway-Cook A. Locomotor training using body-weight support on a treadmill in conjunction with ongoing physical therapy in a child with severe cerebellar ataxia. Phys Ther. 2008;88(1):88–97.

[121] Vaz DV, Schettino Rde C, Rolla de Castro TR, Teixeira VR, Cavalcanti Furtado SR, de Mello Figueiredo E. Treadmill training for ataxic patients: a single-subject experimental design. Clin Rehabil. 2008;22(3):234–241.

[122] Baram Y, Miller A. Auditory feedback control for improvement of gait in patients with Multiple Sclerosis. J Neurol Sci. 2007;254(1–2):90–94.

[123] Goulipian C, Bensoussan L, Viton JM, Milhe-De Bovis V, Ramon J, Delarque A. Orthopedic shoes improve gait in Friedreich's ataxia: a clinical and quantified case study. Eur J Phys Rehabil Med. 2008;44(1):93–98.

[124] Filmer HL, Dux PE, Mattingley JB. Applications of transcranial direct current stimulation for understanding brain function. Trends Neurosci. 2014;37(12):742–753.

[125] Adeyemo BO, Simis M, Macea DD, Fregni F. Systematic review of parameters of stimulation, clinical trial design characteristics, and motor outcomes in non-invasive brain stimulation in stroke. Front Psychiatry. 2012;3:88.

[126] Wessel MJ, Zimerman M, Hummel FC. Non-invasive brain stimulation: an interventional tool for enhancing behavioral training after stroke. Front Hum Neurosci. 2015;9:265.

[127] Koganemaru S, Mima T, Thabit MN, Ikkaku T, Shimada K, Kanematsu M, et al. Recovery of upper-limb function due to enhanced use-dependent plasticity in chronic stroke patients. Brain. 2010;133(11):3373–3384.

[128] Fujimoto S, Kon N, Otaka Y, Yamaguchi T, Nakayama T, Kondo K, et al. Transcranial direct current stimulation over the primary and secondary somatosensory cortices transiently improves tactile spatial discrimination in stroke patients. Front Neurosci. 2016;10:128.

[129] Werhahn K, Taylor J, Ridding M, Meyer B, Rothwell J. Effect of transcranial magnetic stimulation over the cerebellum on the excitability of human motor cortex. Electroencephalogr Clin Neurophysiol. 1996;101(1):58–66.

[130] Fierro B, Giglia G, Palermo A, Pecoraro C, Scalia S, Brighina F. Modulatory effects of 1 Hz rTMS over the cerebellum on motor cortex excitability. Exp Brain Res. 2007;176(3):440–447.

[131] van Dun K, Bodranghien F, Manto M, Marien P. Targeting the cerebellum by noninvasive neurostimulation: a review. Cerebellum. 2016.

[132] Shah B, Nguyen TT, Madhavan S. Polarity independent effects of cerebellar tDCS on short term ankle visuomotor learning. Brain Stimul. 2013;6(6):966–968.

[133] Dutta A, Paulus W, Nitsche MA. Facilitating myoelectric-control with transcranial direct current stimulation: a preliminary study in healthy humans. J Neuroeng Rehabil 2014;11:13.

[134] Galea JM, Vazquez A, Pasricha N, de Xivry JJ, Celnik P. Dissociating the roles of the cerebellum and motor cortex during adaptive learning: the motor cortex retains what the cerebellum learns. Cereb Cortex. 2011;21(8):1761–1770.

[135] Block H, Celnik P. Stimulating the cerebellum affects visuomotor adaptation but not intermanual transfer of learning. Cerebellum. 2013;12(6):781–793.

[136] Hardwick RM, Celnik PA. Cerebellar direct current stimulation enhances motor learning in older adults. Neurobiol Aging. 2014;35(10):2217–2221.

[137] Zuchowski ML, Timmann D, Gerwig M. Acquisition of conditioned eyeblink responses is modulated by cerebellar tDCS. Brain Stimul. 2014;7(4):525–531.

[138] Cantarero G, Spampinato D, Reis J, Ajagbe L, Thompson T, Kulkarni K, et al. Cerebellar direct current stimulation enhances on-line motor skill acquisition through an effect on accuracy. J Neurosci. 2015;35(7):3285–3290.

[139] Grimaldi G, Manto M. Anodal transcranial direct current stimulation (tDCS) decreases the amplitudes of long-latency stretch reflexes in cerebellar ataxia. Ann Biomed Eng. 2013;41(11):2437–2447.

[140] Grimaldi G, Oulad Ben Taib N, Manto M, Bodranghien F. Marked reduction of cerebellar deficits in upper limbs following transcranial cerebello-cerebral DC stimulation: tremor reduction and re-programming of the timing of antagonist commands. Front Syst Neurosci. 2014;8:9.

[141] Benussi A, Koch G, Cotelli M, Padovani A, Borroni B. Cerebellar transcranial direct current stimulation in patients with ataxia: a double-blind, randomized, sham-controlled study. Mov Disord. 2015;30(12):1701–1705.

7

# Clinical Application of Motor Imagery Training

Tsubasa Kawasaki

**Abstract**

Motor imagery training is applied to a rehabilitation program based on previous studies regarding neuroscience and behavioral science. Motor imagery training is useful because it can be applied to almost all patients in clinical settings. However, because motor imagery training has some shortcoming, clinicians need to consider its shortcoming. The objective of this chapter is to promote understanding about using motor imagery effectively.

**Keywords:** motor imagery, motor learning, rehabilitation

## 1. Introduction

Motor imagery is defined as the process of mentally rehearsing a motor act without overt body movement [1]. Motor imagery basically involves an experience as of movement of body part and action, meaning that the motor imagery is influenced with based on motor representations internally by working memory [2].

Motor imagery is called first-perspective imagery (1PP imagery), that is, image originates from the same viewpoint experienced at encoding [3], different from visual imagery (third-person perspective imagery or 3PP imagery) which is imagining physical movement from an external viewpoint as though observing other people's body movements as an onlooker. In comparison to brain activation during visual imagery, brain activation in the motor-related area (e.g., pre-supplementary area, precuneus, and inferior parietal lobule) was great during 1PP imagery [4].

Many previous studies have shown that neural plasticity and brain activation during motor imagery training are similar to that of actual physical practice of motor learning. Most previous studies demonstrated brain activation in the supplementary motor area, premotor cortex [5–7], and parietal cortex [6]. Additionally, as with changes in the motor neuron, enhancing cortico-spinal excitability during motor imagery led to an increase in the motor-evoked potential (MEP) by using transcranial magnetic stimulation [8, 9]. In behavioral data, there is a similarity between motor imagery and actual performance. Motor imagery is widely recognized as an effective method to enhance motor performance. Currently, motor imagery training is applied in rehabilitation programs in clinical settings. This training, which can be made available to all patients because it does not impose a physical load on patients, was confirmed through clinical evidence from meta-analysis. However, there are some problems with using motor imagery training for elderly people or stroke patients with reduced motor imagery ability and cognitive function. Based on this fact, physical therapists would be recommended to assess patients' motor imagery ability and to apply motor imagery training following the assessment. This chapter (a) addresses the effects of simple motor imagery training for patients such as those who have suffered a stroke and (b) offers three recommendations for resolving the problem of administering the training to patients with reduced cognitive function.

## 2. Motor imagery training

The biggest advantage of motor imagery training is that, unlike general physical training, there is no limitation on the patient's ability to execute motions because motor imagery is a cognitive activity and does not require physical exertion. Because of this advantage, motor imagery training is currently applied for a wide range of body functions.

For example, Hamel et al. reported the availability of motor imagery training for postural control. This study used imagery intervention for 6 months to enable patients to autonomously maintain a straight standing position, without body sway [10]. In a more recent study, Yasuda et al. reported the beneficial effect of decreased body sway after performing only 20 repetitions of imagining one's own body movement (dorsiflexion-plantarflexion) [11]. For chronic post-stroke patients, Cho et al. demonstrated that postural balances (Fugl-Meyer score (FMS)), functional reach (distance), and gait ability (time required for up-and-go and 10-m walk test) were improved after motor imagery training for normal gait [12].

Previous studies have also shown improved upper extremity function after stroke. Page and his colleagues have demonstrated that motor imagery training has beneficial effects on upper extremity function as measured by the FMS of motor recovery, motor activity log, and action research arm (ARA) test in subacute [13] and chronic patients [14–16]. Particularly, Page's works used randomized control trial to verify the availability of motor imagery training, which contributed to demonstrate high clinical evidence for the enhancement of upper extremity function, measuring ARA test, motor assessment scale, and the FMS in stroke patients [17]. According to Langhorne's report, mental practice (motor imagery training) seems most effective for upper extremity function when conducting meta-analysis. Therefore, this report has shown that motor imagery training had a greater effect than other interventions in established clinical evidence, such as constraint-induced movement therapy [18–21] (where patients are asked to use an affected limb (execute a task) for a long time and for a large number of repetitions under the condition that the intact limb is constrained), robot-assisted therapy [22, 23] (where robotic devices can assist patients' affected limb use in high-intensity, repetitive, specific task by digital control), and electrical interface [24] (where electrostimulation can deliver electric impulses to the muscle through the skin surface and elicit muscle contraction by simulating the neuromuscular system; the intensity, frequency, and patterns of impulse delivery can be selected depending on the patient's condition). The reports investigating the effects of motor imagery training are increasing; however, it must be considered that there are still a very few number of reports verifying the beneficial effects of motor imagery training. This means that additional studies are necessary to establish and accumulate clinical evidence of availability of motor imagery training for improvement of upper extremity by high-evidence level study design. Based on the clinical evidence, motor imagery training is a potential interventional approach for stroke disability [25]. In this report, intervention via motor imagery is an important tool to promote information processing for the improvement of actual motor function.

In almost all previous studies investigating the effects of motor imagery training on motor performance, subjects imagined their body movements while sitting or lying in a relaxed position, with eyes closed. This means that the effects of motor imagery training are influenced by the environmental context and participants' emotional condition. Considering these factors, Holmes and Collins devised the PETTLEP model as a guideline for applying motor imagery training for athletes [26]. PETTLEP is an acronym (Physical, Environment, Task, Timing, Learning, Emotion, and Perspective), with each letter representing an important factor for practitioners to consider when conducting motor imagery training.

The author suggests that the PETTLEP model can be used for some patients in rehabilitation settings considering clinical application. Although PETTLEP model was originally proposed for improving athlete's performance using motor imagery training, athletes in sports settings and patients in clinical settings are in common that both of them improve motor performance via motor-learning process, Therefore, contents in terms of clinical patients will be stated below. *Physical* refers to patients' physical experience when they imagine action (including body position, clothing, and sports equipment specific to the task/situation). In order to produce effective imagery intervention, patients should attempt to physically replicate as much as possible their actual performance. *Environment* refers to the surroundings when the patients imagine their own movement. The surroundings should be replicas of the actual environment of action. *Task* refers to the identicalness of the task imaging to the actual task. This detail would need to be updated regularly as the patient's skill improves. *Timing* refers to the congruence between times for actual action and imagery of the action. Decety et al. reported the temporal coupling and the same neural substrate between actual and simulated movements measured by mental chronometry (refers to inferring the time course of information processing in the nervous system [2, 27]). Therefore, patients have to imagine the action as if they have temporal consistency between the two. *Learning* in the PETTLEP model refers to updating and reflecting the contents of their imagery with improvement of the skill. Some previous studies reported that the structural and functional changes are shown by improving motor skills or practice [28, 29]. Because of that, patients have to refine the contents of their imagery in association with learning processes instead of routine contents of imagery throughout their improvement of the skill. *Emotion* refers to the emotions with which patients perform the actual action. While patients are imagining action, they should attempt to accompany this with the emotions and arousal associated with the typical physical performance. *Perspective* refers to the direction from which the imagery is viewed. 1PP imagery is commonly used for motor imagery training because 1PP imagery involves shared neural mechanisms and functional equivalence, suggesting that 1PP imagery training would be most beneficial. However, some research has demonstrated that 3PP imagery training is more beneficial [30, 31]. Based on these studies, Holms and Collins stated that individuals should combine 3PP imagery with 1PP imagery [26]. These elements of the PLTTEP model would be most important to the improvement of motor function; therefore, clinicians should consider them when applying motor imagery training.

Although it would be certain that the effects of motor imagery training would be influenced by the elements of PETTLEP model, because motor imagery is simple cognitive activity, it would have difficulty for precise and vividness motor imagery in some individuals. Binder pointed out that the clinician cannot comprehend how patients imagine their body movements, and the most concerning limitation of motor imagery is that it is not easy to objectively assess how the subject vividly imagines his or her action. Thus, indirect assessment methods were commonly used as a self-rating scale, for example, MIQ-RS [32, 33], KVIQ [34], mental chronometry, and a mental rotation (MR) task (see below for detail). In particular, some disease conditions involving the central nervous system (CNS) are affected to imagine their body movements. For example, Personnier et al. showed that elderly people decline in motor imagery ability by using mental chronometry of various walking tasks (i.e., subjects actually or mentally walked (walking distance: 5 m) along three paths having different widths (15, 25, and 50 cm)) [35]. In the report, functional changes in the aging brain cause reduced motor imagery ability in elderly people. Patients having upper limb motor dysfunction due to stroke have difficulty imagining their own body movement. Li et al. measured the motor imagery ability of stroke patients by having them imagery performing a sequence of three kinds of movement and then choose from among four options (photograph) of the final posture of the three-sequence movement. The result showed that 1PP imagery was disturbed in stroke patients, but 3PP imagery was not. This suggested that it is difficult for stroke patients to imagine their own actions (1PP imagery) [36]. Also, Decety et al. investigated motor imagery in patients with stroke and spinal cord injuries by measuring mental chronometry. Incongruence between the duration of actual body movement and its motor imagery was shown in stroke patients [37]. Moseley et al. demonstrated that patients with complex regional pain (refractory chronic pain) decrease low motor imagery ability by measuring MR task of hand stimuli. Notably, in the report, the low motor imagery ability is shown at affected body parts but not the unaffected limb. This means that patients who have difficulty imagining their body movement, such as stroke and chronic pain patients, may not benefit from motor imagery training. In fact, motor imagery does not enhance motor recovery in early post-stroke patients [38]. Timmermans et al. reported that video-based motor imagery training was not effective for subacute stroke patients, as measured by the FMS, Frenchay arm test, Wolf motor function test, and accelerometry [39]. Although Page et al. showed the improvement of hand function by motor imagery in acute stroke patients, Ietwaart et al. and Timmermans et al. reported no effect of the training. A possible reason for the inconsistency in results would be different in affected lesion due to brain stroke. The critical lesion site responsible for imagining one's own body movement was the inferior parietal lobule [40]. In this study, subjects were administered transcranial magnetic stimulation (TMS) using theta-burst stimulation to inhibit activity in the left inferior parietal lobule before they performed an implicit sequence-learning task. In comparison with the sham stimulation (control condition), the inhibition of the left IPL impaired the acquisition of motor skills. This study revealed the contribution of the left inferior parietal lobule to motor imagery. Moreover, patients with stroke-disturbed motor imagery were investigated for responsible brain lesions to identify the area responsible for motor imagery. The results showed that stroke patients were damaged in the fronto-parietal network, the left putamen, the left ventral premotor cortex, and long association fibers linking parieto-occipital regions with the dorsolateral premotor and prefrontal areas. In addition to the results of brain activation in the left IPL resulting by Kraeutner's study, these areas indicated a responsible lesion for motor imagery. In any case, these previous studies provide the clinicians with valuable information about the importance of the left brain area during motor imagery. This indicates that the clinicians should consider some possibility of impaired motor imagery ability in patients with left brain damage when the clinicians apply motor imagery training to these patients.

More practical strategies using motor imagery rather than simple motor imagery were verified for some patients having difficulty with motor imagery using a brain machine interface. Mihara et al. measured the changes in hemodynamic responses (associated with neuron behavior reflecting brain activity) using near infrared spectroscopy during motor imagery [41]. In this study, subjects were delivered information on the changes in hemodynamic responses in real time while subjects imagine the finger movements. The hemodynamic changes (i.e., brain activity) in real-time monitoring were greater than in baseline and sham information. This result suggested that the neuro-feedback approach, such as real-time monitoring using near infrared spectroscopy, would enhance brain activity, which was to be expected that subjects can perform mental imagery effectively by using this neuro-feedback approach.

## 3. Mental rotation task

In order to overcome the shortcomings mentioned above (some patients find it difficult to imagine their body movement precisely and vividly), one idea was to use a mental rotation (MR) task. MR refers to the ability to imagine the rotation of an object in space [42]. In a seminal study by Shepard and Metzler [42], participants were required to judge whether the pairs of three-dimensional objects were the same or different (**Figure 1a**, **b**). The results showed that the time required for the judgment (the MR reaction time) increased as the angle of rotation

### 3.1. Mental rotation of body parts for motor imagery

An MR task using a visual stimulus of a body part (typically a hand or a foot) requires participants to judge the laterality of a rotated body part (i.e., whether the stimulus is the right or the left hand/foot) (**Figure 2**).

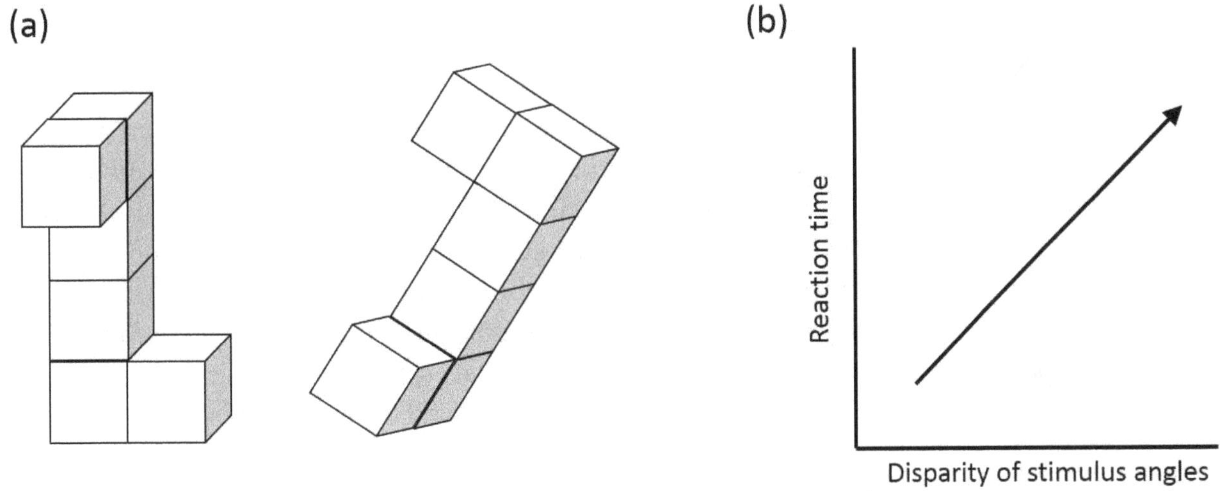


**Figure 1.** (a) MR task for three-dimensional objects: same-different judgment task. (b) The schematic liner relationship between reaction times (vertical axis) disparity angle of two objects (horizontal axis) [42].

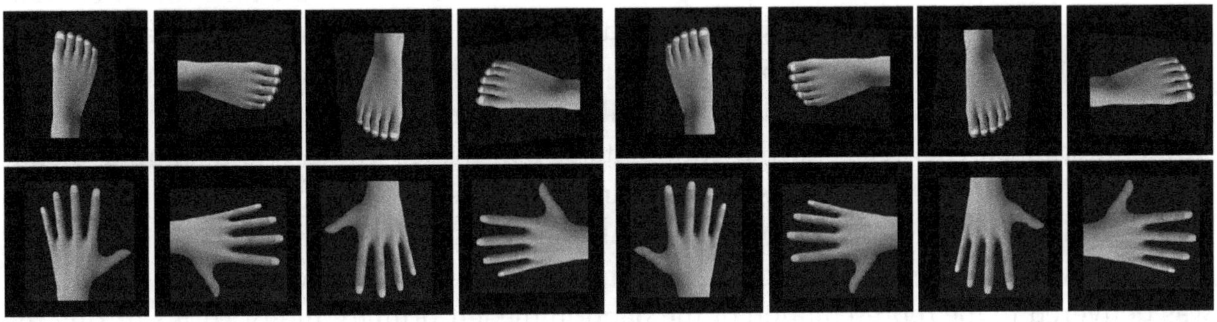

**Figure 2.** The MR task of body parts stimuli: making judgment of right or left parts.

In an MR task using body part stimuli, the time required for laterality judgment increased with the increasing rotation angle of the stimuli (**Figure 4**, unpublished work) as reaction times for MR task using object stimuli [42]. On the other hand, the time required for the simple reaction in the same MR task using body part stimuli was not significantly different. This suggested that the subject would imagine their own body movement of body parts of MR stimuli during MR task using body part stimuli. More directly, Parsons indicated that the MR of body parts involves cognitive processes used for both motor imagery and motor execution. The author reported that times required for the laterality judgment (i.e., the reaction time) of hand and foot stimuli were related to the times required for actual hand movement [43]. Participants were instructed to (a) judge the laterality as quickly and accurately as possible and (b) execute a hand/foot movement in a stimulus orientation. As a result, the reaction times for the hand/foot and the times required to execute these movements are nearly equivalent (e.g., the reaction time for 180° is similar to the time of actual hand movement of 180°). Parsons concluded that participants mentally rotate their own body image into congruence with the rotating stimuli during the MR task. Therefore, that study indicated that the MR of body parts can determine the ability to operate one's body image (i.e., the ability to operate motor imagery) by measuring the reaction time.

A more recent study by Ionta et al. showed that, during the MR of body parts, individuals simulate to move their own body image so as to match the observed stimulus [44]. They compared the MR reaction times for hand and foot stimuli in two postural conditions: (a) an anatomical posture (i.e., participants positioned their hands on their knees) and (b) an unusual posture (i.e., they positioned their hands behind their back, with fingers intertwined). The results showed that the MR reaction times for hand stimuli, but not for foot stimuli, were delayed in the unusual posture condition. Even if a stimulus was presented with no rotation, the reaction time was delayed when individuals kept their hands behind their back, so that the orientation of the hands was different from that of the stimuli. Ionta et al. concluded that the MR of body parts was a cognitive task in which individuals simulate moving a specific body part image from its actual posture to that of the same observed or imagined body part [45].

Other previous studies investigating brain science strengthen the evidence that the MR of a body part promotes motor imagery involving the MR stimuli. Many previous reports demonstrated that execution-related motor areas were activated during the MR of body parts (typically the hand). More specifically, brain activation in premotor area and parietal cortex was shown during the MR of body parts. Kawamichi et al. examined the time course of brain activation during the MR of body part (hand) stimuli. This article reported that neuronal activity in the visual cortex was observed approximately 100–200 ms from stimulus onset. Brain activation in the inferior parietal lobe followed (after 200 ms). Notably, brain activation in the inferior parietal lobe showed contralateral dominance in the visual stimulus hemifield. Then premotor area activity started the inferior parietal lobe activity [46]. Moreover, to clarify the importance of the motor area's contribution to the MR of body parts, Ganis et al. examined whether MR performance (reaction time) was hindered when single-pulse TMS was delivered to the representation of the hand in the left primary motor cortex during the MR of pictures of hands and feet [47]. The results showed that the response times for the judgment (MR performance) were slower when TMS was delivered, as compared with a peripheral magnetic stimulation (control stimulation). It was striking that the interference was obtained delivered at 650 ms after hand-picture stimulus onset, and the effects were greater for hand stimuli in comparison with the foot-picture stimulus. These findings indicated that the primary motor cortex is involved in the MR of body parts. In particular, the involvement of the primary motor cortex is (a) relatively late in the processing of MR and (b) stimulus specificity like a physical representation of the human body, located within the brain (the cortical homunculus). This physiological study directly revealed that the cortico-spinal tract (central nervous system in the primary motor cortex to the spinal cord) plays an essential role in performing MR.

Brain activity during MR has been investigated in many previous studies. Zacks investigated brain activity in a meta-analysis of neuroimaging study during MR. This reports showed brain activity in the superior parietal cortex, the motor region in the precentral cortex, and the lateral inferior prefrontal cortex when subjects were performing the MR of body parts [48]. These results support the view that MR depends on motor simulation of the body part stimulation in some situations. Enhanced cortico-spinal excitability during the MR of hand stimuli indicates that the excitement of the motor area is involved in performing the MR of body parts [47]. However, since some studies show no brain activity in the primary motor area, its involvement remains unclear, that is, it is necessary to determine the involvement of primary motor area during the MR of body parts.

### 3.2. Intervention of mental rotation

Including the author's previous works, it is indicated that the intervention of the MR of body part stimuli would promote improvement of physical function. Kawasaki et al. showed that the reaction time for the MR of foot stimuli (see **Figure 3**) was related to the postural displacement of one foot while standing (the length of body sway), but there was no relationship between that and the reaction time for the MR of hand and car stimuli [49]. Jansen showed similar results in elderly people [50]. These results suggested the availability of an MR task using foot stimuli for the improvement of challenging postural stability, such as one-foot standing, through motor imagery of feet of individuals themselves.

Based on previous research investigating neuroscientific mechanisms during the MR of body parts, the availability of MR using foot stimuli has immediate beneficial effects on postural stability during a challenging posture, such as standing on one foot, but not during bipedal standing. Notably, when the subject performed MR using hand stimuli, these beneficial effects were not obtained. After the report, the beneficial effects of the MR of foot stimuli on the postural stability while standing on one foot for a relatively long time (60 min <) were demonstrated. The long-term effects would be helpful for a discussion about the mechanism of the effects of MR intervention. As stated above, Ganis determined the involvement of cortico-spinal excitability performing the MR of body parts [47]. According to previous reports, the duration of the enhanced cortico-spinal excitability is for a maximum of 30 min after finger movement [51, 52]. Therefore, the long-term beneficial effects for a long time were not completely explained. A possible explanation is motor consolidation, as previous studies have shown that motor memory was

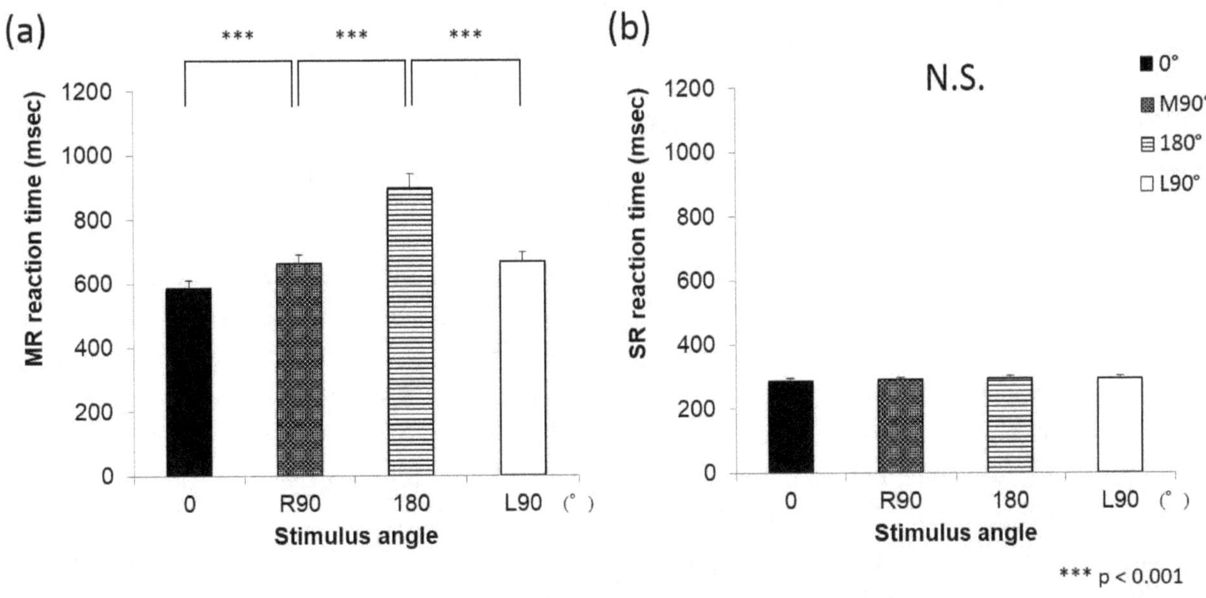


**Figure 3.** Time required for (a) MR task using foot stimuli and (b) simple reaction for the foot stimuli. The reaction times for MR task using foot stimuli were delayed with rotation angle, but not simple reaction time.

consolidated for more than 24 h after repetitive motor imagery intervention [53]. Considering the findings, the beneficial effects of the MR of foot stimuli on postural stability are ascribed to factors such as the enhancement of cortico-spinal excitability and memory consolidation.

## 4. Action observation therapy

Action observation therapy refers to learning through observing the behavior of another person as a model; this can be used in clinical settings to encourage motor performance without any physical activity. Action observation therapy involves bottom-up processing based on visual information, which is different from motor imagery training (top-down using a conscious cognitive process) [54]. Several previous studies have reported that observational learning is effective for younger participants [55, 56], and it has also been shown to improve motor performance in patients hospitalized due to stroke with upper or lower extremity hemiplegia [57–59] and in patients with Parkinson's disease [60, 61]. Thus, observational learning has been used for many kinds of patients in clinical settings.

The effect of observing the behavior of another person upon overt motor performance is most commonly attributed to the demonstration of brain activity in the ventral premotor areas, sulcus temporalis superior, and inferior parietal lobe (i.e., mirror neuron system) during action observation [62, 63]. Historically, electrical activity in the rostral part of the inferior area 6 (area F5) of two macaque monkeys was shown both when the monkeys performed a given action and when they observed a similar action performed by the experimenter [64]. Particularly, the F5 area acutely responses to both the observation and execution of actions in terms of the goal (e.g., grasping) and how the goal is achieved (e.g., a precision grip). Human data also revealed that these areas are involved in imitating the actions of others [65–67] and understanding the intention of others' actions [63, 68]. When the beneficial effects of action observation are gained, high activation in the observer's mirror neuron system would be expected to create first-person perspective (1PP) imagery [57, 76], that is, the mental process of the movement without any body movement [69–71]. Ertelt et al. reported that after the action observation therapy, brain activation in the mirror neuron system was increased [57], meaning that such activation is strongly related to the effects of action observation therapy.

Basically, action observation therapy has beneficial effects on motor performance through the activation of the central nervous system (CNS), which is involved in movement by first-person perspective imagery. Actually, there is some condition for more effective activation of the CNS when applying action observation therapy. Based on a previous study by Gallese investigating the mirror neuron in monkeys, one condition is the observation of a goal-oriented action. Fadiga et al. demonstrated that increasing MEP was shown when subjects observed the grasping of objects (observing movement of finger) compared with when they observed (a) the objects, (b) arm movement of the grasping objects, (c) and sham [72]. Muthukumaraswamy et al. examined whether mu rhythm modulates during observation of grasping to an object-directed [73]. The electroencephalographic mu rhythm is an 8–13-Hz rhythm generated by the sensorimotor cortex that is most prominent when subjects are resting and are attenuated or abolished when subjects move or observe biological movements [74, 75]; therefore, the hypothesis of the examination was to attenuate or abolish an 8–13-Hz rhythm during these action observations. Consistent with the hypothesis, the result showed a lower mu rhythm magnitude for the object-grip condition than for the empty-grip condition. This result is fully reasonably taken together with the studies by Fadiga and Muthukumaraswamy, which suggested that the observation of movement with intention, such as tool manipulation or daily activities, can lead to brain modulation, and as a result, these observations would be expected to be more effective for motor learning.

Another way of the effective condition was that patients imagine body movement while they observed model's action (i.e., combined action observation and motor imagery). Vogt suggested that action observation with motor imagery is more effective for motor performance than action observation therapy or motor imagery training alone [76]. Tsukazaki et al. demonstrated that the MEP amplitude was significantly increased by observing a video clip of three-ball cascade juggling combined with motor imagery of it for novel motor learning [77]. This suggested the effectiveness of action observation combined with motor imagery. By contrast, they reported that for expert subjects increased the MEP amplitude when motor imagery only (without observation). This suggested that motor imagery alone is more effective than action observation therapy combined with motor imagery for novel motor learning. As evidence of the effectiveness of action observation plus motor imagery, in neuroscience data, Taube et al. have shown that greater activation in the mirror neuron system was obtained when subjects observed the movement of others during which time subjects imagined their own body movement in terms of the model's movement [78].

In addition, previous work has been focused on observing the model's skill. According to the studies mentioned above, although the beneficial effects of action observation therapy are robust, opinions vary as to the optimal model for observers (learners). For a typical example, previous studies have shown that motor learning was promoted both with a skilled model demonstrating movement quickly without error [56, 79, 80] and with an unskilled model demonstrating slowly with error [81–83]. Taken together, the effective model's skill has not been inconsistent among the previous studies, meaning that there is no evidence for promoting a model in terms of skill for a long time. Kawasaki et al. have begun to demonstrate effective learning with action observation therapy. To date, they have conducted two investigations in young people. The results of the study were that the unskilled model demonstrating movement slowly with error was more effective than a skilled model demonstrating quickly without error [84]. Considering the clinical applications of action observation therapy, it is important to verify a model to promote for elderly persons for whom clinicians have many opportunities to care in clinical settings, because previous studies did not examine clinical settings. The ability to imagine their own body movements [35, 85] and to imitate movements after observation declines in elderly people [86]. Visual information processing of dynamic movement also declines with aging [87, 88]. Based on the previous study showing changes in body function with aging, Kawasaki and colleague investigated whether the unskilled model was effective for motor learning as the author's previous research in young people. Consistent with the hypothesis, the unskilled model showing quickness with some error has the advantage to acquire new motor skills (under review). Moreover, almost all of the subjects gained acquiring higher motor skills in subjects observed unskilled model than in subjects observed skilled model regardless of individuals' motor imagery ability; in other words, unskilled model provides observer (patients or learners) with positive effects on the motor learning with or without impairment of motor imagery ability. This suggested that motor imagery ability is not necessary when the clinicians use action observation therapy and unskilled models are readily available. In this research, positive information can be provided to apply action observation to elderly people in clinical settings.

Recently, the beneficial effects of action observation therapy have been established and applied in clinical settings. However, note that the effects of action observation therapy may be influenced by an individual's motor imagery ability. Lawrence et al. showed the effectiveness of gymnastic movement performance after observation of the movement. Additionally, the improved gymnastic movement performance in subjects having high motor imagery ability was greater than in subjects having low motor imagery ability, suggesting that the effects of action observation on motor performance are moderated by imagery ability [89]. Considering that the effects of action observation are based on imagining the individual's body movement, using the PETTPEP model would provide an advantage and lead to beneficial effects when using action observation therapy.

## 5. Verbalizing motor skills

To address the difficulty of motor imagery training mentioned above, verbalizing motor skills is also an effective tool for improving motor performance. Verbalizing motor skills promote to imagine own body movement because the process of verbalizing one's own motor skills would be induced by internal language [90, 91] through recalling one's own motor skills and, as a result, promoting motor imagery. The left frontal lobe is activated not only during the recalling of one's own body movement [92] but also when inducing internal language [93]. Additionally, the left frontal lobe is involved in motor programming [94]. This means that the neural circuit of verbalizing motor skill and its motor execution was shared, therefore, it is with regard to strangeness closeness relationship between verbalizing motor skill and its motor execution [95–97]. In fact, using verbal expression motor behavior leads to improved motor control and accuracy of hand grasp [98]. Considering these previous studies, we hypothesized that verbalizing of own body skills involves a process of promoting motor imagery through recalling own motor performance, as a result, the verbalizing motor skills might improve motor learning.

Based on previous knowledge, we hypothesized that the effects of verbalizing motor skills provide the subject with improved motor performance. One examination was conducted to investigate the effect of verbalizing motor skills after practicing a ball-rotation task compared with scientific read aloud (i.e., no verbalizing). The results showed the beneficial effects of verbalizing motor skills on acquiring the motor skill of finger coordination (under review, **Figure 4**). This showed that verbalizing would be effective for acquiring and improving motor skills. The author considered that verbalizing motor skills provide subjects' motor skills with beneficial effects through motor imagery. Further study is needed to analyze contents of subjects' verbalizing (qualitative research) as well as quantitative research, such as present data.

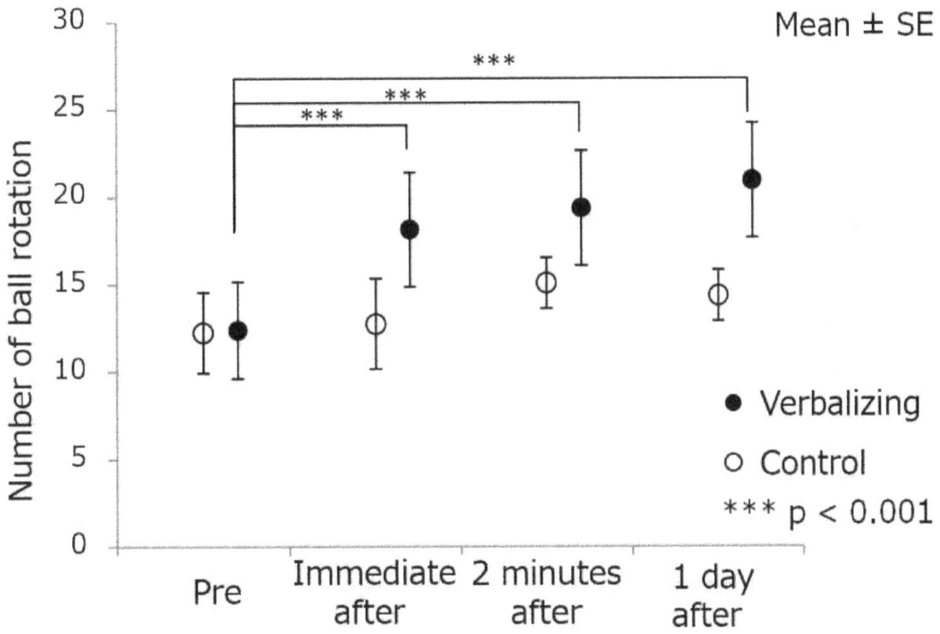


**Figure 4.** The changes in the number of ball rotation in all sessions. Results showed improvement of motor skills only after verbalizing.

## 6. Summary

There are some interventions and ideas to compensate for the shortcoming of traditional motor imagery training. This chapter studied that investigating methods of applied motor imagery training is important to develop clinical rehabilitation settings because the suggesting interventions and ideas are commonly based on motor imagery. Therefore, it is necessary to more deeply investigate motor imagery (e.g., the most effective procedure and method for individual disease characteristics), expecting that this will lead to future development of motor imagery training.

## Acknowledgements

Part of this work was supported by JSPS KAKENHI Grant Number 15K16402.

## Author details

Tsubasa Kawasaki

Address all correspondence to: kawasaki.283@gmail.com

Department of Physical Therapy, Faculty of Health Science, Ryotokuji University, Urayasu, Chiba, Japan

## References

[1] Jeannerod M. Mental imagery in the motor context. Neuropsychologia. 1995;33(11): 1419–1432.

[2] Decety J. Do imagined and executed actions share the same neural substrate? Brain Research Cognitive Brain Research. 1996;3(2):87–93.

[3] Rice HJ, Rubin DC. I can see it both ways: First-and third-person visual perspectives at retrieval. Consciousness and Cognition. 2009;18(4):877–890.

[4] Ruby P, Decety J. Effect of subjective perspective taking during simulation of action: a PET investigation of agency. Nature Neuroscience. 2001;4(5):546–550.

[5] Dechent P, Merboldt K-D, Frahm J. Is the human primary motor cortex involved in motor imagery? Cognitive Brain Research. 2004;19(2):138–144.

[6] Mizuguchi N, Nakata H, Hayashi T, Sakamoto M, Muraoka T, Uchida Y, et al. Brain activity during motor imagery of an action with an object: a functional magnetic resonance imaging study. Neuroscience Research. 2013;76(3):150–155.

[7] Lorey B, Pilgramm S, Walter B, Stark R, Munzert J, Zentgraf K. Your mind's hand: motor imagery of pointing movements with different accuracy. Neuroimage. 2010;49(4):3239–3247.

[8] Kasai T, Kawai S, Kawanishi M, Yahagi S. Evidence for facilitation of motor evoked potentials (MEPs) induced by motor imagery. Brain Research. 1997;744(1):147–150.

[9] Fadiga L, Buccino G, Craighero L, Fogassi L, Gallese V, Pavesi G. Corticospinal excitability is specifically modulated by motor imagery: a magnetic stimulation study. Neuropsychologia. 1998;37(2):147–158.

[10] Hamel MF, Lajoie Y. Mental imagery. Effects on static balance and attentional demands of the elderly. Aging Clinical and Experimental Research. 2005;17(3):223–228.

[11] Yasuda K, Kawasaki T, Higuchi T. Intervention of self-monitoring body movement has an immediate beneficial effect to maintain postural stability. Journal of Novel Physiotherapies. 2012;2(118).

[12] Cho H-y, Kim J-s, Lee G-C. Effects of motor imagery training on balance and gait abilities in post-stroke patients: a randomized controlled trial. Clinical Rehabilitation. 2013;27(8):675–680.

[13] Page SJ, Levine P, Sisto S, Johnston MV. A randomized efficacy and feasibility study of imagery in acute stroke. Clinical Rehabilitation. 2001;15(3):233–240.

[14] Page SJ. Imagery improves upper extremity motor function in chronic stroke patients: a pilot study. OTJR: Occupation, Participation and Health. 2000;20(3):200–215.

[15] Page SJ, Levine P, Leonard A. Mental practice in chronic stroke results of a randomized, placebo-controlled trial. Stroke. 2007;38(4):1293–1297.

[16] Page SJ, Levine P, Leonard AC. Effects of mental practice on affected limb use and function in chronic stroke. Archives of Physical Medicine and Rehabilitation. 2005;86(3):399–402.

[17] Langhorne P, Coupar F, Pollock A. Motor recovery after stroke: a systematic review. The Lancet Neurology. 2009;8(8):741–754.

[18] Page SJ, Sisto S, Johnston MV, Levine P. Modified constraint-induced therapy after subacute stroke: a preliminary study. Neurorehabilitation and Neural Repair. 2002;16(3):290–295.

[19] Page SJ, Sisto S, Levine P, McGrath RE. Efficacy of modified constraint-induced movement therapy in chronic stroke: a single-blinded randomized controlled trial. Archives of Physical Medicine and Rehabilitation. 2004;85(1):14–18.

[20] Page SJ, Levine P, Leonard AC. Modified constraint-induced therapy in acute stroke: a randomized controlled pilot study. Neurorehabilitation and Neural Repair. 2005;19(1):27–32.

[21] Page SJ, Levine P, Leonard A, Szaflarski JP, Kissela BM. Modified constraint-induced therapy in chronic stroke: results of a single-blinded randomized controlled trial. Physical Therapy. 2008;88(3):333–340.

[22] Amirabdollahian F, Loureiro R, Gradwell E, Collin C, Harwin W, Johnson G. Multivariate analysis of the Fugl-Meyer outcome measures assessing the effectiveness of GENTLE/S robot-mediated stroke therapy. Journal of NeuroEngineering and Rehabilitation. 2007;4(1):1–16.

[23] Volpe BT, Lynch D, Rykman-Berland A, Ferraro M, Galgano M, Hogan N, et al. Intensive sensorimotor arm training mediated by therapist or robot improves hemiparesis in patients with chronic stroke. Neurorehabilitation and Neural Repair. 2008;22(3):305–310.

[24] Cauraugh J, Light K, Kim S, Thigpen M, Behrman A. Chronic motor dysfunction after stroke recovering wrist and finger extension by electromyography-triggered neuromuscular stimulation. Stroke. 2000;31(6):1360–1364.

[25] Sharma N, Cohen LG. Recovery of motor function after stroke. Developmental Psychobiology. 2012;54(3):254–262.

[26] Holmes PS, Collins DJ. The PETTLEP approach to motor imagery: A functional equivalence model for sport psychologists. Journal of Applied Sport Psychology. 2001;13(1):60–83.

[27] Malouin F, Richards CL, Durand A, Doyon J. Reliability of mental chronometry for assessing motor imagery ability after stroke. Archives of Physical Medicine and Rehabilitation. 2008;89(2):311–319.

[28] Pascual-Leone A, Nguyet D, Cohen LG, Brasil-Neto JP, Cammarota A, Hallett M. Modulation of muscle responses evoked by transcranial magnetic stimulation during the acquisition of new fine motor skills. Journal of Neurophysiology. 1995;74(3):1037–1045.

[29] Wright DJ, Holmes P, Di Russo F, Loporto M, Smith D. Reduced motor cortex activity during movement preparation following a period of motor skill practice. PloS One. 2012;7(12):e51886.

[30] Hardy L, Callow N. Efficacy of external and internal visual imagery. Journal of Sport & Exercise Psychology. 1999;21:95–112.

[31] White A, Hardy L. Use of different imagery perspectives on the learning and performance of different motor skills. British Journal of Psychology. 1995;86(2):169–180.

[32] Gregg M, Hall C, Butler A. The MIQ-RS: a suitable option for examining movement imagery ability. Evidence-Based Complementary and Alternative Medicine. 2010;7(2):249–257.

[33] Butler AJ, Cazeaux J, Fidler A, Jansen J, Lefkove N, Gregg M, et al. The movement imagery questionnaire-revised, (MIQ-RS) is a reliable and valid tool for evaluating motor imagery in stroke populations. Evidence-Based Complementary and Alternative Medicine. 2012;2012:Article ID 497289.

[34] Malouin F, Richards CL, Jackson PL, Lafleur MF, Durand A, Doyon J. The Kinesthetic and Visual Imagery Questionnaire (KVIQ) for assessing motor imagery in persons with physical disabilities: a reliability and construct validity study. Journal of Neurologic Physical Therapy. 2007;31(1):20–29.

[35] Personnier P, Kubicki A, Laroche D, Papaxanthis C. Temporal features of imagined locomotion in normal aging. Neuroscience Letters. 2010;476(3):146–149.

[36] Li C-sR. Impairment of motor imagery in putamen lesions in humans. Neuroscience Letters. 2000;287(1):13–16.

[37] Decety J, Boisson D. Effect of brain and spinal cord injuries on motor imagery. European Archives of Psychiatry and Clinical Neuroscience. 1990;240(1):39–43.

[38] Ietswaart M, Johnston M, Dijkerman HC, Joice S, Scott CL, MacWalter RS, et al. Mental practice with motor imagery in stroke recovery: randomized controlled trial of efficacy. Brain. 2011;134(5):1373–1386.

[39] Timmermans AA, Verbunt JA, van Woerden R, Moennekens M, Pernot DH, Seelen HA. Effect of mental practice on the improvement of function and daily activity performance of the upper extremity in patients with subacute stroke: a randomized clinical trial. Journal of the American Medical Directors Association. 2013;14(3):204–212.

[40] Kraeutner SN, Keeler LT, Boe SG. Motor imagery-based skill acquisition disrupted following rTMS of the inferior parietal lobule. Experimental Brain Research. 2015 ;234(2): 397–407.

[41] Mihara M, Miyai I, Hattori N, Hatakenaka M, Yagura H, Kawano T, et al. Neurofeedback using real-time near-infrared spectroscopy enhances motor imagery related cortical activation. PloS One. 2012;7(3):e32234.

[42] Shepard R, Metzler J. Mental rotation of three-dimensional objects. Science. 1971;171 (3972):701–703.

[43] Parsons LM. Temporal and kinematic properties of motor behavior reflected in mentally simulated action. Journal of Experimental Psychology: Human Perception & Performance. 1994;20(4):709–730.

[44] Fiorio M, Tinazzi M, Ionta S, Fiaschi A, Moretto G, Edwards MJ, et al. Mental rotation of body parts and non-corporeal objects in patients with idiopathic cervical dystonia. Neuropsychologia. 2007;45(10):2346–2354.

[45] Ionta S, Fourkas AD, Fiorio M, Aglioti SM. The influence of hands posture on mental rotation of hands and feet. Experimental Brain Research. 2007;183(1):1–7.

[46] Kawamichi H, Kikuchi Y, Endo H, Takeda T, Yoshizawa S. Temporal structure of implicit motor imagery in visual hand-shape discrimination as revealed by MEG. Neuroreport. 1998;9(6):1127–1132.

[47] Ganis G, Keenan JP, Kosslyn SM, Pascual-Leone A. Transcranial magnetic stimulation of primary motor cortex affects mental rotation. Cerebral Cortex. 2000;10(2):175–180.

[48] Zacks JM. Neuroimaging studies of mental rotation: a meta-analysis and review. Journal of Cognitive Neuroscience. 2008;20(1):1–19.

[49] Kawasaki T, Yasuda K, Fukuhara K, Higuchi T. Relationship between mental rotation of body parts and postural stability during quiet stance. Journal of Imagery Research in Sport and Physical Activity. 2014;9(1):39–46.

[50] Jansen P, Kaltner S. Object-based and egocentric mental rotation performance in older adults: The importance of gender differences and motor ability. Aging, Neuropsychology, and Cognition. 2013;4(ahead-of-print):1–21.

[51] Kawasaki T, Higuchi T. Mental rotation intervention using foot stimuli has lasting effect on postural stability during quiet stance: a randomized controlled study. Journal of Motor Behavior. 2016;48(357–364):357–364.

[52] Classen J, Liepert J, Wise SP, Hallett M, Cohen LG. Rapid plasticity of human cortical movement representation induced by practice. Journal of Neurophysiology. 1998;79(2):1117–1123.

[53] Gentili R, Han CE, Schweighofer N, Papaxanthis C. Motor learning without doing: trial-by-trial improvement in motor performance during mental training. Journal of Neurophysiology. 2010;104(2):774–783.

[54] Holmes P, Calmels C. A neuroscientific review of imagery and observation use in sport. Journal of Motor Behavior. 2008;40(5):433–445.

[55] Aglioti SM, Cesari P, Romani M, Urgesi C. Action anticipation and motor resonance in elite basketball players. Nature Neuroscience. 2008;11(9):1109–1116.

[56] Heyes C, Foster C. Motor learning by observation: Evidence from a serial reaction time task. The Quarterly Journal of Experimental Psychology: Section A. 2002;55(2):593–607.

[57] Ertelt D, Small S, Solodkin A, Dettmers C, McNamara A, Binkofski F, et al. Action observation has a positive impact on rehabilitation of motor deficits after stroke. Neuroimage. 2007;36(Suppl 2):T164–T173.

[58] Franceschini M, Ceravolo MG, Agosti M, Cavallini P, Bonassi S, Dall'Armi V, et al. Clinical relevance of action observation in upper-limb stroke rehabilitation a possible role in recovery of functional dexterity. A randomized clinical trial. Neurorehabilitation and Neural Repair. 2012;26(5):456–462.

[59] Hwang S, Jeon H-S, Yi C-h, Kwon O-y, Cho S-h, You S-h. Locomotor imagery training improves gait performance in people with chronic hemiparetic stroke: a controlled clinical trial. Clinical Rehabilitation. 2010;24(6):514–522.

[60] Pelosin E, Avanzino L, Bove M, Stramesi P, Nieuwboer A, Abbruzzese G. Action observation improves freezing of gait in patients with Parkinson's disease. Neurorehabilitation and Neural Repair. 2010;24(8):746–752.

[61] Pelosin E, Bove M, Ruggeri P, Avanzino L, Abbruzzese G. Reduction of bradykinesia of finger movements by a single session of action observation in Parkinson disease. Neurorehabilitation and Neural Repair. 2013;27(6):552–560.

[62] Rizzolatti G, Craighero L. The mirror-neuron system. Annual Review of Neuroscience. 2004;27:169–192.

[63] Iacoboni M. Neural mechanisms of imitation. Current Opinion in Neurobiology. 2005;15(6):632–637.

[64] Gallese V, Fadiga L, Fogassi L, Rizzolatti G. Action recognition in the premotor cortex. Brain. 1996;119(2):593–609.

[65] Watanabe R, Higuchi T, Kikuchi Y. Imitation behavior is sensitive to visual perspective of the model: an fMRI study. Experimental Brain Research. 2013;228(2):161–171.

[66] Koski L, Iacoboni M, Dubeau M-C, Woods RP, Mazziotta JC. Modulation of cortical activity during different imitative behaviors. Journal of Neurophysiology. 2003;89(1):460–471.

[67] Jackson PL, Meltzoff AN, Decety J. Neural circuits involved in imitation and perspective-taking. Neuroimage. 2006;31(1):429–439.

[68] Iacoboni M, Molnar-Szakacs I, Gallese V, Buccino G, Mazziotta JC, Rizzolatti G. Grasping the intentions of others with one's own mirror neuron system. PLoS Biology. 2005;3(3):e79.

[69] Malouin F, Richards CL. Mental practice for relearning locomotor skills. Physical Therapy. 2010;90(2):240–251.

[70] Parsons LM. Integrating cognitive psychology, neurology and neuroimaging. Acta Psychologica (Amst). 2001;107(1–3):155–181.

[71] Jeannerod M. The representing brain: Neural correlates of motor intention and imagery. Behavioral and Brain Sciences. 1994;17(2):187–245.

[72] Fadiga L, Fogassi L, Pavesi G, Rizzolatti G. Motor facilitation during action observation: a magnetic stimulation study. Journal of Neurophysiology. 1995;73(6):2608–2611.

[73] Muthukumaraswamy SD, Johnson BW, McNair NA. Mu rhythm modulation during observation of an object-directed grasp. Cognitive Brain Research. 2004;19(2):195–201.

[74] Babiloni C, Carducci F, Cincotti F, Rossini PM, Neuper C, Pfurtscheller G, et al. Human movement-related potentials vs desynchronization of EEG alpha rhythm: a high-resolution EEG study. Neuroimage. 1999;10(6):658–665.

[75] Pineda JA, Allison B, Vankov A. The effects of self-movement, observation, and imagination on μ rhythms and readiness potentials (RP's): toward a brain-computer interface (BCI). IEEE Transactions on Rehabilitation Engineering. 2000;8(2):219–222.

[76] Vogt S, Rienzo FD, Collet C, Collins A, Guillot A. Multiple roles of motor imagery during action observation. Frontiers in Human Neuroscience. 2013;7:807.

[77] Tsukazaki I, Uehara K, Morishita T, Ninomiya M, Funase K. Effect of observation combined with motor imagery of a skilled hand-motor task on motor cortical excitability: difference between novice and expert. Neuroscience Letters. 2012;518(2):96–100.

[78] Taube W, Mouthon M, Leukel C, Hoogewoud HM, Annoni JM, Keller M. Brain activity during observation and motor imagery of different balance tasks: An fMRI study. Cortex. 2014;64c:102–114.

[79] Bird G, Heyes C. Effector-dependent learning by observation of a finger movement sequence. Journal of Experimental Psychology: Human Perception and Performance. 2005;31(2):262.

[80] Hodges NJ, Chua R, Franks IM. The role of video in facilitating perception and action of a novel coordination movement. Journal of Motor Behavior. 2003;35(3):247–260.

[81] Buchanan JJ, Ryu YU, Zihlman K, Wright DL. Observational practice of relative but not absolute motion features in a single-limb multi-joint coordination task. Experimental Brain Research. 2008;191(2):157–169.

[82] Buchanan JJ, Dean NJ. Specificity in practice benefits learning in novice models and variability in demonstration benefits observational practice. Psychological Research PRPF. 2010;74(3):313–326.

[83] Black CB, Wright DL. Can observational practice facilitate error recognition and movement production? Research Quarterly for Exercise and Sport. 2000;71(4):331–339.

[84] Kawasaki T, Aramaki H, Tozawa R. An Effective Model for Observational Learning to Improve Novel Motor Performance. Journal of Physical Therapy Science. 2015; 27(12):3829–3832.

[85] Mulder T, Hochstenbach JB, van Heuvelen MJ, den Otter AR. Motor imagery: the relation between age and imagery capacity. Human Movement Science. 2007;26(2):203–211.

[86] Maryott J, Sekuler R. Age-related changes in imitating sequences of observed movements. Psychology and Aging. 2009;24(2):476.

[87] Muiños M, Ballesteros S. Sports can protect dynamic visual acuity from aging: A study with young and older judo and karate martial arts athletes. Attention, Perception, & Psychophysics. 2015;77(6):2061–2073.

[88] Ishigaki H, Miyao M. Implications for dynamic visual acuity with changes in age and sex. Perceptual and Motor Skills. 1994;78(2):363–369.

[89] Lawrence G, Callow N, Roberts R. Watch me if you can: imagery ability moderates observational learning effectiveness. Frontiers in Human Neuroscience. 2013;7:522.

[90] Suwa M. Meta-cognition as a tool for storytelling and questioning what design is. Bulletin of Japan Society for the Science of Design. 2009;16(2):21–26.

[91] Suwa M. A cognitive model of acquiring embodied expertise through meta-cognitive verbalization. Transactions of the Japanese Society for Artificial Intelligence 2008;23(3):141–150.

[92] Morin A, Hamper B. Self-reflection and the inner voice: activation of the left inferior frontal gyrus during perceptual and conceptual self-referential thinking. The Open Neuroimaging Journal. 2012;6:78–79.

[93] Duffau H, Capelle L, Denvil D, Gatignol P, Sichez N, Lopes M, et al. The role of dominant premotor cortex in language: a study using intraoperative functional mapping in awake patients. Neuroimage. 2003;20(4):1903–1914.

[94] Rizzolatti G, Camarda R, Fogassi L, Gentilucci M, Luppino G, Matelli M. Functional organization of inferior area 6 in the macaque monkey. Experimental Brain Research. 1988;71(3):491–507.

[95] Pulvermüller F, Hauk O, Nikulin VV, Ilmoniemi RJ. Functional links between motor and language systems. European Journal of Neuroscience. 2005;21(3):793–797.

[96] Pulvermüller F, Fadiga L. Active perception: sensorimotor circuits as a cortical basis for language. Nature Reviews Neuroscience. 2010;11(5):351–360.

[97] Pulvermüller F. Brain mechanisms linking language and action. Nature Reviews Neuroscience. 2005;6(7):576–582.

[98] Fargier R, Ménoret M, Boulenger V, Nazir TA, Paulignan Y. Grasp it loudly! Supporting actions with semantically congruent spoken action words. PLoS One. 2012;7(1):e30663.

# 8

# Application of Robotics for Therapeutic Exercise of Neural Disorder

Yasuhiko Hatanaka, Kazuki Yamaguchi,
Koichi Saito and Satomi Tada

**Abstract**

**Background:** The application of robots for rehabilitation has been developing over the past decade. In neuro-rehabilitation, motor learning has become an important topic. To maximize the effect of motor learning, we need to clarify the key muscle and adequate intensity.

**Objective:** Examination of a new method of robotic rehabilitation that employs a motion capture system and ground reaction force platforms to calculate kinematic and kinetic parameters.

**Design:** A cross-sectional study of healthy subjects and individual cerebral palsy and stroke patients as case studies.

**Methods:** We employed a motion capture system and ground reaction force platforms to calculate kinematic and kinetic parameters of healthy volunteers, a cerebral palsy patient, and a stroke patient in both gait and active movement assessments. This method allows the comparison of motor performances before and after exercise. A hybrid assistive limb (HAL) was employed for the exercise. HAL is a humanoid exoskeletal robot that uses bioelectrical signals as triggers.

**Results:** Immediate and after effects on gait velocity, step length, and hip extensional moments were observed in healthy subjects and the stroke patient. The cerebral palsy patient showed improvement in range of movement in a practised movement.

**Keywords:** robotics, neuro-rehabilitation, motor learning, stroke, cerebral palsy

## 1. Introduction

The application of robotics and mechatronics for medical rehabilitation has been developed over the past decade. In particular, the power assistive apparatus may affect neuro-rehabilitation based on the brain cell plasticity. In 1992, prior to the beginning of the applications of the robotic, Wernig advocated the weight support treadmill (WST) for gait exercise in paraplegic patients [1]. He reported that some patients showed recovery of EMG of the lower extremities, or actual gait function remarkably after 5–20 months. For the WST, two physical therapists are required to guide the movement of the lower extremities manually. In 1999, Hocoma Corporation (Volketswil, Switzerland) developed Lokomat, which is a WST that does not require physical therapists assistance [2]. In the last 15 years, 600 Lokomats have been used in the world. There are two uses of robots in medical rehabilitation. One is the use as a supportive device in daily living such as orthoses. The other is the use in therapeutic exercise. For functional recovery of the patients with neural disorder, motor learning is necessary. For appropriate motor learning, appropriate repetitions and appropriate difficulty of the task are necessary. For the appropriate difficulty of the task, feedback is the key. However, we have no good tool that can control the feedback gain easily. We suggest that hybrid assistive limb (HAL): Cyberdyne Inc., Japan) may be a solution HAL, which is controlled by surface EMG of flexor and extensor of the hip and knee. However, the effects of therapeutic exercise using HAL for patients with neural disorder are unclear. In this study, we clarify the effects of therapeutic exercise using HAL.

## 2. Method

### 2.1. Hybrid assistive limb

HAL was employed for the therapeutic exercise [3]. HAL is a powered exoskeleton bionic device that is controlled by surface EMG of the hip flexor, hip extensor, knee flexor, and knee extensor muscle of the subject. HAL consists of a CPU, interface units, surface EMG, plantar pressure sensors, four motor units, a lithium polymer battery, and exoskeletal of lower body (**Figure 1**).

### 2.2. Motor learning and its effect on development of gait function

We focused on the activation of the gluteus maximus muscle. Subjects demonstrated good feedback from surface EMG. The tasks were squatting and walking. The numbers of the exercises were 500 repetitions and 500 steps (**Figure 2**).

We had conducted the exercise programs once a week for three times for patients (2.3.2, 1.3.3). Furthermore, we conducted the exercise programs once a week for three times for healthy subjects to investigate the after-effect (1.3.1).

### 2.3. Assessments of gait and motor performance

Before and after exercise, gait or throwing motion was captured. Infrared reflectors attached on the bilateral acromion, lateral epicondyle of humerus, styloid process of the radius, the

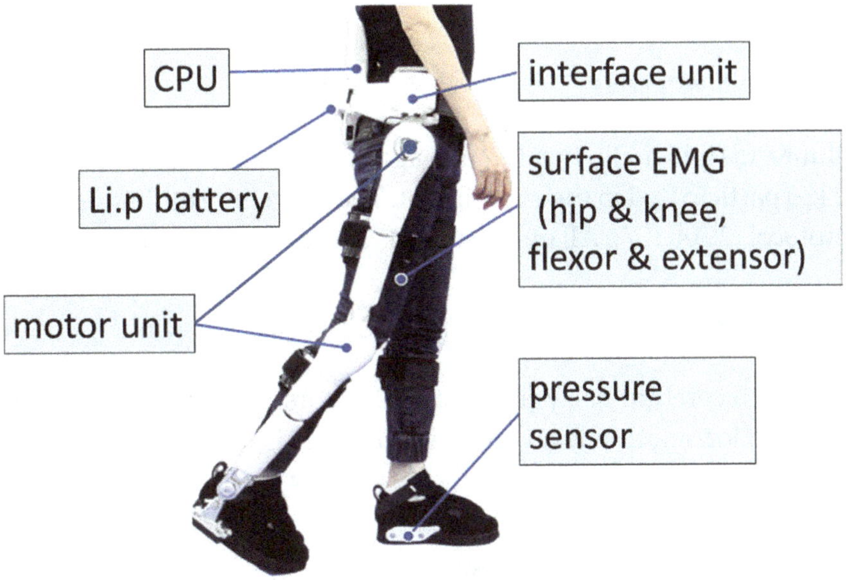


**Figure 1.** The structure of HAL.

head of the third metacarpal bone, greater trochanter, lateral edge of the femoral bone, lateral malleolus, and the head of the fifth metatarsal bone. A three-dimensional motion capture system (VICON 612: Vicon Motion Systems Ltd., UK) was employed to measure the spatial coordinates of the body joints, which were substituted into the numerical model with human dynamic constants. Joint angles, angular velocities, linear velocities, trunk inclinational angle, and deviation of the center of gravity were calculated. Simultaneously, five ground reaction force platforms (OR6-6: AMTI Inc., USA) were employed to measure the ground reaction force and the displacement of center of pressure during walking. Inverse dynamics was applied to calculate the joint moment of the hip.

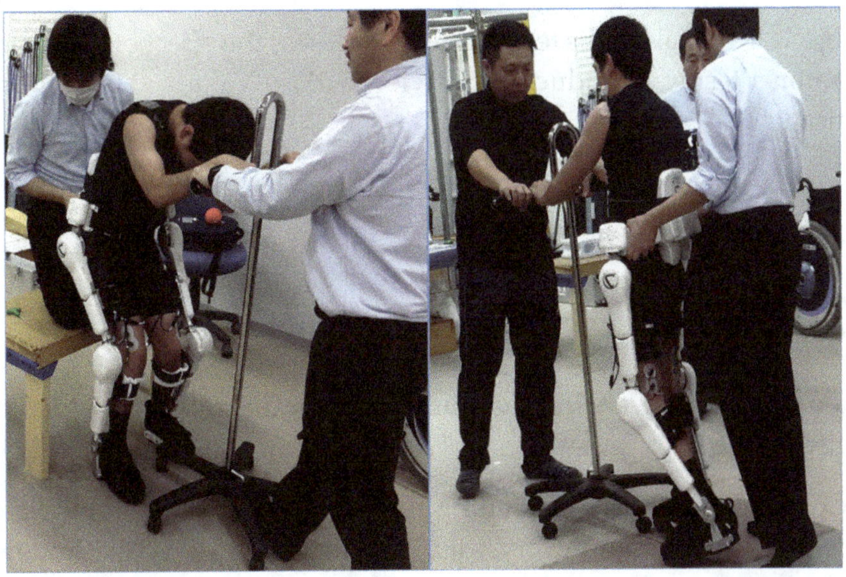

**Figure 2.** The setting of exercise with HAL (left, squatting; right, walking).

### 2.4. Subjects

#### 2.4.1. *Experiment of healthy subjects*

Ten healthy volunteers (five male, five female, age, 20–22 years old, height, 1.61–1.71 m, body weight, 51.2–62 kg) participated in the experiment. The university ethic committee approved the experimental protocol (2014-177). All of the subjects signed the consent form before experiment.

#### 2.4.2. *Experiment of electric wheelchair user with cerebral palsy*

One boccia player with cerebral palsy (male; age, 22 years; height, 1.51 m; body weight, 52 kg; type, spastic diplegia; locomotion level, electric wheelchair; Boccia level, BC2) participated in the study.

#### 2.4.3. *Experiment of wheelchair user with stroke*

One volunteer with stroke (female; age, 67 years old; height, 1.61 m; body weight, 48 kg; type, cerebral infarction; affected side, right, post stroke, 17 years; Brunnstrom recovery stage, upper extremity 2 and lower extremity 3; locomotion level, wheelchair; complications and higher brain dysfunctions, negative) participated in the study. Until the beginning of the exercise program, the stroke volunteer could not hold a standing posture by herself. She could not walk at all without an ankle foot orthosis, a T-cane, and support of a care giver. At initial contact, rapid hip flexion, trunk anterior bending, and posterior withdraw of the pelvis were observed. During the single limb support phase, extensional thrust of the knee was observed. During terminal stance, heel-off was not observed. We accessed her main issue as insufficiency of gluteus maximus activation.

### 2.5. Statistical analysis

For healthy subjects, Kruskal-Wallis test was used to assess the effect of exercise. When appropriate, Tukey-Kramer test was conducted (Statview 5.01). $p$-Values $<0.05$ were considered statistically significant.

## 3. Results

### 3.1. Healthy subjects

Gait velocity and step length were increased immediately after exercise and after 1 h compare to before exercise (**Table 1**).

Maximal hip extensional moment in loading response was greater immediately after exercise compare to before exercise in every trial. Maximal hip extensional moment in loading response after one hour was greater than that before exercise in three subjects. The difference in the hip joint angle in terminal stance before and after exercise was not significant.

| | Day 1 | | | Day 2 | | | Day 3 | | |
|---|---|---|---|---|---|---|---|---|---|
| | **Before** | **After** | **1 h** | **Before** | **After** | **1 h** | **Before** | **After** | **1 h** |
| Step length (m) | 1.16 ± 0.15 | 1.37 ± 0.21* | 1.29 ± 0.18* | 1.17 ± 0.18 | 1.24 ± 0.18* | 1.21 ± 0.1* | 1.16 ± 0.12 | 1.25 ± 0.14* | 1.24 ± 0.1* |
| Velocity (m/s) | 1.20 ± 0.14 | 1.34 ± 0.16* | 1.25 ± 0.14* | 1.16 ± 0.16 | 1.21 ± 0.18* | 1.23 ± 0.09* | 1.18 ± 0.1 | 1.22 ± 0.31* | 1.23 ± 0.11* |
| Hip moment (Nm/kg) | 0.45 ± 0.08 | 0.61 ± 0.14* | 0.57 ± 0.11 | 0.42 ± 0.12 | 0.55 ± 0.15* | 0.52 ± 0.11 | 0.50 ± 0.12 | 0.66 ± 0.1* | 0.61 ± 0.15 |

*$p < 0.05$.

**Table 1.** Comparison of gait parameter before and after exercise.

### 3.2. Electric wheelchair user with cerebral palsy

Boccia ball velocity at release after exercise was greater than that before exercise (**Figure 3**).

The range of motion of the shoulder during throwing after exercise was greater than that before exercise (**Figure 4**).

In contrast, range of motion of the anterior inclination of the trunk during throwing after exercise was less than that before exercise (**Figure 5**).

### 3.3. Wheelchair user with stroke

Gait velocity and step length after exercise were greater than that before exercise (**Figure 6**).

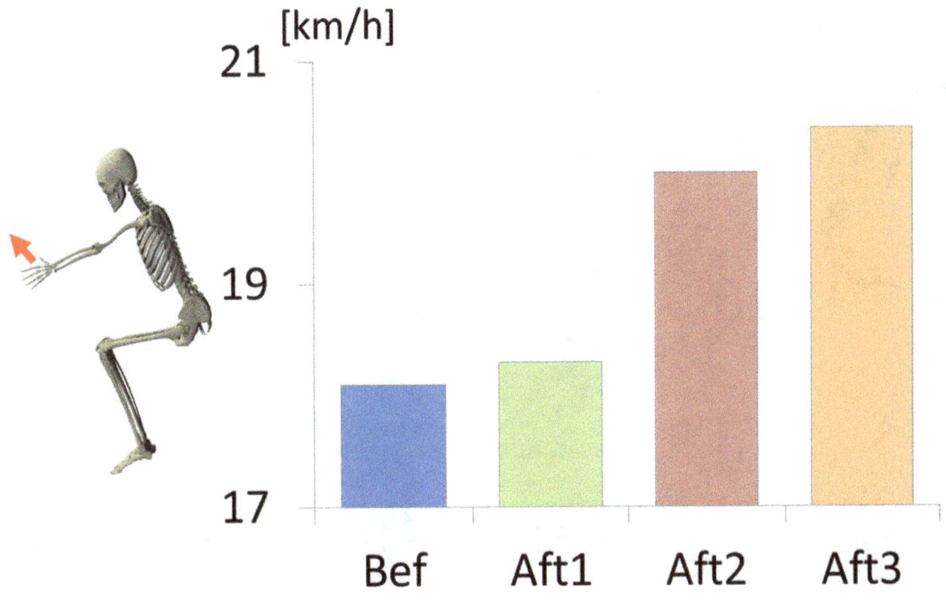


**Figure 3.** Ball velocity at release second before and after exercise. Bef, before exercise; Aft, after exercise.

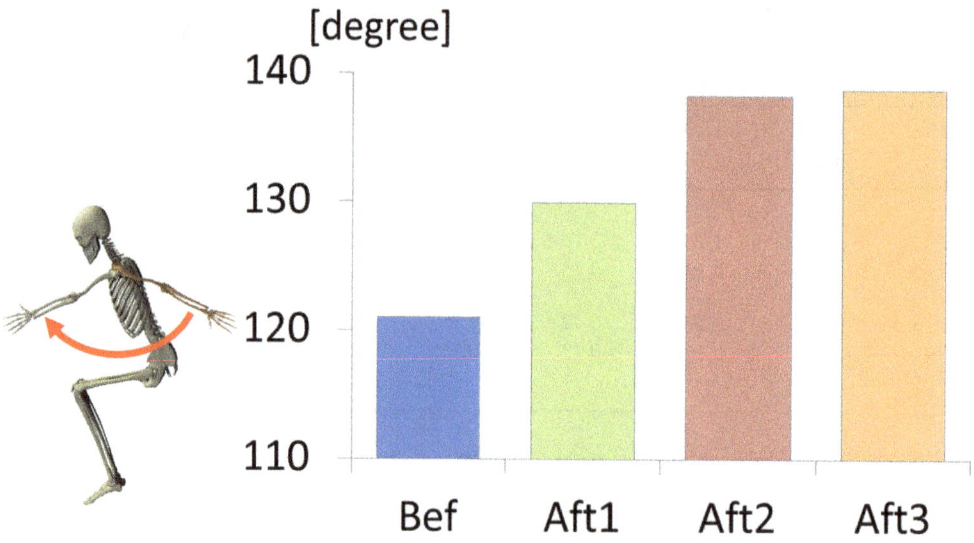


**Figure 4.** The range of motion of the shoulder during throwing before and after exercise. Bef, before exercise; Aft, after exercise.

The hip joint angle and the anterior inclination of the trunk at initial contact after exercise were less than that before exercise (**Figure 7**).

Maximal hip extensional moment in loading response after exercise was greater than that before exercise (**Figure 8**).

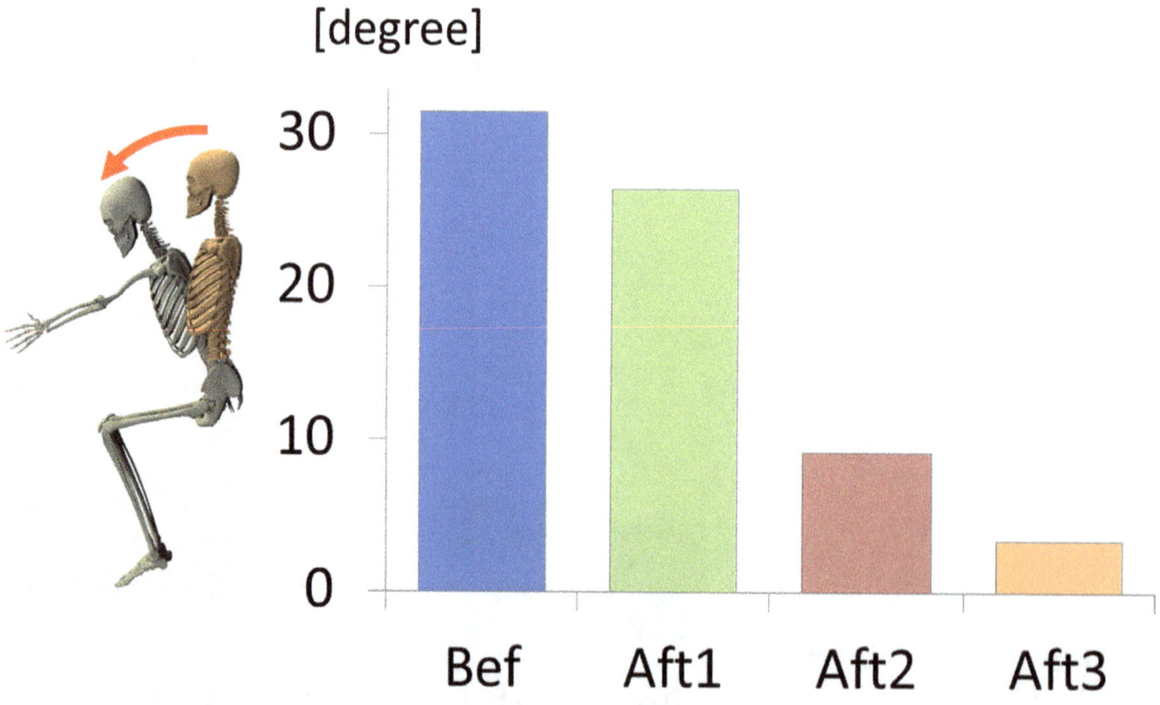


**Figure 5.** Range of motion of the anterior inclination of the trunk during throwing before and after exercise. Bef, before exercise; Aft, after exercise.

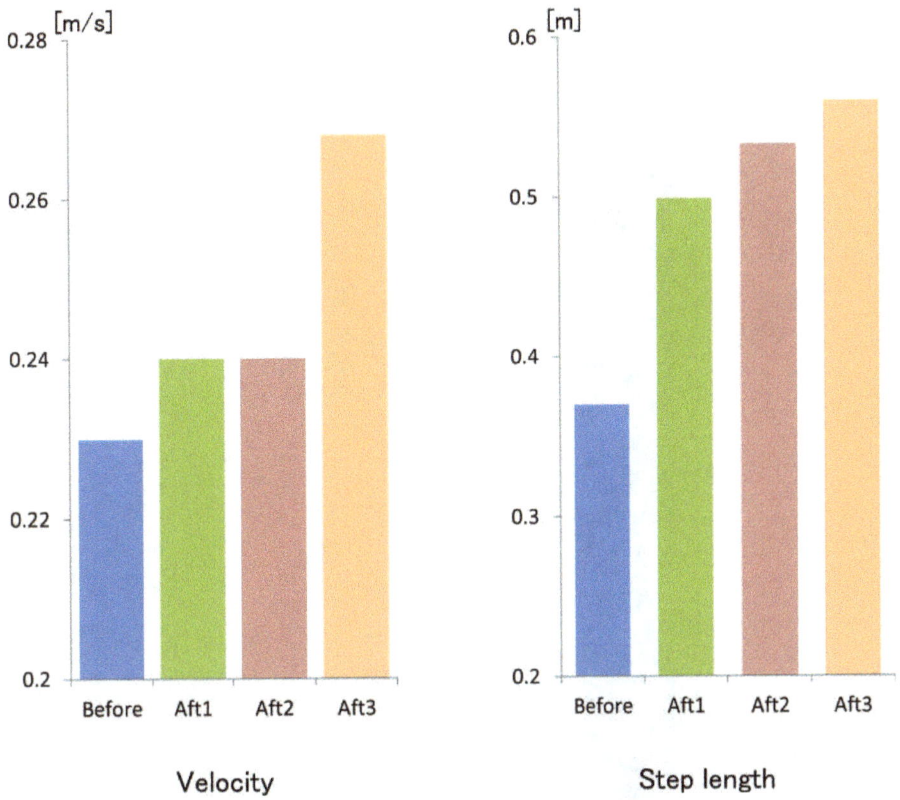


**Figure 6.** Gait velocity and step length of before and after exercise. Bef, before exercise; Aft, after exercise.

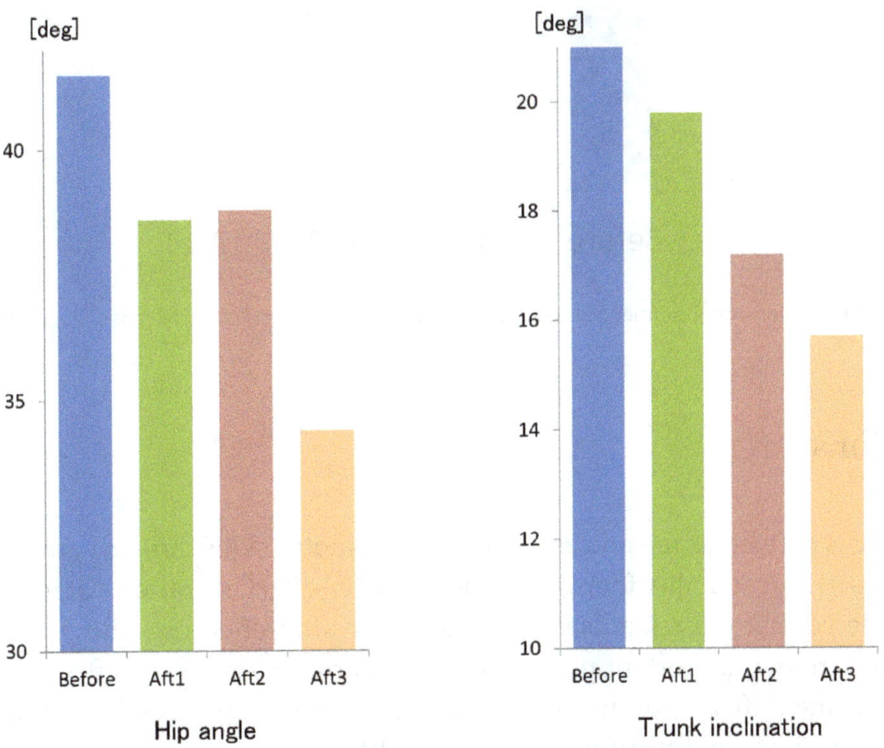


**Figure 7.** The hip joint angle and the anterior inclination of the trunk at initial contact of before and after exercise. Bef, before exercise; Aft, after exercise.

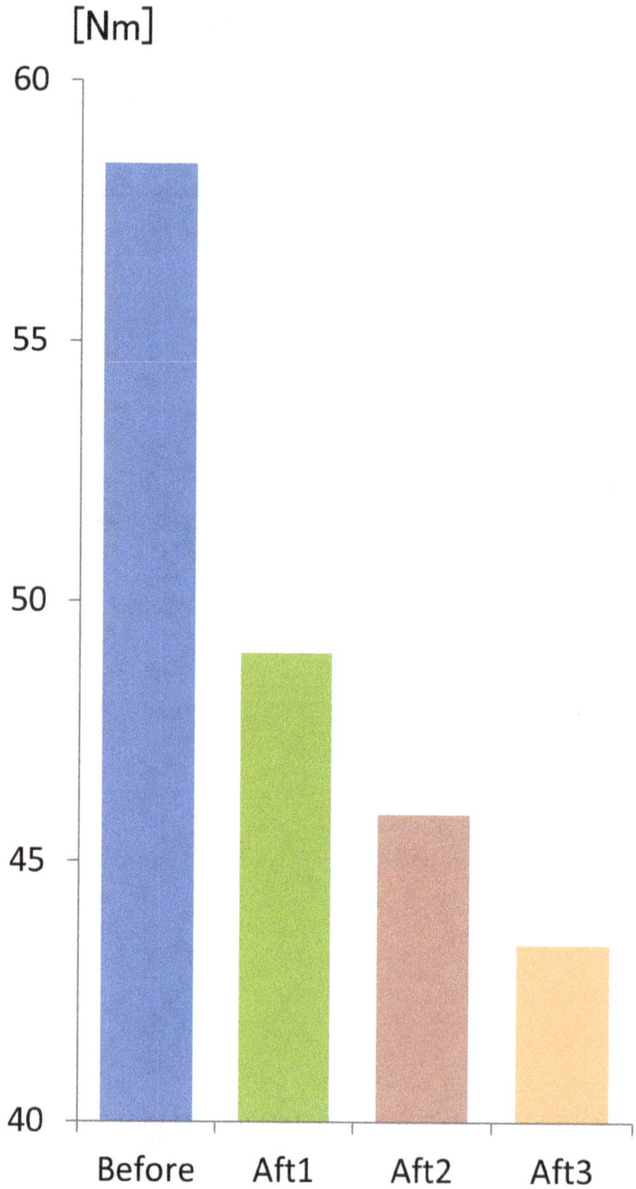


**Figure 8.** Maximal hip extensional moment in loading response of before and after exercise. Bef, before exercise; Aft, after exercise.

## 4. Discussions

Motor learning is defined as the process of improving motor skills through practice, with long-lasting changes in the capability for responding [4]. After-effect is a process of motor adaptation [5]. We considered that these kinematic changes were after-effects resulting from the robotic exercise. There are two important points in motor learning, one is the effect with repetition, and the other is the difficulty of the task. Prism adaptation requires 500 repetitions for motor reference. An appropriate difficulty of the task, not too hard and not too easy, is also necessary for motor reference. Thus, the load in motor learning, especially in early phase, should be quite different from that in muscle training. Because body weight may be excessive for weak muscles, wheelchair users may have little chance to activate their hip muscles. For the normal subjects, the difficulty of the task is easy so that there is no difference in hip moment between before and after exercise. However, it is too difficult for wheelchair users to walk 500 steps without support. The exoskeletal structure of HAL stabilized the lower body of the subjects, and the power assist in the hip in loading response allows the upper body to be upright and advances the contralateral leg forward. Furthermore, triggering of EMG increases the visual and the somatosensory feedback (normal sensation of "muscle activation-joint motion"). As a result, the difficulty of the task can be reduced to appropriate level. With only three times of exercise, wheelchair users showed a tremendous effect of our proposed exercise. This result suggests that wheelchair users learned how to activate the gluteus maximus during walking or throwing.

## 5. Conclusions

Our results suggest that the application of the HAL for motor learning may improve motor function in subjects with neural disorders.

## Acknowledgements

This work was supported by JSPS KAKENHI Grant Number 26350799.

## Author details

Yasuhiko Hatanaka*, Kazuki Yamaguchi, Koichi Saito and Satomi Tada

*Address all correspondence to: hatanaka@suzuka-u.ac.jp

Suzuka University of Medical Science, Suzuka, Mie, Japan

## References

[1] Wernig A, Müller S. Laufband locomotion with body weight support improved walking in persons with severe spinal cord injuries. Paraplegia. 1992;30:229–238. doi:10.1038/sc.1992.61

[2] Colombo G, Wirz M, Dietz V. Driven gait orthosis for improvement of locomotor training in paraplegic patients. Spinal Cord. 2001;39:252–256. doi:10.1038/sj.sc.3101154

[3] Kubota S, Nakata Y, Eguchi K, Kawamoto H, Kamibayashi K, Sakane M, Sankai Y. Feasibility of rehabilitation training with a newly developed wearable robot for patients

with limited mobility. Archives of Physical Medicine and Rehabilitation. 2013;94:1080–1087. doi:10.1016/j.apmr.2012.12.020

[4] Schmidt RA. Motor schema theory after 27 years: reflections and implications for a new theory. Res Q Exerc Sport. 2003;74: 366–375. doi:10.1080/02701367.2003.10609106

[5] Trempe M. Distinct consolidation outcomes in a visuomotor adaptation task: Off-line leaning and persistent after-effect. Brain Cogn. 2010;73:135–45. doi:10.1016/j.bandc.2010.04.005.

# 9

# Motor Imagery and Action Observation as Effective Tools for Physical Therapy

Hideki Nakano and Takayuki Kodama

**Abstract**

Motor imagery and action observation facilitate motor recovery of patients because both the motor imagery and the action observation share the activation of cortical neural networks implicated in movement execution. Specifically, imagery, observation, and execution activate the medial parietal area of the brain located between the parieto-occipital sulcus and the posterior end of the cingulate sulcus. This chapter reviews the neural mechanisms and clinical studies of motor imagery and action observation and discusses the applications in physical therapy.

**Keywords:** action observation, motor imagery, physical therapy

## 1. Introduction

Motor imagery and action observation have been proven as effective tools in rehabilitation [1]. Motor imagery is a cognitive process in which a subject only imagines completing a movement, without tensing any muscles (**Figure 1(a)**) [2]. While motor imagery alone can improve motor performance [3], it is particularly effective when associated with physical practice [4] as compared to physical practice alone. Hétu et al. reported the neural network of motor imagery using ALE meta-analysis [5]. The meta-analysis examined the general pattern of consistent activations during motor imagery and revealed several large clusters of activated tissue spanning over both hemispheres of the brain. In the frontal lobes, the bilateral inferior frontal gyri (IFG, including the pars opercularis), precentral gyrus (PcG), middle

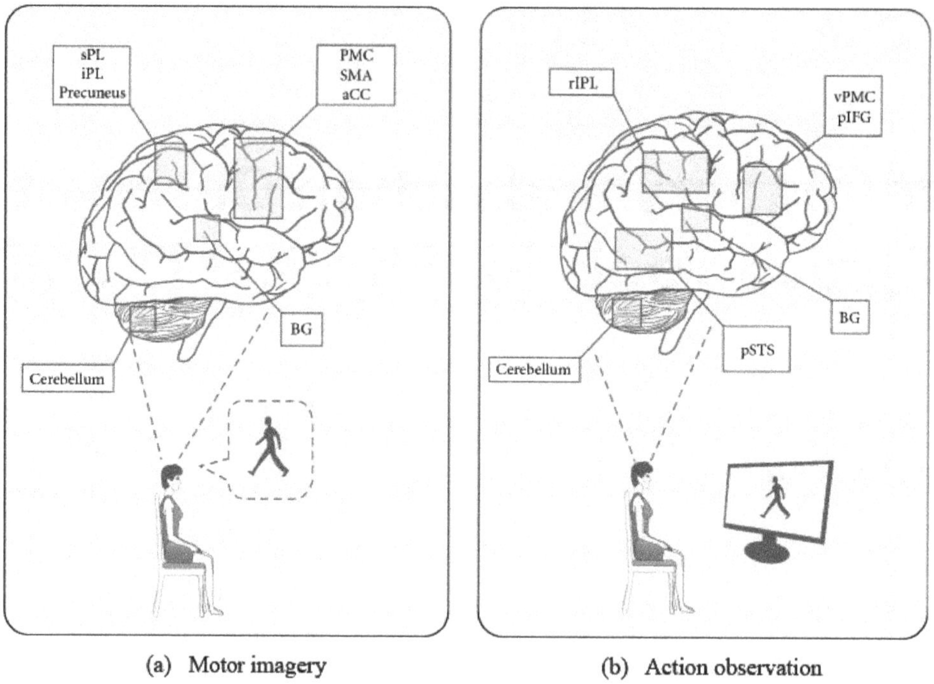


**Figure 1.** Motor imagery and action observation [2]. Human brain activity during motor imagery (a) and action observation (b). (a) Brain areas activated during kinesthetic and visual motor imagery. The pattern of activity includes the following regions: ventral and dorsal part of the premotor cortex (PMC); the supplementary motor area (SMA); anterior cingulate cortex (aCC); superior parietal lobule (sPL) and inferior parietal lobule (IPL); precuneus; basal ganglia (BG); and cerebellum. (b) The complex brain network ("mirror neuron system") involved in action observation: the ventral premotor cortex (vPMC), posterior part of the inferior frontal gyrus (pIFG), rostral part of the inferior parietal lobule (rIPL), and posterior superior temporal sulcus (pSTS).

frontal gyrus (MfG), supplementary motor area (SMA), and regions of the anterior insula were regions consistently activated during motor imagery. In the parietal lobes, the bilateral superior parietal lobule (SPL), supramarginal gyrus (SMG), and left inferior parietal lobule (IPL) and, in the subcortical regions, the left putamen, right thalamus, and pallidum were activated. Finally, the areas VI (bilateral) and the vermis of the cerebellum (CB) were also found to be consistently activated.

When a subject observes a specific action being performed, activation of the same neural structures used for the movement pattern is also repeated in the subject (**Figure 1(b)**) [2]. The neurophysiological basis of action observation is represented by the discovery of mirror neurons in the cerebral cortex of monkeys [6, 7]. These neurons discharge during both the execution of goal-directed actions and the observation of other individuals performing similar movements. The definition of the mirror neuron system (MNS) is the area that comprises the cerebral areas containing mirror neurons. Evidence with the use of transcranial magnetic stimulation (TMS) and functional magnetic resonance imaging (fMRI) suggested that MNS is also present in the human brain [8]. Some studies suggest a similar learning effect of action observation and physical practice [9–11]. Caspers et al. reported the neural network of action observation using ALE meta-analysis [12]. Brain regions showing consistent activation across action observation experiments were observed symmetrically across both hemispheres in frontal areas BA 44/45, lateral dorsal premotor cortex (dPMC, BA 6), supplementary motor area (SMA, BA 6), rostral IPL (area PFt), primary somatosensory cortex (SI, BA 1/2), SPL (area 7A), intraparietal cortex (IPS, area hIP3), posterior middle temporal gyrus (pMTG) at the transition to visual area V5, and the fusiform face area/fusiform body area (FFA/FBA). Both motor imagery and action observation share the activation of cortical neural networks as implicated in movement execution (**Figure 2**) [13]. Moreover, we reported that brain activity during movement observation, imagery, and execution uses different pathways according to the sensory modality (**Figure 3**) [14]. This chapter discusses the clinical results of motor imagery and action observation studies and rehabilitation applications.

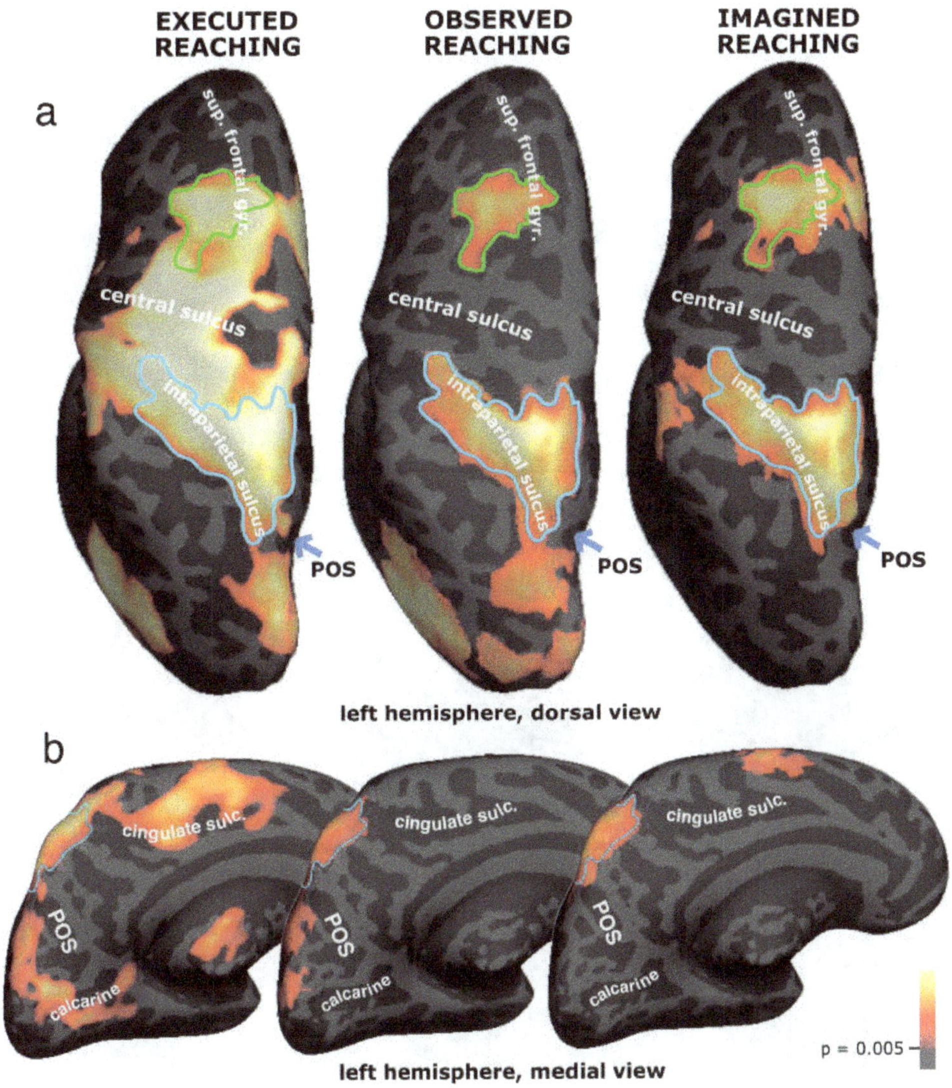


**Figure 2.** Outline of the overlap between executed, observed, and imagined reaching in the left dorsal premotor (superior frontal sulcus and gyrus) and left posterior parietal areas [13]. The overlaps in the premotor and parietal regions served as regions of interest in the percent signal change analysis. (a) Dorsal view of the left hemisphere. (b) Medial view of the left hemisphere. Executed, observed, and imagined reaching all activated a medial parietal area located in-between the parieto-occipital sulcus and the posterior end of the cingulate sulcus, outlined in light blue. Sup. frontal gyr., superior frontal gyrus; POS, parieto-occipital sulcus; calcarine, calcarine sulcus; cingulate sulc., cingulate sulcus.

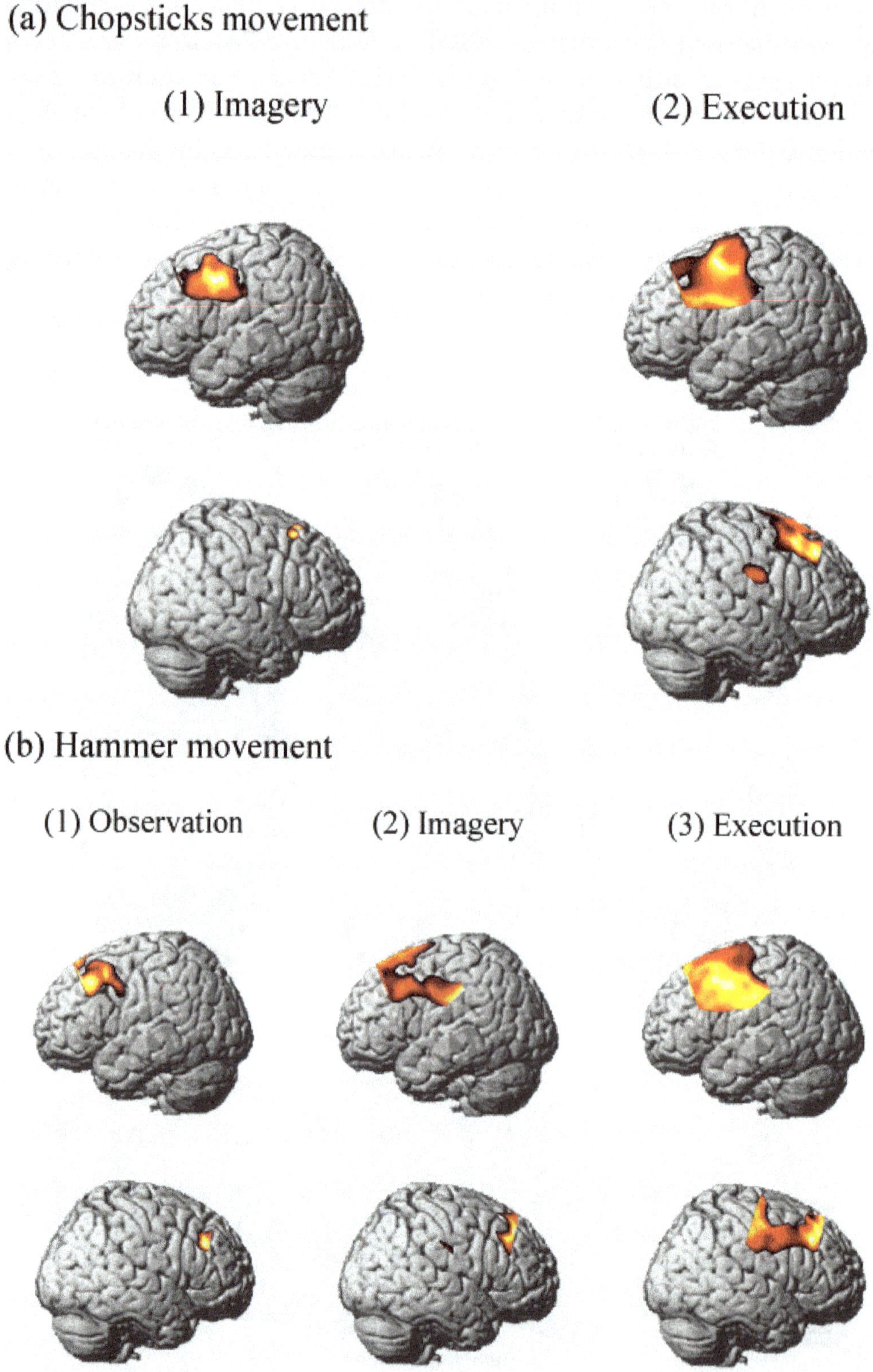


**Figure 3.** Brain activity during observation, imagery, and execution of tool use [14]. The top row of the images shows the left side of the brain, whereas the bottom row of the images shows the right side of the brain. (a) Brain regions where a significant increase in the oxyhemoglobin (oxyHb) levels was detected during (1) imagery and (2) execution of the chopsticks movement. No significant differences in the oxyHb levels were detected during observation of the chopsticks movement. (b) Brain regions where a significant increase in the oxyHb levels was detected during (1) observation, (2) imagery, and (3) execution of the hammer movement.

## 2. Clinical studies of motor imagery

Motor imagery studies were conducted on several diseases relating to the central nervous system and acute injuries involving orthopedics such as subacute stroke [15–19], chronic stroke [20–22], traumatic brain injury [23], multiple sclerosis [23], shoulder impingement syndrome [24], postsurgical anterior cruciate ligament [25], postsurgical flexor tendon repair [26], burn injury [27], phantom limb pain [28], complex regional pain syndrome [28, 29], and motor coordination problems [30]. **Table 1** lists motor imagery clinical studies found in PubMed. "Motor imagery" which did not include "Brain Computer Interface (BCI)" or "Brain Machine Interface (BMI)" was used as a finding keyword, and the searched article type was "Randomized Controlled Trial (RCT)."

Nearly all studies reported that the effectiveness of motor imagery in orthopedic diseases was significant. Hoyek et al. investigated the effect of motor imagery on a range of motion and pain in patients with stage II shoulder impingement syndrome [24] and found positive results in the intervention group compared to the control group. This indicates that motor imagery contributes to a range of motion improvements and pain reductions in patients with stage II shoulder impingement syndrome. Lebon et al. investigated the effect of motor imagery on muscle activity in patients with a postsurgical anterior cruciate ligament [25]. The results showed that the intervention group significantly improved compared to the control group, which states that motor imagery improves motor recovery in patients after anterior cruciate ligament surgery. Stenekes et al. examined the effect of motor imagery on hand function during immobilization after flexor tendon repair [26]. The results showed that increased preparation time significantly reduced after the immobilization period in the intervention group compared with the control group. This study disclosed that motor imagery improves hand functions in patients after surgical flexor tendon repair.

The effectiveness of motor imagery in patients with pain is also significant. Moseley et al. investigated the effect of graded motor imagery on pain and swelling in patients with complex regional pain syndrome [24]. The results showed that the neuropathic pain scale and finger circumference both significantly improved after training in the intervention group compared to the control group. Moreover, the improvement was observed for 12 weeks. Another study by Moseley et al. indicated that a motor imagery program for patients with complex regional pain syndrome not displaying a limp was effective. Moseley et al. reported the effect of graded motor imagery on pain and disability in patients with phantom limb pain or complex regional pain syndrome, and the results indicated that pain and disability significantly improved through motor imagery after training in the intervention group compared with the control group. In addition, the effect of the training lasted for 6 months [28].

On the other hand, some studies indicate that motor imagery has both effective and ineffective results for motor recovery in stroke patients. The effects of motor imagery were observed in upper extremity function in subacute [16] and chronic [23] stroke patients, gait function in subacute [15, 18] and chronic [20–22] stroke patients, and balance functions in chronic stroke patients [22]. Motor imagery used for motor recovery showed a lack of results in subacute stroke patients with limited upper extremity function [19], stroke patients struggling with goal attainment and

| References | Study design | Type of patients | N | Intervention | Treatment period | Outcome measures and results |
|---|---|---|---|---|---|---|
| Oostra et al. [15] | RCT | Patients with subacute stroke | 44 | MI + standard rehab vs muscle relaxation + standard rehab | 6 weeks | MIQ-RS visual (−)<br>MIQ-RS kinesthetic (+)<br>Imagery walking time/actual walking time (−)<br>10-m walk test (+)<br>FMA-LE (−)* |
| Hoyek et al. [24] | RCT | Patients with stage II shoulder impingement syndrome | 16 | MI + standard rehab vs standard rehab | 4 weeks | Constant score (+)<br>ROM (+)<br>Pain VAS (+) |
| Dickstein et al. [20] | RCT | Patients with chronic stroke | 23 | Integrated MI practice vs upper extremity rehab | 4 weeks | 10-m walk test (+)<br>Community ambulation (steps) (−)<br>Community ambulation (maximal activity) (−)<br>Falls efficacy scale (+)* |
| Sun et al. [21] | RCT | Patients with severe chronic stroke | 18 | MI + standard rehab vs standard rehab | 4 weeks | FMA-UE (+)<br>fMRI |
| Mihara et al. [16] | RCT | Patients with subacute stroke | 20 | Real-neurofeedback with MI + standard rehab vs sham-neurofeedback with MI + standard rehab | 2 weeks | FMA (+)<br>Action research arm test (−)<br>Motor activity log (−)<br>KVIQ-10 (+) |
| Cho et al. [22] | RCT | Patients with chronic stroke | 28 | MI + gait training vs gait training | 6 weeks | Functional reach test (+)<br>Timed up-and-go test (+)<br>10-m walk test (+)<br>FMA (+) |
| Schuster et al. [17] | RCT | Patients with subacute stroke | 39 | MI embedded into physiotherapy vs MI added to physiotherapy vs physiotherapy | 2 weeks | Motor task (time) (+)*<br>Motor task (help) (+)*<br>KVIQ visual (−)<br>KVIQ kinesthetic (−)<br>Imaprax visual (−)<br>Berg balance scale (−)<br>Activities-specific balance confidence scale (−)<br>Wellbeing VAS (−) |

| References | Study design | Type of patients | N | Intervention | Treatment period | Outcome measures and results |
|---|---|---|---|---|---|---|
| Lebon et al. [25] | RCT | Patients with anterior cruciate ligament injury | 20 | MI + standard rehab vs standard rehab | 5 weeks | Quadriceps EMG activity (+)<br>Pain VAS (+)*<br>Anthropometric data (−)<br>Lower extremity functional scale test (−) |
| Verma et al. [18] | RCT | Patients with subacute stroke | 30 | Task-oriented circuit class training with MI vs standard rehab | 2 weeks | Functional ambulation classification (+)<br>Rivermead visual gait assessment (+)<br>Step length asymmetry (+)<br>Stride length asymmetry (−)<br>Cadence (−)<br>Comfortable walking speed (−)<br>Maximal walking speed (−)<br>6-minute walk test (−) |
| Ietswaart et al. [19] | RCT | Patients with subacute stroke | 121 | MI + standard rehab vs Attention-Placebo Control + standard rehab vs Normal Care Control | 4 weeks | Action research arm test (+)*<br>Grip strength (−)<br>Timed manual dexterity task (−)<br>Barthel index (−)<br>Functional limitations profile (−) |
| Bovend'Eerdt et al. [23] | RCT | Patients with stroke, traumatic brain injury, multiple sclerosis | 30 | Integrated MI program vs standard rehab | 5 weeks | Goal attainment scaling (+)*<br>Barthel index (+)*<br>Rivermead mobility index (+)*<br>Nottingham extended ADL index (+)*<br>Action research arm test (+)* |
| Guillot et al. [27] | RCT | Patients with severe hand burn injury | 14 | MI + standard rehab vs standard rehab | 2 weeks | Spellcaster wrist movement (extension) (+)<br>Spellcaster wrist movement (flexion) (−)<br>Finger opposition task (+)<br>Finger flexion task (+) |

| References | Study design | Type of patients | N | Intervention | Treatment period | Outcome measures and results |
|---|---|---|---|---|---|---|
| Stenekes et al. [26] | RCT | Patients after surgical flexor tendon repair | 28 | MI + standard rehab vs standard rehab | 6 weeks | Preparation time (+)<br>Michigan hand outcome questionnaire score (−)<br>Hand function VAS (−)<br>Kinematic analysis (−)<br>Active total motion (−)<br>Grip strength (−) |
| Moseley et al. [28] | RCT | Patients with phantom limb pain, CRPS1 | 51 | Graded MI vs standard rehab | 6 weeks | Pain VAS (+)<br>Function NRS (+) |
| Moseley et al. [29] | RCT | Patients with chronic CRPS1 | 13 | Graded MI vs ongoing medical management | 6 weeks | Neuropathic pain scale (+)<br>Finger circumference (+) |
| Wilson et al. [30] | RCT | Children with motor coordination problems | 54 | MI training vs Traditional Perceptual-Motor Training vs No-treatment | 5 weeks | Total movement assessment battery for children scores (+)* |

*Significant within-subject factor of time ($P < 0.05$) but no significant between-subject factor of group or interaction time × group ($P > 0.05$).

RCT, Randomized Controlled Trial; CRPS1, Complex Regional Pain Syndrome type 1; MI, Motor Imagery; MIQ-RS, Movement Imagery Questionnaire-Revised, Second Edition, FMA-UE/LE, Fugl-Meyer Assessment Upper Extremity/Lower Extremity; ROM, Range of Motion; VAS, Visual Analogue Scale, fMRI, functional Magnetic Resonance Imaging; KVIQ, Kinesthetic and Visual Imagery Questionnaire; EMG, Electromyogram; NRS, Numerical Rating Scale.

**Table 1.** Representative clinical studies of motor imagery.

task performance [17], and those with traumatic brain injury and multiple sclerosis [23]. A possible reason for the different effects of motor imagery is the decline of cognitive function after a patient experiences a stroke. A previous study reported that not only motor function but also cognitive function declines after a stroke [31]. Moreover, cognitive function is largely associated with the ability to execute motor imagery [32]. Therefore, the cognitive function level in stroke patients influences the outcome of motor imagery training.

## 3. Clinical studies of action observation

Clinical studies of action observation were also conducted on a wide range of diseases, such as central nervous system diseases and orthopedic events that include acute stroke [33], subacute stroke [34], chronic stroke [35], Parkinson's disease [36, 37], cerebral palsy [38], and orthopedic surgery [39]. **Table 2** lists clinical studies of action observations found in PubMed. "Action observation" was used as a finding keyword, and "Randomized Controlled Trial (RCT)" was the article type that was searched.

The first clinical study of action observation was reported by Ertelt et al. [35]. This study examined the effect of action observation therapy on motor recovery in chronic stroke patients using motor

| References | Study design | Type of patients | N | Intervention | Treatment period | Outcome measures and results |
|---|---|---|---|---|---|---|
| Sale et al. [34] | RCT | Patients with subacute stroke | 67 | AO + standard rehab vs sham-AO + standard rehab | 4 weeks | FMA (+)<br>BBT (+) |
| Pelosin et al. [36] | RCT | Patients with Parkinson's disease | 38 | AO vs ACOUSTIC vs sham-AO vs AO (on, off) | 1 day | Self-paced movement rate (+)<br>Intertapping interval (+)<br>Touch duration (+)* |
| Buccino et al. [38] | RCT | Children with cerebral palsy | 15 | AO + standard rehab vs sham-AO + standard rehab | 3 weeks | Melbourne Assessment Scale (+) |
| Franceschini et al. [33] | RCT | Patients with acute stroke | 102 | AO + standard rehab vs sham-AO + standard rehab | 4 weeks | FMA-UE (+)*<br>FAT (−)<br>BBT (+)<br>Modified ashworth scale (−)<br>Functional independence measure motor items (+)* |
| Bellelli et al. [39] | RCT | Patients after orthopedic surgery | | AO + standard rehab vs sham-AO + standard rehab | 3 weeks | FIM scores (+)<br>FIM motor subscores (+)<br>Tinetti scores (+)<br>Dependence on walking aids (+) |

| References | Study design | Type of patients | N | Intervention | Treatment period | Outcome measures and results |
|---|---|---|---|---|---|---|
| Pelosin et al. [37] | RCT | Patients with Parkinson's disease | 20 | AO + standard rehab vs landscape + standard rehab | 4 weeks | FOG Questionnaire (+)*<br>Number of FOG episodes (total) (+)<br>Number of FOG episodes (start walking) (+)<br>Number of FOG episodes (turn) (+)<br>Number of FOG episodes (obstacle) (−)<br>Timed up and go test (+)*<br>10-meter walking test (+)*<br>Tinetti scale (part I) (+)*<br>Berg balance scale (+)*<br>Tinetti scale (part II) (+)*<br>39-item PD questionnaire (+)* |
| Ertelt et al. [35] | RCT | Patients with chronic stroke | 16 | AO + standard rehab vs sham-AO + standard rehab | 4 weeks | FAT (+)<br>Wolf motor function test (+)<br>Stroke impact scale (+)<br>fMRI (+) |

*Significant within-subject factor of time ($P < 0.05$) but no significant between-subject factor of group or interaction time × group ($P > 0.05$).

RCT, Randomized Controlled Trial; AO, Action Observation; FMA-UE, Fugl-Meyer Assessment Upper Extremity; BBT, Box and Block Test; FAT, Frenchay Arm Test; FIM, Functional Independence Measure; FOG, Freezing of Gait; fMRI, functional Magnetic Resonance Imaging.

**Table 2.** Representative clinical studies of action observation.

function outcome and functional magnetic resonance imaging (fMRI). The results showed that motor function after a four-week training significantly improved. Moreover, the improvement was retained for 8 weeks post-training. fMRI during the sensorimotor task of object manipulation showed that significant activations in the bilateral ventral premotor cortex (vPMC), bilateral superior temporal gyrus, supplementary motor area, and the contralateral supramarginal gyrus were observed in the intervention group compared to the control group. This study indicated that action observation has positive effects for motor recovery in stroke patients. Similarly, other studies reported that action observation is effective for motor recovery of upper extremity function in acute stoke patients [33] and for the improvement of motor function in subacute stroke patients [34].

Action observation is also helpful in patients with Parkinson's disease. Pelosin et al. investigated the effect of action observation on gait-freezing (GF) [37]. The results showed that the GF functional score after training significantly improved in both the intervention and control groups. In addition, retention was observed after the four-week training period in only the intervention group. This study indicated that action observation had a positive effect on the walking ability in Parkinson's disease patients displaying GF. In the same manner, another study reported that action observation improved finger function in patients with Parkinson's disease [36].

Action observation is also a useful tool for postsurgical orthopedic patients. Bellelli et al. reported the effect of action observation treatment on motor function in patients who underwent hip arthroplasty, knee arthroplasty, and hip fracture repair [39]. The functional score after training was significantly higher in the intervention group than the control group. This revealed that action observation treatment is effective for postsurgical orthopedic patients.

These studies suggest that the effect of action observation is improved not only in central nervous system diseases but also in orthopedic diseases and events.

## 4. Application of motor imagery and action observation to physical therapy

As described above, motor imagery and action observation have positive effects on central nervous system diseases, as well as in patients who experienced orthopedic diseases and events.

Kim and Lee reported the comparison of the effects of both action observation and motor imagery training on motor recovery of chronic stroke patients [40]. The results showed significant improvements in a timed up-and-go test, gait speed, cadence, and single limb support of the affected side in motor imagery and action observation groups after training. Although no significant difference was observed between action observation and motor imagery groups, the action observation group showed significant improvement compared with the control group. This study indicated that action observation had positive effects on dynamic balance and gait abilities compared with motor imagery.

The different effects between motor imagery and action observation are associated with the degree of difficulty in training methods. Specifically, action observation uses a bottom-up approach based on sensory information. Human motor control has high dependence on visual information; therefore, as action observation uses the sense of vision, the level of difficulty is lower compared with motor imagery. Additionally, action observation can influence human movement easily. On the other hand, motor imagery uses a top-down approach based on cognitive information. The cognitive function is greatly associated with cognitive information processing. Therefore, the level of difficulty is higher in motor imagery than action observation, especially for stroke patients who see a decline in cognitive function [31]. How then are action observation and motor imagery used for physical therapy?

Gatti et al. revealed that action observation is superior to motor imagery in the early stages of new complex motor learning, as shown by behavioral [41] and EEG data [42]. As described above, motor imagery is influenced by the environment, personal imaging ability, and mental effort. In contrast, action observation is easier to apply, despite activation of the same neural network as motor imagery [43]. In addition, Conson et al. revealed that action observation had an effect of promoting motor imagery [44]. According to these studies, it is recommended that strategies should transfer from action observation performed in the early stages of motor learning to motor imagery performed during the later stages of motor learning.

Graded motor imagery is a similar therapeutic approach that consists of three specific levels of increasing complexity in terms of time and difficulty, which is thought to reflect graded activation of cortical networks [45]. Graded motor imagery includes three consecutive steps: implicit motor imagery, explicit motor imagery, and mirror therapy [46]. Polli et al. investigated the feasibility and clinical effects of graded motor imagery in motor function recovery after a stroke [47]. The results showed that the Wolf Motor Function Test and Fugl-Meyer Assessment after training in the intervention group significantly improved compared to the control group. This study demonstrated that graded motor imagery is a feasible treatment for stroke patients to provide better outcomes than conventional therapy.

Thus, gradually increasing the difficulty level of treatment strategy is recommended. However, motor imagery and action observation are just tools for modulating brain states [48]. Therefore, it is important to choose the appropriate treatment strategy according to functional characteristics and recovery phases of patients in the clinical setting [49].

## Acknowledgements

This work was supported by JSPS KAKENHI (Grant Number JP26750208) and ASTEM RI/KYOTO.

## Author details

Hideki Nakano* and Takayuki Kodama

*Address all correspondence to: nakano-h@tachibana-u.ac.jp

Department of Physical Therapy, Faculty of Health Science, Kyoto Tachibana University, Kyoto, Japan

## References

[1] Mulder T. Motor imagery and action observation: Cognitive tools for rehabilitation. J Neural Transm (Vienna). 2007;114(10):1265–78.

[2] Abbruzzese G, Avanzino L, Marchese R, Pelosin E. Action observation and motor imagery: Innovative cognitive tools in the rehabilitation of Parkinson's disease. Parkinsons Dis. 2015;2015:1–9.

[3] Gentili R, Han CE, Schweighofer N, Papaxanthis C. Motor learning without doing: Trial-by-trial improvement in motor performance during mental training. J Neurophysiol. 2010;104(2):774–83.

[4] Gentili R, Papaxanthis C, Pozzo T. Improvement and generalization of arm motor performance through motor imagery practice. Neuroscience. 2006;137(3):761–72.

[5] Hétu S, Grégoire M, Saimpont A, Coll MP, Eugène F, Michon PE, Jackson PL. The neural network of motor imagery: An ALE meta-analysis. Neurosci Biobehav Rev. 2013;37(5):930–49.

[6] Gallese V, Fadiga L, Fogassi L, Rizzolatti G. Action recognition in the premotor cortex. Brain. 1996;119(Part 2):593–609.

[7] Rizzolatti G, Fadiga L, Gallese V, Fogassi L. Premotor cortex and the recognition of motor actions. Brain Res Cogn Brain Res. 1996;3(2):131–41.

[8] Fabbri-Destro M, Rizzolatti G. Mirror neurons and mirror systems in monkeys and humans. Physiology (Bethesda). 2008;23:171–9.

[9] Hayes SJ, Elliott D, Bennett SJ. General motor representations are developed during action-observation. Exp Brain Res. 2010;204(2):199–206.

[10] Heyes CM, Foster CL. Motor learning by observation: Evidence from a serial reaction time task. Q J Exp Psychol A. 2002;55(2):593–607.

[11] Vinter A, Perruchet P. Implicit motor learning through observational training in adults and children. Mem Cognit. 2002;30(2):256–61.

[12] Caspers S, Zilles K, Laird AR, Eickhoff SB. ALE meta-analysis of action observation and imitation in the human brain. Neuroimage. 2010;50(3):1148–67.

[13] Filimon F, Nelson JD, Hagler DJ, Sereno MI. Human cortical representations for reaching: Mirror neurons for execution, observation, and imagery. Neuroimage. 2007;37(4):1315–28.

[14] Nakano H, Ueta K, Osumi M, Morioka S. Brain activity during the observation, imagery, and execution of tool use: An fNIRS/EEG study. J Nov Physiother. 2012;S1:009.

[15] Oostra KM, Oomen A, Vanderstraeten G, Vingerhoets G. Influence of motor imagery training on gait rehabilitation in sub-acute stroke: A randomized controlled trial. J Rehabil Med. 2015;47(3):204–9.

[16] Mihara M, Hattori N, Hatakenaka M, Yagura H, Kawano T, Hino T, Miyai I. Near-infrared spectroscopy-mediated neurofeedback enhances efficacy of motor imagery-based training in poststroke victims: A pilot study. Stroke. 2013;44(4):1091–8.

[17] Schuster C, Butler J, Andrews B, Kischka U, Ettlin T. Comparison of embedded and added motor imagery training in patients after stroke: Results of a randomised controlled pilot trial. Trials. 2012;13:11.

[18] Verma R, Arya KN, Garg RK, Singh T. Task-oriented circuit class training program with motor imagery for gait rehabilitation in poststroke patients: A randomized controlled trial. Top Stroke Rehabil. 2011;18(Suppl 1):620–32.

[19] Ietswaart M, Johnston M, Dijkerman HC, Joice S, Scott CL, MacWalter RS, Hamilton SJ. Mental practice with motor imagery in stroke recovery: Randomized controlled trial of efficacy. Brain. 2011;134(Part 5):1373–86.

[20] Dickstein R, Deutsch JE, Yoeli Y, Kafri M, Falash F, Dunsky A, Eshet A, Alexander N. Effects of integrated motor imagery practice on gait of individuals with chronic stroke: A half-crossover randomized study. Arch Phys Med Rehabil. 2013;94(11):2119–25.

[21] Sun L, Yin D, Zhu Y, Fan M, Zang L, Wu Y, Jia J, Bai Y, Zhu B, Hu Y. Cortical reorganization after motor imagery training in chronic stroke patients with severe motor impairment: A longitudinal fMRI study. Neuroradiology. 2013;55(7):913–25.

[22] Cho HY, Kim JS, Lee GC. Effects of motor imagery training on balance and gait abilities in post-stroke patients: A randomized controlled trial. Clin Rehabil. 2013;27(8):675–80.

[23] Bovend'Eerdt TJ, Dawes H, Sackley C, Izadi H, Wade DT. An integrated motor imagery program to improve functional task performance in neurorehabilitation: A single-blind randomized controlled trial. Arch Phys Med Rehabil. 2010;91(6):939–46.

[24] Hoyek N, Di Rienzo F, Collet C, Hoyek F, Guillot A. The therapeutic role of motor imagery on the functional rehabilitation of a stage II shoulder impingement syndrome. Disabil Rehabil. 2014;36(13):1113–9.

[25] Lebon F, Guillot A, Collet C. Increased muscle activation following motor imagery during the rehabilitation of the anterior cruciate ligament. Appl Psychophysiol Biofeedback. 2012;37(1):45–51.

[26] Stenekes MW, Geertzen JH, Nicolai JP, De Jong BM, Mulder T. Effects of motor imagery on hand function during immobilization after flexor tendon repair. Arch Phys Med Rehabil. 2009;90(4):553–9.

[27] Guillot A, Lebon F, Vernay M, Girbon JP, Doyon J, Collet C. Effect of motor imagery in the rehabilitation of burn patients. J Burn Care Res. 2009;30(4):686–93.

[28] Moseley GL. Graded motor imagery for pathologic pain: A randomized controlled trial. Neurology. 2006;67(12):2129–34.

[29] Moseley GL. Graded motor imagery is effective for long-standing complex regional pain syndrome: A randomised controlled trial. Pain. 2004;108(1–2):192–8.

[30] Wilson PH, Thomas PR, Maruff P. Motor imagery training ameliorates motor clumsiness in children. J Child Neurol. 2002;17(7):491–8.

[31] Arsic S, Konstantinovic Lj, Eminovic F, Pavlovic D, Popovic MB, Arsic V. Correlation between the quality of attention and cognitive competence with motor action in stroke patients. Biomed Res Int. 2015;2015:823136.

[32] Munzert J, Lorey B, Zentgraf K. Cognitive motor processes: The role of motor imagery in the study of motor representations. Brain Res Rev. 2009;60(2):306–26.

[33] Franceschini M, Ceravolo MG, Agosti M, Cavallini P, Bonassi S, Dall'Armi V, Massucci M, Schifini F, Sale P. Clinical relevance of action observation in upper-limb stroke rehabilitation: A possible role in recovery of functional dexterity. A randomized clinical trial. Neurorehabil Neural Repair. 2012;26(5):456–62.

[34] Sale P, Ceravolo MG, Franceschini M. Action observation therapy in the subacute phase promotes dexterity recovery in right-hemisphere stroke patients. Biomed Res Int. 2014;2014:1–7.

[35] Ertelt D, Small S, Solodkin A, Dettmers C, McNamara A, Binkofski F, Buccino G. Action observation has a positive impact on rehabilitation of motor deficits after stroke. Neuroimage. 2007;36(Suppl 2):T164–73.

[36] Pelosin E, Bove M, Ruggeri P, Avanzino L, Abbruzzese G. Reduction of bradykinesia of finger movements by a single session of action observation in Parkinson disease. Neurorehabil Neural Repair. 2013;27(6):552–60.

[37] Pelosin E, Avanzino L, Bove M, Stramesi P, Nieuwboer A, Abbruzzese G. Action observation improves freezing of gait in patients with Parkinson's disease. Neurorehabil Neural Repair. 2010;24(8):746–52.

[38] Buccino G, Arisi D, Gough P, Aprile D, Ferri C, Serotti L, Tiberti A, Fazzi E. Improving upper limb motor functions through action observation treatment: A pilot study in children with cerebral palsy. Dev Med Child Neurol. 2012;54(9):822–8.

[39] Bellelli G, Buccino G, Bernardini B, Padovani A, Trabucchi M. Action observation treatment improves recovery of postsurgical orthopedic patients: Evidence for a top-down effect? Arch Phys Med Rehabil. 2010;91(10):1489–94.

[40] Kim JH, Lee BH. Action observation training for functional activities after stroke: A pilot randomized controlled trial. NeuroRehabilitation. 2013;33(4):565–74.

[41] Gatti R, Tettamanti A, Gough PM, Riboldi E, Marinoni L, Buccino G. Action observation versus motor imagery in learning a complex motor task: A short review of literature and a kinematics study. Neurosci Lett. 2013;540:37–42.

[42] Gonzalez-Rosa JJ, Natali F, Tettamanti A, Cursi M, Velikova S, Comi G, Gatti R, Leocani L. Action observation and motor imagery in performance of complex movements: Evidence from EEG and kinematics analysis. Behav Brain Res. 2015;281:290–300.

[43] Buccino G. Action observation treatment: a novel tool in neurorehabilitation. Philos Trans R Soc Lond B Biol Sci. 2014;369(1644):20130185.

[44] Conson M, Sarà M, Pistoia F, Trojano L. Action observation improves motor imagery: Specific interactions between simulative processes. Exp Brain Res. 2009;199(1):71–81.

[45] Moseley GL. Is successful rehabilitation of complex regional pain syndrome due to sustained attention to the affected limb? A randomised clinical trial. Pain. 2005;114(1–2):54–61.

[46] Bowering KJ, O'Connell NE, Tabor A, Catley MJ, Leake HB, Moseley GL, Stanton TR. The effects of graded motor imagery and its components on chronic pain: A systematic review and meta-analysis. J Pain. 2013;14(1):3–13.

[47] Polli A, Moseley LG, Gioia E, Beames T, Baba A, Agostini M, Tonin P, Turolla A. Graded motor imagery for patients with stroke: A non-randomised controlled trial of a new approach. Eur J Phys Rehabil Med. 2017;53(1):14–23.

[48] Vogt S, Di Rienzo F, Collet C, Collins A, Guillot A. Multiple roles of motor imagery during action observation. Front Hum Neurosci. 2013;7:807.

[49] Hatem SM, Saussez G, Della Faille M, Prist V, Zhang X, Dispa D, Bleyenheuft Y. Rehabilitation of motor function after stroke: A multiple systematic review focused on techniques to stimulate upper extremity recovery. Front Hum Neurosci. 2016;10:442.

# 10

# Neuromuscular Diseases and Rehabilitation

Yasemin Parlak Demir

**Abstract**

Neuromuscular diseases (NMDs) are a heterogeneous group of diseases that are inherited or acquired, resulting from an abnormality in the anterior horn motor cells, peripheral nerves, neuromuscular junctions, or muscles.

In NMDs, evaluation is performed to monitor the progression of the disease, to determine the appropriate treatment methods, to investigate the efficacy of treatment methods, and to predict and prevent possible complications. Evaluation methods should include evaluation of respiratory functions, muscle testing, normal joint movement, evaluation of flexibility, evaluation of motor functions and functional capacities, functional posture, and gait analysis.

The aim of physiotherapy approaches is to improve the quality of life of patients and their families. The rehabilitation program should include the protection of the functional level of the patient and the physical and psychological functions, increasing the physical and mental capacity of the patient, and slowing the progress of the disease symptoms. The rehabilitation program should include the preservation of muscle strength, an exercise program for the prevention of contractures, increasing respiratory function and aerobic capacity, gait and balance training, fall prevention, walking aid training, psychosocial approach, vocational counseling, ergotherapy processes and nutrition expert support.

**Keywords:** neuromuscular diseases, physiotherapy, rehabilitation, ICF, assessment

## 1. Introduction

### 1.1. Identification and classification of NMD

Neuromuscular diseases (NMDs) are a heterogeneous group of diseases that are inherited or acquired, resulting from an abnormality in the anterior horn motor cells, peripheral nerves, neuromuscular junctions, or muscles [1]. The most common neuromuscular diseases are motor neuron diseases, neuropathies, neuromuscular junction diseases, and muscular diseases based on anatomic localization [2].

Motor neuron diseases are a group of diseases that progress with lower and/or upper motor neuron involvement in motor neurons in the anterior horn of medulla spinalis. They are characterized by muscle weakness associated with fasciculation and atrophy that differs with respect to the location and function of the affected motor neurons. Hereditary spinal muscular atrophy (SMA) is the most common motor neuron disease. SMA is caused by the degeneration of the anterior horn cells in the spinal cord and brain stem and by the activation of the corticospinal tract. Progressive symmetrical weakness, hypotonia, hyporeflexia or areflexia, muscle atrophy, fasciculation typically affecting the tongue, and postural tremor in the fingers are typical signs and symptoms of SMA. Spasticity may also be seen as a disease-specific finding in patients with upper motor neuron involvement such as amyotrophic lateral sclerosis (ALS) [3].

Neuropathies are peripheral nerve diseases with sensory and motor symptoms. The observation of sensory changes in addition to muscle weakness distinguishes peripheral nerve diseases from diseases of other components of the motor unit. It causes demyelination in the nerve and axonal degeneration in the nerve by affecting the nerve myelin sheath and/or axon [4]. The most common neuropathies are hereditary, but there are also different syndromes such as inflammatory, toxic, and infectious neuropathies [2]. The loss of muscular strength and muscular atrophy is observed starting from feet and legs in the lower extremity and hands in the upper extremity, while paresthesia/dysesthesia is observed in a stocking-glove distribution [5]. The most common Charcot-Marie-Tooth (CMT) disease or hereditary motor and sensory neuropathy constitutes a genetically heterogeneous group of diseases affecting the peripheral nervous system. CMT, which is characterized by the abnormal development or degeneration of the peripheral nerve, has different genetic pattern transitions. The disease begins during infancy in many cases. Symptoms include inadequate gait, muscular atrophy and weakness progressing from the distal to proximal extremities, foot deformities such as cavus deformity, deep tendon reflex loss, and sensory loss in the distal extremities. Inappropriate gait may be evident as walking with jumping and there may be a prone to falling [6–8]. Hereditary neuropathies are diseases affecting peripheral nerves and classified as hereditary motor and sensory neuropathies (HMSNs), hereditary motor neuropathies, hereditary sensory neuropathies, and hereditary sensory and autonomic neuropathies. Autonomic neuropathies include loss of sweating, bladder dysfunction, constipation, and impotence in males [5, 9].

Neuromuscular junction diseases are autoimmune diseases that result from the destruction, impairment, or absence of one or more proteins during neuromuscular transmission. Most neuromuscular junction diseases are acquired and occur associated with presynaptic, synaptic, and postsynaptic disorders. Myasthenia gravis (MG), the result of a postsynaptic disorder, is the most common neuromuscular transmission disorder [10, 11]. MG has two clinical forms: ocular and generalized. Weakness in the ocular form is limited to the eyelids and extraocular muscles. In generalized myasthenic patients, however, there is also a weakness in the bulbar, extremity, and respiratory muscles in varying degrees due to the cranial involvement. As a result, ptosis, diplopia, dysphagia, and dysarthria are observed. Myasthenic weakness typically fluctuates during the day, usually the least in the morning, and worsens as the day progresses with prolonged use of muscles, especially those that are stiff [12–15].

The main problem in muscle diseases involves the degeneration in muscle rather than in the nerve. It is a group of genetic diseases proceeding with progressive muscle weakness that causes subsequent limitation of joint movements, shortness of muscles, a decrease in respiratory capacity, and posture disorders. The loss of function in the body and in the upper and lower limb, impairment of organization of postural reactions, fatigue, loss of cardiopulmonary adjustment, and disturbed psychosocial condition are among the clinical and functional problems encountered [16, 17]. Different functional levels and clinical characteristics may be observed ranging from minimal influence to being confined to bed depending on the type of disease, the age of onset, and the location of the affected muscle group (proximal and/or distal). Bed confinement is observed in the early period in Duchenne musculoskeletal dystrophy (DMD) and Becker muscular dystrophy (BMD). However, facioscapulohumeral musculoskeletal dystrophy (FSHMD) and limb-girdle muscular dystrophy (LGMD) progress slowly and decrease the patient's functional ability and quality of life by causing scoliosis, wing scapula, difficulty in going up or down the stairs, toe walking and lordotic posture, difficulty in standing up from a sitting or squatting position, and Gower's sign. Gower's sign indicates the weakness of the proximal muscles, namely those of the lower limb. The sign describes a patient that has to use their hands and arms to "walk" up their own body from a squatting position due to lack of hip and thigh muscle strength, and contractures are observed [18]. In many types of diseases, the decreased pulmonary function is due to the respiratory muscle weakness and spinal deformities (kyphoscoliosis), which leads to respiratory tract infections and respiratory disorders. Cardiomyopathy and arrhythmia lead to cardiac failure and this cardiorespiratory complications cause death [19]. In the literature, various classifications were done according to the rate of progression of the disease, the affected area, and the body part involved, but the most recent classification was done according to the Belgian Neuromuscular Disease Registry [20]. The classification of neuromuscular diseases is given in **Table 1**.

According to the international classification of health, function, and disability (ICF) by the World Health Organization (WHO), neuromuscular disorders are associated with disability in body structure and function, resulting in problems with activity and participation [21]. These problems in muscle diseases can be addressed in two parts: primary and secondary. Primary disorders are muscular pain, atrophy, pseudohypertrophy, myotonia, and the loss of postural control, while the secondary ones are fatigue, difficulty in transfer activities and mobility problems, exercise intolerance, contractures, respiration, and psychological problems. The problems observed in the patient are related to the type of disease, pathogenesis, and progression of illness [22].

| 1. Muscular dystrophies | 2. Myotonic and relaxation disorders | 3. Myopathies | 4. Disorder of the neuromuscular transmission | 5. Disorder of the motor neurons | 6. Neuropathies |
|---|---|---|---|---|---|
| 1. Congenital muscular dystrophy | 1. Thomsen-type myotonia congenita | **a. Congenital myopathies** | 1. Myasthenia gravis | 1. Amyotrophic lateral sclerosis | **a. Hereditary** |
| 2. Duchenne muscular dystrophy | 2. Becker-type myotonia congenita | 1. Central core disease | 2. Congenital myasthenia | 2. Primary muscular atrophy | 1. Hereditary motor and sensory neuropathy |
| 3. Becker muscular dystrophy | 3. Paramyotonia congenita | 2. Multiminicore disease | 3. Lambert-Eaton syndrome | 3. Postpolio syndrome | 2. Hereditary neuropathy with liability to pressure palsies |
| 4. Dystrophinopathy | 4. Familial periodic paralysis | 3. Nemaline myopathy | 4. Other disorders of neuromuscular transmission | 4. Primary lateral sclerosis | 3. Hereditary sensory & autonomous neuropathy |
| 5. Facioscapulohumeral dystrophy | 5. Other myotonic disorders | 4. Myotubular | | 5. Werdnig-Hoffman spinal muscular atrophy | **b. Inflammatory** |
| 6. Limb girdle muscular dystrophy | | **b. Myopathy** | | 6. Intermediate spinal muscular atrophy | 4. Guillain-Barré syndrome |
| 7. Emery-Dreifuss muscular dystrophy | | 5. Centronuclear myopathy | | 7. Kugelberg-Welander spinal muscular atrophy | 5. Chronic inflammatory demyelinating polyneuropathy |
| 8. Distal myopathy | | 6. Fiber-type disproportion myopathy | | 8. Adult spinal muscular atrophy | 6. Multifocal motor neuropathy |
| 9. Oculopharyngeal muscular dystrophy | | 7. Metabolic myopathies | | 9. X-linked bulbo-spinal muscular atrophy or Kennedy's disease | 7. Vasculitis |
| 10. Myotonic dystrophy type 1 | | 8. Muscle glycogenoses | | 10. Distal spinal muscular atrophy | 8. Neuropathy associated with paraproteinemia |
| 11. Myotonic dystrophy type 2 | | 9. Disorders of fatty acid metabolism mitochondrial myopathy | | 11. Hereditary spastic paraplegia | 9. Neuropathy associated with plasma cell dyscrasia |
| 12. Other muscular dystrophies | | **c. Inflammatory myopathies** | | 12. Other disorders of motor neurons | 10. Amyloisdosis |
| | | 10. Polymyositis | | | 11. Neuropathy in systemic disease |
| | | 11. Dermatomyositis | | | 12. Other neuropathies |
| | | 12. Inclusion body myositis | | | 7. Hereditary ataxias and others |
| | | 13. Other myopathies | | | |

**Table 1.** Classification of neuromuscular diseases [20].

## 2. Body structure and function disorders in NMD according to the international classification of function

### 2.1. Loss of strength

The progressive loss of strength, severity of which changes depending on the type of the disease, is one of the leading problems that constitute the deficiencies seen in neuromuscular diseases. The functional deficiencies seen in neuromuscular diseases vary depending on the localization of affected muscle groups and secondary outcomes caused by muscle weakness vary depending on the type and progression of the disease but it should be remembered that the severity of the disease may vary due to the individual differences among the patients [23]. The loss of strength can be seen in the distal and/or proximal region. Also, the loss of strength can also be seen in the neck and mimic muscles. The reason for the progressive loss of muscle strength in neuromuscular diseases varies according to the nature of the disease. It is due to the reduction in the number and size of intrinsic contractile fibers in muscle diseases that are followed by replacement of these fibers by fat infiltration and connective tissue. These changes are caused by the disturbance in the nerve stimulation and transmission pathways necessary for muscle contraction [7, 18]. Also, the decrease in the optimal length of the muscle and deterioration of the sarcomere structure resulting from decreased physical activity secondary to the disease is among the causes of the development of immobilization. It has been shown in the literature that the muscle ceasing to the contraction has lost half of its strength after 3–5 weeks [24]. For example, patients with FSMD typically show weakness around the shoulder and facial muscles, thereby weakening the activities involving the upper extremity for function, while DMD typically shows weakness around the hips of the patients. Thus, patients have difficulty in activities involving the lower extremities [23, 25]. Approximately 75% of muscle patients have muscle strength loss in the proximal limb of the extremity, 20% in the facioscapulohumeral, and 4% in the scapuloperoneal part of the body [26, 27]. However, in acquired diseases (such as inflammatory myopathy), a loss of strength occurs subacutely. Some neuromuscular diseases affect specific muscles. FSHMD should be considered if there is asymmetric loss of strength in the muscles around the scapula, humerus, facial, and mimic muscles. Myotonic dystrophy (MD) should primarily be considered if there is involvement of the frontal and facial muscles, as well as the sternocleidomastoid muscle and the distal (especially tibialis anterior) muscles [26].

In CMT disease, in which foot and ankle problems and especially muscle weakness are commonly seen, weakness typically begins in the intrinsic muscles of the foot and follows the peroneus brevis and longus, tibialis anterior, extensor digitorum longus, and extensor hallucis longus muscles. This weakness pattern causes the muscle imbalance; while the plantar flexors remain relatively strong, the dorsiflexors weaken and consequently leads to the contraction of the Achilles tendon. As a secondary to this muscle imbalance, together with calcaneus inversion, forefoot adduction, and claw toe, pes cavus deformity develops typically in CMT disease [28, 29]. Also, symptoms such as drop head, ptosis, dysphagia, and dysarthria can be seen in oculopharyngeal muscular dystrophy [18]. In patients with peripheral neuropathy, however, the loss of muscle strength has been shown to be more prominent in the foot dorsiflexors, knee extensors, and hip flexor muscles [30].

### 2.2. Postural control and balance problems

The strength necessary for the movement of the extremities is generated, collected, and transferred to the upper extremity from the lower extremity by the postural control. Thus, the segments from the proximal to distal that are independent of each other operate in a specific interaction and concordance during functional activities [31].

The efferent system is composed of the structures necessary for postural control including vestibular, visual, and somatosensory inputs. The somatosensory input disorders can disrupt the postural control and lead to falls in neuromuscular diseases, which causes various conditions such as the weakness of the proximal or distal extremity (like patients with myopathy), axial weakness (myositis or amyotrophic lateral sclerosis), stiffness (myotonia), slow muscle contraction (nemaline myopathy), intermittently varying weakness (myasthenia gravis), sensory polyneuropathic end-effector proprioceptive (myasthenia gravis), and sensory polyneuropathy resulting in proprioceptive insufficiency [32–34]. While the efferent system is also necessary to maintain a similar upright stabilization, it provides effective postural correction after perturbations during posture. The inadequacy of the efferent system can disrupt balance control and cause falls [35].

One of the problems that threaten postural control in neuromuscular diseases is the progressive nature of muscle weakness; the other is the inactivity due to the loss of ambulation following the progression. In both cases, spinal stabilization is affected due to the motor and postural reasons, leading to spinal problems. In cases where the ambulation continues despite the decrease in muscular strength, many postural problems such as lordosis, kyphosis, scoliosis, and wing scapula are observed due to the increase in the compensatory responses in the body [32, 36].

Scoliosis develops before the loss of ability to walk in 30% of muscle patients. The restriction of the paraspinal muscles causing the lordotic sitting posture in extension emerges as a result of locking of the posterior facets of the vertebral bone and the vertebral bones remaining flattened [37]. In addition, kyphotic sitting position is also preferred by patients as a result of the weakened paraspinal muscles. This kyphotic position prevents the locking of the posterior facets of the vertebral bones and causes the opening of the joint faces, vertebral rotation, and lateral curve formation. Finally, the functional scoliosis develops as a result of the inability of the vertebrae to resist to the gravity, the multifaceted adverse influencing of the posture, and difficulty in controlling this effect [38–40].

One of the major problems in the clinical postural control is pelvic obliquity. It affects the sitting balance and causes increased pressure on the lower ischial tuberosity, making the sitting position uncomfortable [41]. Also, the hip joint left on the higher side in the pelvic obliquity tends to be subluxated. Subluxation of the hips may also be observed secondary to progressive muscle weakness [42]. The increasing pelvic obliquity affects spinal stabilization. This condition affects the sitting balance of the patients and causes complaints of pain [43].

Hip movements are an important factor in correcting lateral balance; hence, proximal muscle weakness can disrupt the ability to balance during external shocks. Distal muscle weakness can lead to falls through different ways; the obstacles that do not look dangerous in normal barrier-free environments can cause the patients with dropped foot to stumble and lose balance, increasing the risk of falls. In studies, it is emphasized that the rotations and movements of the ankles during standing is essential for maintaining and correcting the balance [44–47].

The wing scapula is observed in patients due to power loss in the shoulder girdle. Wing scapula adversely affects upper extremity functions [48]. Kyphosis and dropped head syndrome have been reported in some myopathies, particularly due to loss of strength in the neck extensor muscles. Patients with dropped head syndrome experience severe walking difficulty with loss of spinal smoothness [49, 50].

Proprioception plays an important role in stabilizing the body during both comfortable posture and unexpected postural perturbations. Therefore, patients with peripheral neuropathy are unstable when their eyes are closed during standing. In addition, reflex responses to postural perturbations are either delayed or decreased in amplitude or both [51–53].

In addition to the above-mentioned findings that are directly related to postural control, postural control plays an important role in many activities such as stair climbing, wheelchair activities, writing, bathing, makeup, shaving, eating, toilet needs, and in-bed mobility [54, 55].

### 2.3. Atrophy

In this disease group that proceeds with progressive muscle weakness, the patients become more inactive and sedentary in time because the muscles are the active structures responsible for movement in the body. It is stated in the literature that atrophy develops between 14 and 17% of muscle fiber after 72 h of immobilization [56]. Atrophy in muscular diseases develops later compared to peripheral nerve diseases. Selective atrophy of certain muscles may be associated with disease-specific disorders [27].

### 2.4. Pseudohypertrophy

Pseudohypertrophy is a false hypertrophy seen in the muscle. The hypertrophic appearance of fibrils in the affected muscles results from the replacement of the fibrils by the fat and connective tissue. It does not cause a real increase in the strength of the muscle even though the muscle volume increases [57]. The hypertrophy in the muscle fibers that have not yet been lost is accompanied by the increase in the fat and connective tissue, and thus muscle mass increases. It is most commonly seen in the gastrocnemius-soleus muscle group, occasionally in quadriceps, biceps brachii, and deltoid muscles. In addition, the presence of atrophic muscles around the muscles of the pseudohypertrophy may exaggerate this enlarged image [26].

### 2.5. Myotonia

Clinically, myotonia refers to any condition that prevents the relaxation of the muscles after contraction. The relaxation difficulty is evident in the first movement of the muscle after its resting position. Relaxation difficulty is reduced when the same movement is repeated after which the movements become easier. Although this is the only symptom in some diseases, in myotonic dystrophy it is associated with permanent muscle strength loss [26]. Myotonia seen in MD and ALS is a factor affecting patients' lives negatively in activities such as handshaking and jar opening.

### 2.6. Pain

Pain is an important problem in most of NMDs, but it is not typically a direct consequence of disease, and now researchers agree that chronic pain is a common symptom that can be seen in all forms of NMDs [58]. In a study on 511 NMPs involving DMD, BMD (myotonic musculoskeletal dystrophy (MMD), metabolic myopathy, FSHMD, and MG), Guy-Coichard et al. evaluated the frequency, characteristics, and effects of pain; they found that the pain was moderate to severe in NMDs and emphasized that pain should be regularly assessed in this patient group [59]. Pain observed in neuromuscular diseases is the result of progressive muscle weakness, fatigue, ligament laxity or stretching, and abnormality of walking and posture [60]. In neuropathic conditions, however, pain-causing mechanisms are neurogenic inflammation, abnormal involvement of the sympathetic nervous system, and the neuroplasticity changes in the central nervous system. In a study aiming to determine the structure and location of pain in muscle patients, 73% of the patients complained of pain, and 27% of them were found to have severe pain [58]. In another study involving the evaluation of pain in 125 patients with neuromuscular disease from different groups, 73% complained of pain, 62% had chronic pain, and 15% had severe pain. The localization of the pain was reported to be spinal column in 81%, shoulder girdle in 54%, hip in 47%, and knee in 47%. In addition, 67% of these patients reported an increase in pain with walking and 68% with standing [60].

### 2.7. Contracture

Joint contractures, subluxations, and dislocations are common problems in NMDs [61, 62]. When the strength of the muscles around the same joint is different from each other, the joint tends to remain at a certain position, the corresponding muscle becomes shortened, and this position of the joint is fixed in time, resulting in the formation of contracture. The development of contracture occurs in patients with NMDs in time. The stiffness, which develops in the tendon and increases until contracture occurs, can be prevented or reduced by exercise or splints holding the joint in the opposite position [22, 26].

Flexion contracture is seen in hip joint with loss of strength of the hip extensor. The lumbar lordosis is increased so that the upright posture can be sustained and the loss of strength can be compensated. However, the progression of the weakness in the muscles of the pelvic girdle causes the knee flexion contracture to develop [62]. The increasingly apparent loss of strength in the gluteus maximus and quadriceps muscle leads to an excessively increased lordosis. As the patient tries to stabilize hips in the extension, lordosis becomes more pronounced. As the muscles weaken, the patient tries to increase stabilization by pulling the arms back and increasing the lordosis to pull the center of gravity behind the hip joint. Due to the loss of dorsiflexor muscle strength, plantar flexion contracture develops in the ankle joint, resulting in toe walking [48].

### 2.8. Cardiopulmonary problems

Neuromuscular diseases cause respiratory problems mainly due to the inadequacy of the respiratory muscles, namely upper airway muscles (mouth and tongue muscles), external intercostal muscles, diaphragm, and abdominal muscles. The restrictive type of respiratory problem is observed in particular. Along with the involvement of the primary respiratory muscles in Becker MD and FSHMD, respiratory problems are encountered. The compliance of the chest wall is reduced, and then, there becomes a decrease in the total lung capacity. The disease may also cause kyphoscoliosis that increases the respiratory problem. Muscle fatigue in MG bears respiratory problems, whereas bulbar involvement in ALS causes increased secretion, inability to close glottis, and decreased respiratory control. In MM dystrophy and congenital myotonic dystrophy, a direct cardiac involvement is in the form of cardiomyopathies observed in addition to respiratory problems [63, 64]. Respiratory disturbances and cardiomyopathy may follow the development of scoliosis [65]. Respiratory muscle strength is insufficient in muscle patients. In particular, the maximal inspiratory (MIP) and expiratory (MEP) pressures are below normal values [66, 67].

The respiratory muscle weakness that emerges in the late stages of any neuromuscular disease results in hypoventilation and hypercapnia. This causes restrictive pulmonary impairment and reduced exercise capacity [68, 69]. Moreover, during terminal stages of all diseases with muscle involvement, the weakness in the respiratory muscles restricts coughing. This problem may result in difficulty in swallowing and aspiration pneumonia. This in turn may cause the mechanical ventilator to be connected [69]. While cardiac involvement is mostly a result of respiratory involvement, it can be primarily seen as cardiac muscle involvement in some NMDs. In patients whose heart muscle is affected, the heart will have difficulty adapting to changes in the body in the event of any increase in physical activity [70, 71].

The presence of cardiomyopathy resulting from a lack of dystrophin in the myocardium and cardiac Purkinje fibers affects the cardiopulmonary response to exercise. Myocardial dysfunction remains silent due to decreased physical activity until the end of the disease process. The effect of cardiomyopathy and restrictive pulmonary disease on physical activity is much greater in NMDs with slower progression [1].

## 3. Activity problems in NMD

Although most neuromuscular disorders have progressive and clinically distinct features, the most important common feature is that they lead to functional problems and activity limitations at various levels [72]. The activity limitations due to the functional deficits vary depending on the localization of the affected region, on the type of the disease with secondary outcomes caused by loss of strength, and even on the patient [22]. The patients with muscle diseases usually go to the doctor with complaints such as difficulty in climbing stairs or a slope, getting up from the sitting position, walking, raising arms and reaching up, and washing the head. The patients may also complain about numbness in feet and hands and not being able to open eyes, and difficulty in swallowing. At the end of the natural progression of the disease, there may be a loss of strength in both the proximal and distal muscles and the inability to perform many activities such as wheelchair activities, writing, bathing, applying makeup, shaving, eating, toilet needs, and mobility within the bed [73].

Fatigue, cardiopulmonary effect, and exercise intolerance cause an increase in fat mass and contractures. It also causes a decrease in the efficient use of locomotion (such as reduced walking space and more energy expenditure), a decreased motivation of the patient, a reduction in support of the social environment for activity, an increase in depression, and social barriers. These restrictions all result in a decline in physical activity performance in NMDs [1]. The progressive muscle weakness present in NMD directly affects the daily activities of the patient. Depending on the degree of muscle weakness in the proximal part of the body, patients may have difficulty in fine hand skills such as self-care, dressing, and hygiene. The patients may also have difficulty in transfers requiring upper extremity support, ambulation activities, reaching to mouth due to the weakness of the distal muscle groups, bilateral use of cutlery, and nail clipping [74]. In a study involving 208 neuromuscular patients, Pieterse et al. have grouped the activities that the patients had difficulty under the following headings: (1) communication, (2) eating and drinking, (3) transfer, (4) walking and moving around, (5) transportation, (6) lifting and carrying, (7) fine hand skill, and (8) use of arms higher than shoulder level [75].

### 3.1. Fatigue

More than 60% of patients with NMD complain about severe fatigue along with muscle weakness and many other problems. Fatigue has a significant effect on exercise limitation and includes the physiological fatigue and the experienced fatigue [76]. The physiological fatigue is defined as an exercise-dependent reduction in maximal voluntary muscle strength while the experienced fatigue is defined as difficulty in initiation and maintenance of voluntary activities [77, 78]. The physiological fatigue is the one with both peripheral and central components, either muscular or related to limitation initiated in the central nervous system (CNS). Many mechanisms may cause this fatigue and exercise limitation [79]. In neuromuscular diseases, there is the fatigue (peripheral fatigue) stemming from the local effects on the muscle function on one side, and there is the fatigue (central fatigue) arising from the level of CNS due to the feedback of the pathological condition in the peripheral nervous system on the other side. This type of fatigue protects the muscle from being damaged in the long term during the improperly set physical activities [77]. This symptom is perceived by patients as a different, abnormal, and feeling of being more tired than before the onset of disease [80]. In a study, which included the neuromuscular disease groups of HMSN, FSHMD, and MG, is indicated that severe fatigue is associated with functional impairment in daily life. The level of fatigue has been found to be significantly related to the muscular strength, the level of physical activity stated by the patient, sleep disorders, and pain. The fatigue level and the physical activity level are mostly associated with functional impairment in daily life [81].

### 3.2. Exercise intolerance and the impact on functional capacity

Exercise intolerance is a type of abnormally severe tiredness that develops with a certain movement in the muscle involved in that movement. In individuals with NMHD, several factors such as loss of functional muscle tissue, unused muscles, injuries due to excessive use, cardiopulmonary involvement, contractures, decreased locomotion adequacy (decreased walking speed and increased energy expenditure), decreased patient motivation, less social participation for activity, increased depression, and increased social barriers lead to a decline in physical activity [1]. Three problems affecting functional capacity and determining the level of physical activity in NMD are often striking. These are muscle weakness, difficulty in exercising, and fatigue. These problems result in a decrease in physical activity and a sedentary lifestyle [1]. Unfortunately, sedentary behavior increases exercise intolerance and causes a decrease in functional capacity in the subsequent periods, resulting in a low quality of life. The occurrence of fatigue is dependent on which of the energy-producing metabolic pathways were used during the activity. For example, if a patient develops exercise intolerance while walking but this patient is not uncomfortable while running fast, this should primarily suggest the impairment of lipid metabolism, which enables slow movements with type-1 muscle fibers. On the other hand, if the same complaint occurs in the arm muscles, for example, in an arm movement such as serial and rapid wiping, it should be primarily considered that the glycogen metabolism used by the type-2 muscle fibers is defective in this case [82]. Individuals who have been diagnosed with NMD are more likely to live a sedentary life when compared to physically healthy people. A person with a lower level of physical activity will later have an increased body weight even with a normal diet. Increased body weight makes the patient more inactive, and this continues in a vicious cycle [83–85]. Therefore, when it is considered that all of the components required for exercise are relatively affected in NMDs, a reduction in exercise capacity in this disease group is inevitable.

### 3.3. Walking and mobility problems

Mobility is defined as the movement of the person around self and transition from one position to another in a safe manner; it is a function that should be carefully observed throughout the course of the disease in NMD [86]. NMDs progress with disorders limiting the patients' mobility and their independence in daily life activities. The reason for this is that the progressive weakness of the muscles affects the functional levels of the patients negatively after a while, leading to the defects in mobility activities such as standing up, walking, running, and stair climbing [87]. In the majority of NMDs, there is a chronic clinical course emerging slowly or progressing with a rapid decline in muscle strength that leads to impaired motor function. Neuromuscular patients suffer from difficulty in standing up from the ground as clinical signs of weakness of hip extensors, quadriceps, and trunk muscles. The increasingly apparent loss of power in the gluteus maximus and quadriceps muscles leads to an excessively increased lordosis. As the patient tries to stabilize hips in extension, lordosis becomes more pronounced. As the muscles weaken, the patient tries to increase stabilization by pulling the arms back and increasing the lordosis to pull the center of gravity behind the hip joint. To expand the area of support while walking, the patient walks like a duck (Trendelenburg gait) [88]. Fracture contracture is seen in hip joint with the loss of strength in hip extensor and the lumbar lordosis is increased so that the upright posture can be sustained and the loss of strength can be compensated. However, the progression of the loss of strength in the muscles of the pelvic girth causes the knee flexion contracture to develop [39]. The weakness of the hip flexor and the eccentric muscle reduces the length of stride. The weakness of the knee extensor reduces the knee flexion moment in the midstance phase. Due to the weakness of dorsiflexion, plantar flexion contracture obstructs the stabilization of the foot during standing as well as the toe-off during the swing phase [22].

Contractures may lead to postural disorders such as kyphoscoliosis and scoliosis, which can interfere with the continuation of sitting and lying activities, and as a result, pain. Furthermore, ortheses that help maintain the force, which reduce the development of contractures and deformities, and surgical medical procedures lead to additional disorders [89]. In the advanced stages of NMDs, various problems are faced such as wheelchair dependence, being confined to bed, difficulty in in-bed transfers, inability to maintain mobility during climbing the stairs without holding to something like railing, not being able to stand up from the sitting position, and falling in and out of home [1]. This makes the patients dependent during their daily life activities.

### 3.4. Psychological and other problems

Even in normal individuals, being ill affects a person psychologically. In a condition such as that of neuromuscular patients where the disease is chronic and has many symptoms, this can make one feel more vulnerable. While some of the patients may cope with the problems associated with the illness and adapt to the social life, some of them respond to these problems with limitations in school, social life, and daily activities. These restrictions manifest themselves as a decrease in independence and self-confidence, limited participation, and social isolation, particularly in youngsters. For example, of two patients with muscular diseases with the same mobility level and the same severity of pain, one may continue to work while the other may quit or even show severe depression. In patients with NMDs, patients with increasing problems are severely affected, and with symptoms such as pain and fatigue, patients may not maintain their psychological well-being [90].

## 4. Participation problems in NMD

It has been shown in the literature that mobility (transfers and walking), which is one of the parameters of social participation, housekeeping, community life, education, work, and leisure activities were affected in NMD [91]. Biomechanical problems present in NMDs lead to participation problems as a result of the increased energy expenditure levels and fatigue [92].

### 4.1. Falling and fear of falling

According to ICF, falling affects participation by deterioration of the affected body structure and body functions [21]. Falling often has a complex form; it is defined as lying on the ground or at a lower level by accident, except conscious positional change for resting on seats, walls, or other objects, and is affected by multiple factors [93–96]. There are different descriptions, such as intrinsic and extrinsic factors, associated with the risk factors of falling [94, 95]. These descriptions include age, duration of illness, presence of prior falls, fear of falling, the number of used medicines, use of antihypertensive medicine, reduction in mobility level, and in-home and out-of-home dangers [97, 98]. Also, risk factors include muscle weakness, the presence of falling history, gait abnormality, balance disorder, the use of assistive device, mobility limitation, visual disturbances, arthritis, depression, cognitive impairment/mental status changes, postural hypotension, vertigo/dizziness, incontinence, and chronic diseases [99, 100]. Prevention and reduction of falling have a positive effect on the patient's activity and participation level [101].

### 4.2. Environmental factors

Participation problems are encountered as a result of the interaction of environmental factors experienced. Slippery floors, bed-chair heights, poor lighting, unsuitable ancillary equipment, improper building designs, and broken or uneven pavements may be listed among the factors [93, 102].

### 4.3. Psychological factors

As the disabilities and difficulties start to be permanent in a patient's life, the patient may lose hope completely. Such people remove themselves from activities and social life, and face many problems including depression as a consequence [103, 104]. Hopelessness, the thought that no one can help them, is a common feeling for neuromuscular patients [105]. In a study of 88 male patients with progressive musculoskeletal dystrophy, it was found that patients had problems in participating in private life and professional life and that more than half of the cases considered themselves to be socially isolated [104]. In his work to assess participation in myotonic dystrophies, Gagnon noted that the participation problems of these patients were about communication, personal care, and interpersonal relationships [106].

In NMD, the restriction of participation occurs in professional life, leisure activities, home, family, community, and social life [104]. Muscle weakness and reduced aerobic capacity may negatively affect participating in the professional life that requires long-term physical activity. Deterioration of interpersonal interaction and relationships is another reason for the restriction of participation. Sometimes, this restriction can lead to extreme consequences such as no communication with people or not being able to eat or drink in public. Participation in the community and social life can also decrease due to depression and fatigue. The psychological burden of having a degenerative and terminal illness affects the participation of the individual. The presence of each of these factors has significant adverse effects on the quality of life [107].

## 5. Assessment methods in rehabilitation of NMD

Nowadays, the key to planning a good rehabilitation program is to know the characteristics of the disease and the problems it will cause in the patient, and to evaluate the patient in detail in light of these features. In NMDs, evaluation is performed to monitor the progression of the disease, to determine the appropriate treatment methods, to investigate the efficacy of treatment methods, and to predict and prevent possible complications. Some evaluation methods are used, in which the disorders of the body structure and function, and the limitations of activity and participation are evaluated. These methods include evaluation of respiratory functions, muscle testing, normal joint movement, evaluation of flexibility, evaluation of motor functions and functional capacities, timed performance tests, functional posture, and gait analysis.

### 5.1. Assessment of muscle strength

Due to the diversity of neuromuscular diseases, it is crucial to determine the pattern or spatial distribution of weakness in the evaluation of muscular weakness to distinguish the etiology. It should be determined whether the loss of strength is general (e.g., bilateral, proximal, distal, or all) or localized [71, 108, 109]. The presence of the weakness predominantly in the proximal muscle groups or the dominance in the distal muscles, its presence on one or both sides of the body, and impairment in a single nerve or a group of nerves reflect the pattern of weakness [70]. In the case of huge weakness, it is determined whether the loss of function is proximal or distal, and which functional activities are limited by muscle weakness [108]. If the patient is having difficulty in standing up (around the hips) or combing the hair (around the shoulders), it indicates proximal muscle weakness, commonly observed among the weaknesses in myopathic diseases. If the weakness is pronounced around the hip, there are difficulties in getting up and down the stairs, standing up from the chair or toilet, or standing up from the ground or squatting position. If there is a weakness in the shoulder, there are many functional difficulties such as lifting heavy objects, reaching to and taking the objects on high shelves, brushing teeth, bathing, dressing, and combing the hair [108–110]. Generally speaking, proximal muscle weakness seen in the form of a limb-girdle pattern in the arms and legs and the muscle group of the shoulder and the hip circumference suggests a myopathic process (process affecting the muscles directly); the presence of distal weakness, however, primarily suggests prevalent polyneuropathy.

However, some myopathies cause distal weakness. This pattern usually cannot be diagnosed and diagnostic errors are possible in relation to the neurogenic feature. The types of myopathic diseases with this atypical distal phenotype are known as distal myopathies and include MD and inclusion body myositis [108–110]. In less frequent cases of distal myopathies and neuropathies, patients complain of distal upper extremity weaknesses that cause difficulty in activities such as opening jars, buttoning, turning the key, and turning the door handle. Patients with distal lower-limb muscle weakness complain about tripping over the pavement edges, having difficulty walking on uneven surfaces, or dragging feet during walking. Patients experience difficulties standing on toes (m. gastrosoleus) or in activities involving hands (intrinsic muscles) [108, 109].

Methods such as manual muscle testing, dynamometric evaluation, isokinetic (eccentric and concentric) evaluation, and surface electromyography (EMG) are used in the clinical evaluation of muscle strength, but manual muscle test (MMT) is the most commonly used method because of its easy application in clinical practice. Static and isometric contractions of the muscles are also measured with cable tensiometers or dynamometers. These measurements are superior methods because they provide numerical data in NMD, are objective, and reflect changes in muscular strength [111]. However, manual muscle strength measurements remain valid today because of the low reliability of dynamometric measures in muscle groups that cannot complete their movements against the gravity or distal muscle groups [112, 113]. Nevertheless, the physiotherapist who will perform the muscle testing in NMD should be able to analyze whether the factors that limit muscle strength stem from weakness, loss of motor control, pain and/or fatigue, or whether the movements completed during manual muscle testing through compensations. Also, the physiotherapist should consider the time and quality of contraction, the range of motion (ROM) of the joint, and patient's ability to maintain contractions. For this reason, the evaluating physiotherapist should have performed a significant number of MMT-related applications in neuromuscular diseases [22]. Another method is to find the maximum weight that a person can lift at once. For this purpose, isokinetic instruments have been developed that measure the maximum force at the specified speed in NMDs. These tools give information about both concentric and eccentric contraction. Studies have shown that it is reliable in good unipolar joints, especially elbows and knees. The use of these instruments is somewhat reliable because it is difficult to isolate the shoulder, wrist, and ankle muscles while measuring their strengths during particular movements. It is stated that it is more suitable to perform the force measurement using hand dynamometers providing better stabilization in these joints [114].

### 5.2. Assessment of range of motion and flexibility

Since there is the loss of muscle fibers in the intrinsic muscle tissue, contractures due to necrosis and fibrosis of the muscle fibers in NMDs, biomechanical analysis of the movement, and normal joint range of the motion and flexibility should be assessed for tracking the disease progression. The range of motion of the joint is monitored objectively by goniometric measurements at regular intervals [115]. The active and passive normal range of the motion should certainly be assessed. The physiotherapist should maintain a record of the presence of limitation and whether the limitation is due to the muscle, the joint capsule, the tendon, or the pain and make a comparison of the agonist-antagonist flexibility. The physiotherapist should consider this situation in the treatment program [22]. In muscle-induced limitations, shortness of muscles should be particularly assessed, particularly since the shortness of hip and knee flexors, plantar flexors, lumbar extensors, latissimus dorsi, pectoral muscles, tensor fascia latae, and quadratus lumborum muscles are considered functional [116].

### 5.3. Assessment of motor function

There are some tests evaluating motor function in NMDs."Motor Function Measurement (MFM)" is a scale with demonstrated validity and reliability developed to evaluate motor function in all NMDs. It was indicated that this is a scale, which evaluates the severity of motor impairment in the NMD group with good psychometric properties. It was indicated that, other scales, MFM is adapted to the severity of deficits at every level in patients who can or cannot walk and that it evaluates all of the head, trunk, lower, and upper extremities [117]. Some of these tests are specific to the disease, while others focus only on one area of the body. The "Spinal Muscle Atrophy Functional Motor Scale" was prepared for SMA patients

[118], the "Amyotrophic Lateral Sclerosis Functional Classification Scale" and the ALS score for patients with ALS [82], and the "Hammersmith Motor Skill Score" for patients with DMD [119]. Among the scales focusing only on one region/function of the body, Trunk Control Test and Trunk Impairment Scale are for the trunk [120, 121], the "Brooke Upper Extremity Scale" is for upper extremity [122], the "Vignos Lower Extremity Scale" is for lower extremity [123], the "North Star Ambulatory Assessment" is for ambulation [124] and the "Jebsen-Taylor Hand Function Test" and "Activlim" are for the hand functions [125, 126].

### 5.4. Performance tests

The timed and controlled tests of the subsequent tests applied to the patient, evaluating the patient's ability to perform a specific activity in a specific time interval. These include some activities such as rolling from the supine to the prone position, rolling from the prone to the supine position, rising to the sitting position from the lying position, standing up without sitting, walking 10 m, climbing 10 steps up and down, and putting on a t-shirt and taking it off [127]. The Minnesota, Purdue pegboard, nine-hole peg test, and Jebsen hand skill tests were developed and are the most frequently used timed tests to assess hand functions [55]. There are no average values for the timed performance tests. The results are interpreted by comparing the clinical findings with the subsequent tests administered to the patient.

### 5.5. Fatigue

Two different methods are used in fatigue evaluations: electrophysiological tests and scales. Since electrophysiological tests are expensive, scales are more commonly used in clinics. The Multidimensional Fatigue Inventory (MFI) [128], the Fatigue Severity Scale [129], the Piper Fatigue Scale (PFS) [129, 130], the Short Fatigue Questionnaire (SFQ) [131], the Chalder Fatigue Scale (CSF) [132], Fatigue Impact Scale (FIS) [133], and Visual Analog Scale (VAS) are among the scales used for assessment of fatigue [134, 135]. While each of these tests has its advantages and disadvantages and is used in a large population of patients, none of the tests have been specifically developed for neuromuscular patients.

### 5.6. Respiratory function

The most commonly used evaluation methods in the clinic are the pulmonary function tests including spirometric measurements of "forced vital capacity (FVC)" and maximum inspiratory and expiratory pressures (MIP, MEP) [136]. Cardiopulmonary exercise tests are the evaluation of respiratory muscle strength, thoracic environment measurements, and assessment of respiratory frequency. In the literature, the recommendations on which respiratory evaluation should frequently be done in neuromuscular disease are given in **Table 2** [137].

### 5.7. Assessment of cardiac functions

Symptoms of heart disease seen in NMDs depend on the severity of skeletal muscle insufficiency and the severity and type of effect. The degree of neuromuscular insufficiency may modulate the symptoms of heart involvement and over time and may sometimes suppress

| Test | Frequency |
|---|---|
| History, physical examination | Six monthly and in acute conditions |
| Lung function test (FVC, FEV1, VC—upright and supine) | Six monthly and after acute conditions |
| MIP, MEP | Six monthly and after acute conditions |
| Cough peak expiratory flow | Six monthly and after acute conditions |
| Polysomnography | At least yearly, symptom oriented and after acute conditions |

*Abbreviations*: FVC, forced vital capacity; FEV1, forced expiratory volume; VC, vital capacity; MIP, maximum inspiratory pressure; MEP, maximum expiratory pressure.

**Table 2.** Respiratory follow-up of patients with NMD [137].

these symptoms [138]. The most commonly used screening test in clinic has two types: resting electrocardiography (ECG) and ambulatory ECG (Holter). Cardiac rhythm, intraventricular state, and ectopic beats can be evaluated noninvasively with ECG [139, 140]. In particular, cardiopulmonary exercise tests in individuals with severe neuromuscular disease generally show a decrease in maximal oxygen consumption, a decrease in pulmonary ventilation, a reduction in work capacity, and an elevation of resting heart rate. These findings reflect respiratory muscle involvement, cardiac decay, and poor physical fitness [69].

### 5.8. Pain

The characteristics of the pain should be recorded, such as localization, type, frequency, day-night difference, factors that increase or decrease the pain, change in pain with movement, and the presence of a response to a pain reliever. It should be established which of the causing factors of the pain are involved such as muscle imbalance, trigger points, joint tension, and muscle spasm. One-dimensional and multidimensional scales are used to assess pain severity. One-dimensional scales are intended to measure pain intensity directly, and the patients make the assessment themselves. They are used especially in the evaluation of acute pain and in monitoring the efficacy of applied pain reliever. Among the one-dimensional scales are the verbal category, numerical and visual comparison scale, and Burford Pain Thermometer [141–147]. Multidimensional scales are thought to be useful in certain cases to assess all aspects of pain in chronic pain [143]. These include the McGill Melzack Pain Questionnaire, the Dartmouth Pain Questionnaire, the West Haven-Yale Multidimensional Pain Inventory, the Memorial Pain Assessment Card, the Wisconsin Brief Pain Inventory, the Pain Perception Profile, and the Behavioral Models [141–147].

### 5.9. Assessment of aerobic (functional) capacity

The purpose of evaluating functional capacity is to assess whether or not the maximal or submaximal activities can be performed in nonclinical settings. The ultimate standard to evaluate the person's aerobic exercise response is maximal increasing cardiopulmonary exercise test [148]. A suitable cardiopulmonary exercise test allows determining the underlying pathophysiological mechanisms. These mechanisms include broad assessment of the exercise response, the objective determination of the functional capacity and impairment, the measurement of the appropriate intensity required for long-term exercise, the amount of factors limiting exercise, and the contribution of various organ systems involved in exercise [149]. Functional capacity is assessed by maximal cardiopulmonary exercise tests, motorized treadmill, and stationary bicycle ergometer. However, submaximal tests are recommended in situations where maximal testing increases the patient's risk status and hinders his/her potential abilities, especially in individuals with significant risk for cardiovascular problems, and in cases where multiple cases are to be tested [148, 150]. The 6- or 12-min walking test is a form of submaximal exercise assessment, finds extensive use in the field, is employed in pulmonary diseases and heart disorders, and evaluates the response to various treatment interventions especially pharmacological treatments and exercise training. The ability to walk at a specified distance is a quick, simple, and inexpensive way to evaluate physical function. Walking is also a critical important component of the quality of life because it is highly necessary to accomplish the daily life activities and reflects patient's capacity [151, 152]. The validity study of the 2-min walk test has been conducted in neuromuscular diseases, and it was put to use in recent years since its period of implementation is short and it does not cause fatigue [153, 154].

### 5.10. Assessment of functional mobility and falling

In clinical practice, the activity and participation problems are also encountered as a result of disorders seen in body structure and function in neuromuscular diseases according to ICF. However, walking emerges as a function related to all of ICF subparameters (body structure and functions, activity, participation, personal and environmental factors). In particular, two important conditions must be considered for mobility evaluation according to ICF: the *capacity* is the ability of an individual to perform a function or a task and what the individual is capable of doing in his/her environment is the *performance* [21].

Functional mobility, bed mobility, transfer, transfer grounds, gait, and wheelchair should be evaluated. The physiotherapist should assess the level of effort to initiate movement, weight transfer, postural alignment, motion timing and motion completion, patient balance, support surface, walking assistance, and energy expenditure level [22]. The Rivearmed Mobility index is also used in mobility analysis [155]. Walking analysis is done by observational and three-dimensional analysis methods. Some parameters and assessments may be used to analyze the gait. These parameters include step-length asymmetry, position of the ankle during heel strike, knee angle in heel strike, knee flexion angle in stance phase, single extremity support, state of foot and ankle in push phase, knee flexion in swing phase, body position, presence of Trendelenburg sign in frontal plane, knee cap in transverse plane, and foot angle and arm posture. The evaluation should be advanced to investigate possible causes in case of detection of a possible impairment in these standards [156]. For three-dimensional analysis, computerized video cameras, passively reflected signal indicators, multicomponent power platforms, dynamic electromyographic analysis, and temporospatial gait analysis systems are used [154]. The timed-up-and-go test, 30-s chair-stand test, the 4-Stage Balance test [157–160], and risk analysis tools such as the Fall Risk Assessment Tool and STRATIFY (St. Thomas

Risk Assessment Tool) may be used for the evaluation of falling in neuromuscular diseases [161–163]. However, there is no specific cutoff value for NMDs in these tests.

### 5.11. Evaluation of activities of daily living (ADL)

Functional level deteriorates due to progressive muscle weakness in NMD, and dependence in ADL increases, while the tests such as Barthel, Katz, and Lawton are used for clinical evaluation of ADL in neurological patients [164]. FIM is the most preferred method for determining the levels of ADL in NMD. The advantage of FIM is that it has proven validity and reliability in evaluating many diseases and that it was found highly reliable by practitioners even when implemented by specialists with varying education and experience [165].

### 5.12. Sensory evaluation

In neuromuscular diseases with sensory involvement, especially in peripheral neuropathy, there is a need for frequent sensory evaluation. Surface sensations such as light touch (cotton), pain (sharp-blunt test), and sense of temperature (with hot-cold) and deep sensations such as vibration sensation, pressure recognition, touch localization, joint position, and motion sense should be evaluated [166].

### 5.13. General health measurements

These measurement methods give a general profile of health such as well-being, functions, social, and emotional health. The most commonly used assessments in NMD in this group are "Nottingham Health Profile (NSP)" and the Short Form SF-36 Quality of Life Survey [167].

## 6. The aim and content of the rehabilitation program

Although there have been some promising studies recently, there is no known curative approach to NMD. Physiotherapy and rehabilitation programs are gaining importance to maintain muscle strength, functional capacity, and quality of life as long as possible and to keep the patient in social life [168]. The lack of therapeutic approaches that can curb the progression of the disease in a large proportion of neuromuscular diseases increases the importance of preventive, supportive, compensatory, and rehabilitative approaches. The aim of physiotherapy rehabilitation approaches is to improve the quality of life of patients and their families. Applications in that direction are to delay muscle weakness or loss of strength, to prevent muscle shortness and distortion in joints, to prevent respiratory problems, to maintain the walking activity for as long as possible, to educate the family, to support and keep the function at different stages of the disease, and to increase functional capacity [169]. The rehabilitation program should include the protection of the functional level of the patient and the physical and psychological functions, increasing the physical and mental capacity of the patient, and slowing the progress of the disease symptoms. Patients have a significant number of clinical problems, so rehabilitation should be done with a multidisciplinary team.

### 6.1. The characteristics of the physiotherapist present in the rehabilitation team of neuromuscular patients

The effectiveness of the rehabilitation program to be administered in NMDs depends on the ability of physiotherapists to assess and analyze the main causes of the patient's problems [22]. As a prominent member of the rehabilitation team, the physiotherapists who will evaluate and implement the rehabilitation in NMD should be specialized for this group of patients and should be able to individualize the rehabilitation program. The physiotherapist should be able to identify the needs of NMD and be able to individualize the treatment program based on needs. The physiotherapist should have knowledge about the pathophysiology of the disorders in the patient and about the progression of the disease. The physiotherapist should be able to serve in different settings (inpatient and outpatient clinics, at home, at home-care facilities, and in workplace arrangements) and various age groups. The physiotherapist should be able to follow up the patient with the short/long-span controls during the planning of research on NMD, the development and implementation of outcome measurements, the setting of treatment interventions, and the natural progression of the disease and should be able to document the process well [22].

The rehabilitation program should include the muscle strength preservation, an exercise program for the prevention of contractures, increasing in respiratory function, increasing the functional (aerobic) capacity, walking and balance training, fall prevention and the stages of deciding walking aids, nutrition expert support, psychosocial approach, vocational counseling, and ergotherapy processes.

### 6.2. Preservation of muscle strength and prevention of contractures

Many international researchers agree on the use of exercise therapy in neuromuscular diseases. There are many physical and psychological benefits of exercise such as muscle strength preservation, prevention of contractures, increased flexibility, reduced energy expenditure, relieving fatigue, reducing pain, depression, social isolation and loneliness, ensuring the participation of the individual active life, sustaining mobility, and increasing the quality of life. However, the number of studies with a high level of evidence about type, intensity, frequency, and speed of the exercise is limited. When deciding on a possible exercise program, the pathophysiology, onset, severity and the progression of the disease, the age and sex of the patient, and the intensity and frequency of the exercise to be given should be considered [170]. In general, there is a consensus on the positive effects of mild to moderate exercise programs on muscular strength without causing significant muscle damage, particularly in the early stages of neuromuscular disease with moderate progress when the muscle strength was not severely affected [171]. Combined use of upper/lower extremity exercises with neck and body exercises is preferred in clinical practice due to the ability to spread force from strong muscles to weak muscles and relieve fatigue [172].

#### *6.2.1. Stretching and normal range-of-motion exercises*

Stretching and normal range-of-motion exercises can prevent the limitation of joint mobility that develops as secondary to the muscle weakness [170]. The static stretching, which is usually used for treatment in NMDs, is performed by proper alignment of the joint and bringing the muscle to its maximum length along the joint during stabilization of the unmovement joints. When the movement reaches the end, the position is held for at least 10 s and repeated. Although healthy individuals are recommended to make one to two repetitions a day or three to seven repetitions per week regarding the frequency of stretching, there is no definite information for neuromuscular patients. Daily stretching exercises are recommended. It has been reported that ROM increases with stretching frequency and the improvement was maintained for 4 weeks after the exercise ends [173]. Surveys show that a little 5-min static stretching causes a change in the muscle-tendon unit [174]. Resting splints can be used during sleep to prevent contractures. When bed confinement has developed, lower extremities can be stretched using the body weight with standing table [175].

### 6.2.2. Strength training

Strength training can be done with resistance exercises. Resistance exercise training is one of the most effective ways to improve the functional capacity of the neuromuscular system. However, the potential benefits and risks of strength training in neuromuscular diseases are still a controversial subject in the literature. Progressive strengthening exercises are also commonly used to increase muscle strength in neuromuscular diseases [170]. Progressive strengthening exercises improve lean body mass, muscle protein mass, contractile strength, strength, and physical function. This improvement varies according to the rate of progression of the disease. There is a consensus in recent years about the benefits of mild to moderate intensity strength training (25–40% of maximum weight) on muscle strength without any deleterious effects, especially for slow-progressing neuromuscular diseases [176]. Considering that the high-intensity (50–70% of maximum weight) eccentric- or concentric-type exercise programs would cause mechanical stress on muscle fibers and increase muscle weakness, they are not recommended for use on dystrophic types with rapid progression and membrane instability (such as Duchenne muscular dystrophy) [170]. However, studies with opposite point of view also exist suggesting that high-intensity training is beneficial with appropriate selection of patients [175]. However, no additional contribution to muscle strength and endurance was shown in a comparison of the maximum intensity weight training to the medium- and low-intensity weight training [171].

Strengthening principles applied especially in healthy muscles should be used carefully here. The level of intensity and resistance, which is above the patient's muscle strength, strain the patient, and cause muscle fatigue, should be avoided. The patient should be recommended to do the exercises in parts during the day so as not to cause fatigue. It should be started with little or no resistance and few repetitions, and the frequency, duration, and resistance of the exercise should be monitored with monthly or tri-monthly evaluations. The intensity and resistance of exercise should be revised if the patient experiences pain, muscle spasms, fasciculations, and excessive fatigue after exercises [177].

Electrical stimulation commonly used in the clinic for strengthening should also be used with caution in NMDs. Since all muscle fibers contract at the same time with electrical stimulation, it can increase degeneration in patients with low muscle fiber counts. For this reason, patients with muscle strength below three should use current types that will not cause fatigue [177].

*6.2.3. In-water exercises (aqua therapy)*

In-water exercises are the most appropriate exercise method for this group of patients. The water lift supports weakened muscles, permits functional movement, and in some cases can also be used as a resistance exercise. Pool exercises treat all muscle groups and maximize the aerobic capacity of the patient. It is particularly effective in a group of patients with limited energy levels. It is recommended in the literature to apply 45 min twice a week. Limitations of pool therapy are lack of accessibility and insurance payment [178].

### 6.3. Aerobic endurance training

Aerobic endurance training generates physiological responses that are different from strength training. Sufficient intensity and duration for aerobic training that involves the use of large muscle groups and will not cause fatigue is 50–85% of VO2max and 30 min. Aerobic training causes stimulation in the heart, the peripheral circulation, and the musculoskeletal system. As a result, circulation of more oxygen in the body leads to an increase in cardiac output, capillary density, and vascular transmission. For this benefit, aerobic exercises such as swimming, walking, and cycling can be performed, which put fewer burdens on the musculoskeletal system [179].

According to the American College of Sports Medicine guidelines, it is adequate to improve cardiorespiratory fitness for most aerobic training when an optimal frequency of 70–85% of maximum heart rate and 60–80% of maximum oxygen consumption are combined with an optimal frequency of 3–5 days per week [180]. A systematic review by Cup et al. suggests that an aerobic training at this intensity can be recommended to the NMD patients with a good functional level. In most of the studies included in the review, the cycling or treadmill exercises done at least three times a week and the use of approximately 70% of the heart rate reserve or the use of an estimated maximum heart rate are recommended. It is stated that the whole program lasting at least 10 weeks for both muscle strengthening and aerobic exercises and regular physical therapist supervision increases the effectiveness and improves the safety and suitability of the exercise [181]. However, in only 30% of all studies involving muscle strengthening and aerobic exercises, training lasted for less than 10 weeks, with an average of 5 weeks. In the literature, it is indicated that the aerobic exercise training in conjunction with muscle strengthening exercises is effective at evidence level of 2 or 3, especially in muscle diseases and neuromuscular patients with heterogeneous features [182].

### 6.4. Development of postural control

The activity of coming to sitting position from the supine position is an important activity of the body against the gravity and is one of the first stages of mobility. During this activity, which is very important for muscle patients also, the anterior trunk muscles contract concentrically while the posterior trunk muscles contract eccentrically. The difficulty of the patient in coming to the sitting position should bring into mind the possibility of encountering mobility problems and that the treatment should involve the precautions related to the trunk [121].

The equilibrium reactions have been tested in patients with isolated muscle weakness, and it was concluded that the muscle weakness is important. Although patients with distal leg weakness are particularly prone to stumble-like stability disorders, the stability has been observed to decrease following the external perturbations of balance in proximal muscle weakness [32]. In previous studies, it has been shown that balance correction strategies assessed by dynamic posturography can vary depending on body parts where muscle weakness is present. Some muscle responses are sensitive to balance perturbations, especially in the sagittal (anterior-posterior) plane, while others are found to be sensitive to the frontal plane or a combination of these two planes. This reveals that the proximal and axial muscles (such as paraspinal or gluteus medius) are more frontal-focused, the lower-limb muscles are more sagittal-focused sensitivity, and the knee muscles have the sensitive role in both directions in muscle response sensitivities following proximal to distal disturbances [183, 184]. Therefore, the patient maintains the balance based on these sided sensitivities, and the question whether the patients with distal muscle weakness are more distressed in the sagittal plane and those with proximal lower extremity weakness are more distressed in the frontal plane should be answered. It is thought that this information can also help in the planning of therapeutic interventions. For example, patients with complete proximal weakness are unstable in balance correction strategies associated with the frontal plane; these patients will need a different intervention than those with complete distal weakness and possibly unstable in strategies associated with the sagittal plane [185].

### 6.5. Increasing respiratory capacity

If there is a coughing weakness in the patient, airway cleaning techniques such as air stacking (glossopharyngeal breathing), mechanical, and manual coughing should be applied as soon as possible [186]. Increasing the pulmonary capacity, breathing exercises, diaphragm breathing exercises, and thoracic expansion exercises aim to maximize the expansion of the patients' lungs and should be taught to the patient.

Pulmonary expansion therapy and maximal insufflation therapy (mask or mechanically assisted hyperinsufflation) increase the forced inspiratory vital capacity. It is reported in the literature that maximum insufflation therapy is important in increasing peak cough flow for neuromuscular patients with vital capacities less than 1500 mL [187]. Manually supported coughing techniques should be continued for maximum expansion. Secretion mobilization can also be provided by a positive expiratory pressure device. With a positive expiratory pressure device, patients breathe freely and breathe against a moderate resistance; air pressure activates secretions, preventing atelectasis. Traditional chest physiotherapy techniques used for airway cleaning should be taught to this patient population. This involves taking the patient to different positions, then clapping on the chest wall, vibrating, and coughing. However, it should be taken into account that Trendelenburg, lateral recumbent, and prone positions are difficult to tolerate in NMDs [186].

*6.5.1. Mechanical insufflation-exsufflation (assisted coughing device)*

The assisted coughing device operates according to the principle of vacuum cleaning. Cleansing of strong expiratory flow and secretions is achieved without tracheostomy by applying negative pressure after maximal insufflation with a positive pressure of the oronasal mask. It is also known to be more effective than aspiration catheters in tracheostomized patients. The use of a peak cough flow below 160 L/min in NMDs is found appropriate. However, in recent publications, a cough flow of at least 300 L/min was used to initiate maximum assisted mechanical cough assistance [187–189]. The assisted coughing device produces an airflow of approximately 10 L/s with pressures between -40 cm $HO_2$ and 40 cm $HO_2$. It is a very vital and efficient device to use in patients using a mechanical ventilator and has reduced coughing ability [190]. Noninvasive mechanical ventilation devices are employed in later stages of NMDs. Indications for noninvasive mechanical ventilation are shown in **Table 3**.

### 6.6. Reduction of pain

The mechanism of pain has not been identified in detail in neuromuscular patients. For this reason, the physiotherapist should choose the appropriate treatment modality based on the pain source he/she has identified. From among the physiotherapy techniques, ultrasound, TENS, hot/cold application, and massage may be used but there are very few studies on the effectiveness of these techniques. There are even contradictory results regarding the increased muscle destruction of the ultrasound and hot application. Physiotherapists should be so cautious in their use. It is thought that TENS is preferred because it uses different ways of inhibiting pain.

In the loss of muscle strength, joint pain can often be associated with improper alignment or excessive stretching of the joint capsule. Pain relief is possible with proper alignment of the joint and removal of excessive tension. However, since the weakness of each NMD patient is seen in different forms, it should be analyzed well before choosing the appropriate treatment. External support such as splints can be used when muscle weakness makes self-stabilization impossible. An external shoulder splint may be utilized for the shoulder pain resulting from shoulder subluxation while an abdominal mattress may be preferred for back pain due to the excessive weakening of the abdominal muscles [22].

Shoulder pain may arise due to the single-point cane, which NMD patients often prefer for cosmetic reasons. In this case, a four-point walker may be used if the patient's energy

- Chronic daytime hypercapnia with $PaCO_2 \geq 45$ mmHg
- Nocturnal hypercapnia with $PaCO_2 \geq 50$ mmHg
- Daytime normocapnia with a rise in $PTcCO_2$ of ≥ 10 mmHg during the night
- A rapid, significant reduction in VC
- MIP <50 $H_2O$ cm or 60% and FVC <40%

*Abbreviations*: $PaCO_2$, partial pressure of carbon dioxide ($CO_2$) in the blood; $PTcCO_2$, transcutaneous carbon dioxide; VC, vital capacity; MIP, maximum inspiratory pressure; FVC, forced vital capacity.

**Table 3.** Indications for noninvasive ventilation in neuromuscular diseases [137].

expenditure level is not increased [154]. If the size of the four-point walker is not suitable for the patient and the patient bends forward, this may be a possible reason for back pain. If the patient has a lack of postural control and the arms carry the whole load when the walker is used, this may be considered as a possible cause of pain in the upper extremity. If the patient's upper extremity strength is unable to carry the weight of the walker and the patient has upper extremity and back pain, then the arm-assisted wheeled walker can be used to reduce pain.

The shoulder pain that occurs in patients using wheelchairs may be due to the improperly positioned inadequate arm support, which prevents the alignment of the humerus in the glenohumeral joint, while the hip and back pain may be caused by improper knee-hip level and foot support. Wheelchair cushions, unsuitable pillows, and the bed should be considered as possible reasons for pain. The preference of a pressure distributing bed is also an important factor in reducing pain in bed dependence [22].

### 6.7. Walking and balance training

Mobility target should be determined according to the evaluation and the progression of the disease. Walking training should include endurance training, teaching the use of walking aids, orthotic approach and fall prevention, learning safe-fall techniques, teaching how to stand up after falling, and teaching energy conservation techniques. In NMDs, the level of energy expenditure during walking increases [191]. For this reason, physiotherapists should choose the most appropriate aerobic exercise for the patient; the disease and exercise tolerance should be closely monitored. Physiotherapists should evaluate and recommend ambulatory assistive devices, transfer supports, and orthoses for improved walking, energy conservation, and safety if the patient develops weakness. However, the use of wrong assistive devices may alter the patient's optimal gait pattern and may prevent gait function or cause new problems in the patient. It has been shown that walking aids affect stability in a negative way in a group of studies in the literature. The reason for stability to be affected is that the upper- and lower-extremity balance reactions, normally used to protect against falls and protective, are restricted by the walking aid [192]. There is also the problem of lower-extremity tripping over the mobility aid. It is stated that the reciprocal movements necessary to use the walking aid in these situations are difficult to achieve. Choosing the right walking aid, using the right size, and training with the walking aid can reduce the risk of falling [193]. Walking aids prevent falls when used safely; it should be kept in mind that they may be the most important reason for falling if misused [154]. When the falling story is evaluated, the frequency of falls, during which activity the fall occurred, the balance, sense, proprioception, the characteristics of the fall area, and the home environment should be evaluated. Balance and proprioception training should be given as a result of these evaluations. Recommendations for orthosis can be made by a physiotherapist, an orthotist, or a doctor. When orthosis advice is given, the desired function, weight, and device tolerance should be considered, and a lightweight material should be used. The articulated orthoses may be granted if the patient has muscular strength to control the dynamic orthosis, fixed orthoses may be given if not. Walking training should be provided with the orthosis given [22].

### 6.8. Training for the activities of daily living and adaptive approach

It has been shown that there is a negative correlation between manual muscle test results and FIM results in studies performed [194]. The manual muscle test score of 3 is a critical threshold value. The average muscle strength value being 3 is an important indicator that the patient is dependent/independent in the activities of daily living or a candidate for dependence [195]. Weakness in the upper extremities causes patients to lose their independence in basic activities of daily living such as dressing, nutrition, and personal hygiene. In addition, muscle weakness around the shoulder in diseases with more pronounced proximal muscle weakness causes difficulty in performing activities such as shaving, makeup, and weight lifting; distal muscle weakness causes difficulty in gripping and increases the functional deficiencies of patients in activities such as writing, turning the faucet on/off, and unlocking the door with the key [127]. It has been found that the activities indicated by the patients as the most challenging are climbing stairs (72%), taking along walk (40%), and getting on or off the bus (18%) [195].

To be able to perform the activities of daily living independently, the functional capacity of the individual and the environmental conditions necessary to carry out the activity should be able to match fully with each other. When there is a discrepancy between these two parameters, problems arise which affect the quality of life of the person negatively. These problems can be solved by increasing the functional capacity of the individual, reducing environmental demands, and adapting the environment to the individual [196]. For example, if a person needs to pick up any item at the top shelf, he/she should be able to lift his/her arms over his/her shoulder. If he/she cannot lift his/her arms, he/she cannot be considered completely independent of this activity. This problem can be solved by strengthening the shoulder muscles to allow the arms to be raised above the head, or by lowering the height of the shelf with a manually adjustable cabinet to the level at which the patient can lift his/her arms [195]. Neuromuscular patients need different aids at various periods of the disease to be able to perform their daily life activities independently as the disease progresses. Assistive devices include tools designed or modified to increase the functional capacities of persons with disabilities that can be considered in a broad spectrum. This equipment can range from simple tools such as jar openers, pen holders, electronic environmental control systems, toilet lifts to prevent fatigue, handlebars, forks, and spoons with thickened stalk, and adjustable beds to complex technological tools. Parallel to the developments in technology, assistive devices are also renewed every day. As the complexity and technology increase, the costs of the assistive devices also increase, making it difficult for patients to obtain these devices. Appropriate devices prescribed to a neuromuscular patient increase the patient's quality of life [195, 197].

## Author details

Yasemin Parlak Demir

Address all correspondence to: fztyasemin@yahoo.com

Hacettepe University, Physiotherapy and Rehabilitation, Ankara, Turkey

## References

[1] McDonald CM. Physical activity, health impairments, and disability in neuromuscular disease. American Journal of Physical Medicine and Rehabilitation. 2002; 81(11 Suppl): 108–20.

[2] Andersson PB, Rando TA. Neuromuscular disorders of childhood. Current Opinion in Pediatrics. 1999; 11: 497–503.

[3] Lunn MR, Wang CH. Spinal muscular atrophy. Lancet. 2008; 21: 2120–33.

[4] Martini R. The effect of myelinating Schwann cells on axons. Muscle & Nerve. 2001; 24(4): 456–66.

[5] Dyck PJ. The causes, classification, and treatment of peripheral neuropathy. New England Journal of Medicine. 1982; 307(5): 283–86.

[6] Casasnovas C, Cano LM, Albertí A, Céspedes M, Rigo G. Charcot-Marie-tooth disease. Foot & Ankle Specialist. 2008; 1: 350–4.

[7] Pareyson D, Marchesi C, Salsano E. Hereditary predominantly motor neuropathies. Current Opinion in Neurology. 2009; 22: 451–9.

[8] Wilmshurst JM, Ouvrier R. Hereditary peripheral neuropathies of childhood: an overview for clinicians. Neuromuscular Disorders. 2011; 21: 763–75.

[9] Parman Y. Hereditary neuropathies. Current Opinion in Neurology. 2007; 20: 542–7.

[10] Vincent A. Immunology of disorders of neuromuscular transmission. Acta Neurologica Scandinavica. 2006; 113: 1–7.

[11] Kaminski HJ. Myasthenia gravis and related disorders. In: Ubogu EE, Ruff RL, editors. Neuromuscular Junction Physiology and Pathophysiology. 2nd ed.Humanan press Springer,USA;2009. pp. 1–12.

[12] Oflazer P, Deymeer F. chap. 37: Kas ve nöromüsküler kavsak hastalıkları. In: Öge E, Baykan B, editors. Nöroloji, 2nd ed. İstanbul Üniversitesi Yayınları, İstanbul; 2011. pp. 729–71.

[13] Ralph JW, Aminoff MJ. chap. 60: Neuromuscular complications of general medical diseases. In: Aminoff MJ, editors. Neurology and General Medicine, 4th ed. Elsevier Health Sciences, Philadelphia; 2008. pp. 1123–25.

[14] Sanders DB, Howard JF. chap. 82: Disorders of neuromuscular transmission. In: Bradley WG, Daroff RB, Fenichel J, editors. Neurology in Clinical Practice, Elsevier Health Sciences, Philadelphia; 2008. pp. 2383–94.

[15] Meriggliolі MN. Myasthenia gravis: immunopathogenesis, diagnosis, and management. Continuum. 2009; 15(1): 35–62.

[16] Tiffreau V, Viet G, Thevenon A. Pain and neuromuscular disease: the results of a survey. American Journal of Physical Medicine and Rehabilitation. 2006; 85(9): 756–66.

[17] Nätterlund B, Ahlström G. Activities of daily living and quality of life in person with muscular dystrophy. Journal of Rehabilitation Medicine. 2001; 33: 206–11.

[18] Manzur AY, Muntoni F. Diagnosis and new treatments in muscular dystrophies. Postgraduate Medical Journal. 2009; 85(1009): 622–30.

[19] Flanigan KM. The muscular dystrophies. Seminars in Neurology. 2012; 32: 255–63.

[20] Roy AJ, Van den Bergh P, Van Damme P, Doggen K, Van Casteren V, The BNMDR Scientific Committee. Early stages of building a rare disease registry, methods and 2010 data from the Belgian Neuromuscular Disease Registry (BNMDR). Acta Neurologica Belgica. 2015; 115(2): 97–104.

[21] Organization WH. International Classification of Functioning, Disability and Health: ICF: World Health Organization. 2001.

[22] Johnson LB, Florence JM, Abresch RT. Physical therapy evaluation and management in neuromuscular diseases. Physical Medicine and Rehabilitation Clinics of North America. 2012; 23(3): 633–51.

[23] Zupan A. Assessment of the functional abilities of the upper limbs in patients with neuromuscular diseases. Disability and Rehabilitation. 1996; 18(2): 69–75.

[24] Porth C. Essentials of pathophysiology: Concepts of altered health states. Lippincott Williams & Wilkins, Philadelphia; 2011.

[25] Yang M, Finkel R. Overview of paediatric neuromuscular disorders and related pulmonary issues: diagnostic and therapeutic considerations. Paediatric Respiratory Reviews. 2010; 11(1): 9–17.

[26] Serdaroğlu PDF. Kas ve nöromüsküler kavsak hastalıkları. Istanbul: Nobel Tıp Kitapevleri. 2004. 28 p.

[27] Dubowitz V, Heckmatt J. Management of muscular dystrophy. Pharmacological and physical aspects. British Medical Bulletin. 1980; 36(2): 139–44.

[28] Refshauge KM, Raymond J, Nicholson G, Van den Dolder PA. Night splinting does not increase ankle range of motion in people with Charcot-Marie-Tooth disease: a randomised, cross-over trial. Australian Journal of Physiotherapy. 2006; 52: 193–9.

[29] Burns J, Redmond A, Ouvrier R, Crosbie J. Quantification of muscle strength and imbalance in neurogenic pes cavus, compared to health controls, using hand–held dynamometry. Foot & Ankle International. 2005; 26: 540–44.

[30] Parlak Demir Y, Kılınç M, Aksu Yıldırım S. Periferik nöropatili olguların düsme ile ilgili özelliklerinin değerlendirilmesi. TAF Preventive Medicine Bulletin. 2013; 12(6): 633–38.

[31] Kibler WB, Press J, Sciascia A. The role of core stability in athletic function. Sports Medicine. 2006; 36(3): 189–98.

[32] Horlings CG, van Engelen BG, Allum J H, Bloem BR. A weak balance: The contribution

of muscle weakness to postural instability and falls. Nature Clinical Practice Neurology. 2008; 4: 504–15.

[33] Creath R, Kiemel T, Horak F, Jeka JJ. Limited control strategies with the loss of vestibular function. Experimental Brain Research. 2002; 145: 323–33.

[34] Nardone A, Galante M, Pareyson D, Schieppati M. Balance control in sensory neuron disease. Clinical Neurophysiology. 2007; 118: 538–50.

[35] Lord J, Behrman B, Varzos N, Cooper D, Lieberman J, Fowler W. Scoliosis associated with Duchenne muscular dystrophy. Archives of Physical Medicine and Rehabilitation. 1990; 71(1): 13–17.

[36] Kinali M, Messina S, Mercuri E, Lehovsky J, Edge G, Manzur A, et al. Management of scoliosis in Duchenne muscular dystrophy: a large 10-year retrospective study. Developmental Medicine and Child Neurology. 2006; 48(6): 513–18.

[37] Zobali G, Mathieu P, Miron M, Bellefleur C, Joncas J, Aubin C. Quantification of fat infiltration in spinal muscles in Duchenne muscular dystrophy. In: International Research Society of Spinal Deformities: Symposium. Vancouver, BC, Canada: 2004.

[38] Gibson DA, Wilkins KE. The management of spinal deformities in Duchenne muscular dystrophy. A new concept of spinal bracing. Clinical Orthopaedics and Related Research. 1975; 108(108): 41–51.

[39] Manzur AY, Kinali M, Muntoni F. Update on the management of Duchenne muscular dystrophy. Archives of Disease in Childhood. 2008; 93(11): 986–90.

[40] Bushby K, Finkel R, Birnkrant DJ, Case LE, Clemens PR, Cripe L, et al. Diagnosis and management of Duchenne muscular dystrophy, part 2: implementation of multidisciplinary care. The Lancet Neurology. 2010; 9(2): 177–89.

[41] Frischhut B, Krismer M, Stoeckl B, Landauer F, Auckenthaler T. Pelvic tilt in neuromuscular disorders. Journal of Pediatric Orthopaedics. Part B. 2000; 9(4): 221–28.

[42] Mubarak SJ, Morin WD, Leach J. Spinal fusion in Duchenne muscular dystrophy-fixation and fusion to the sacropelvis? Journal of Pediatric Orthopaedics. 1993; 13(6): 752–57.

[43] Canavese F, Sussman M. Strategies of hip management in neuromuscular disorders: Duchenne muscular dystrophy, spinal muscular atrophy, Charcot-Marie-tooth disease and arthrogryposis multiplex congenita. Hip International: The Journal of Clinical and Experimental Research on Hip Pathology and Therapy. 2008; 19: 46–52.

[44] Grüneberg C, Bloem B R, Honegger F, Allum JH. The influence of artificially increased hip and trunk stiffness on balance control in man. Experimental Brain Research. 2004; 157: 472–85.

[45] Bloem BR, Allum JH, Carpenter MG, Honegger F. Is lower leg proprioception essential for triggering human automatic postural responses. Experimental Brain Research. 2000; 130: 375–91.

[46] Edwards WT. Effect of joint stiffness on standing stability. Gait & Posture. 2007; 25: 432–39.

[47] Hsu WL, Scholz JP, Schöner G, Jeka JJ, Kiemel T. Control and estimation of posture during quiet stance depends on multi joint coordination. Journal of Neurophysiology. 2007; 97: 3024–35.

[48] İrdesel J. Nöromusküler hastalıklar ve rehabilitasyonu. Turkiye Klinikleri Journal of Internal Medical Sciences. 2007; 3(10): 68–77.

[49] Taniguchi K, Okino I, Yamamoto N, Matsumoto S, Tachibana N, Hamano T. Two cases with dropped head syndrome caused by hypokalemic myopathy. Clinical Neurology. 2011; 51(2): 110–13.

[50] Liao JP, Waclawik AJ, Lotz BP, Salamat SM, Beinlich BR, Brooks BR. Myopathic dropped head syndrome: An expanding clinicopathological spectrum. American Journal of Physical Medicine and Rehabilitation. 2007; 86(12): 970–76.

[51] Nardone A, Grasso M, Schieppati M. Balance control in peripheral neuropathy: Are patients equally unstable under static and dynamic conditions. Gait & Posture. 2006; 23: 364–73.

[52] Fitzpatrick R, McCloskey D I. Proprioceptive, visual and vestibular thresholds for the perception of sway during standing in humans. Journal of Physiology. 1994; 478: 173–86.

[53] Ledin T, Odkvist LM, Vrethem M, Moller C. Dynamic posturography in assessment of polyneuropathic disease. Journal of Vestibular Research. (1990–1991); 1: 123–8.

[54] Mehta J, Gibson M. The treatment of neuromuscular scoliosis. Current Orthopaedics. 2003; 17(4): 313–21.

[55] Hiller LB, Wade CK. Upper extremity functional assessment scales in children with Duchenne muscular dystrophy: a comparison. Archives of Physical Medicine and Rehabilitation. 1992; 73(6): 527–34.

[56] Nigam Y, Knight J, & Jones A. Effects of bedrest 3: musculoskeletal and immune systems, skin and self-perception. Nursing Times. 2009; 105(23): 16–20.

[57] Beenakker EA, de Vries J, Fock JM, van Tol M, Brouwer OF, Maurits NM, et al. Quantitative assessment of calf circumference in Duchenne muscular dystrophy patients. Neuromuscular Disorders. 2002; 12(7–8): 639–42.

[58] Jensen MP, Abresch RT, Carter GT, McDonald CM. Chronic pain in persons with neuromuscular disease. Archives of Physical Medicine and Rehabilitation, 2005; 86(6): 1155–63.

[59] Guy-Coichard C, Nguyen DC, Delorme T, Boureau F. Pain in hereditary neuromuscular disorders and myasthenia gravis: a national survey of frequency, characteristics, and impact. Journal of Pain Symptom Manage. 2008; 35: 40–50.

[60] Abresch RT, Carter GT, Jensen MP, Kilmer DD. Assessment of pain and health-related

quality of life in slowly progressive neuromuscular disease. American Journal of Hospice and Palliative Care. 2002; 19(1): 39–48.

[61] Shapiro F, Bresnan M. Orthopaedic management of childhood neuromuscular disease. part ii: peripheral neuropathies, Friedreich's ataxia, and arthrogryposis multiplex congenita. The Journal of Bone & Joint Surgery. 1982; 64(6): 949–53.

[62] Sussman, M. Duchenne muscular dystrophy. Journal of the American Academy of Orthopaedic Surgeons. 2002; 10(2): 138–151.

[63] Ambrosino N, Carpene N, Gherardi M. Chronic respiratory care for neuromuscular diseases in adults. European Respiratory Journal. 2009; 34(2): 444–51.

[64] Kartaloğlu Z, Okutan OS. Nöromusküler hastalıklardaki solunumsal problemlere güncel yaklasım. Tuberk Toraks. 2012; 60(3): 279–90.

[65] Smith AD, Koreska J, Moseley CF. Progression of scoliosis in Duchenne Muscular Dystrophy. The Journal of Bone & Joint Surgery. 1989; 71(7): 1066–74.

[66] Neder JA, Andreoni S, Lerario M, Nery L. Reference values for lung function tests: i. maximal respiratory pressures and voluntary ventilation. Brazilian Journal of Medical and Biological Research. 1999; 32(6); 719–27.

[67] Mehta S. Neuromuscular disease causing acute respiratory failure. Respiratory Care. 2006; 51(9): 1016–23.

[68] Aboussouan LS. Mechanisms of exercise limitation and pulmonary rehabilitation for patients with neuromuscular disease. Chronic Respiratory Disease. 2009: 6; 231.

[69] Kilmer DD. Response to aerobic exercise training in humans with neuromuscular disease. American Journal of Physical Medicine and Rehabilitation. 2002; 81: 148–50.

[70] Reeves AG, Swenson RS. Disorders of the Nervous System, A Primer Reeves & Swenson Chapter 12—Evaluation of the Patient with Weakness. Dartmouth medical school [internet]. 2008. Available from: https://www.dartmouth.edu/~dons/part_2/chapter_12.html [Accessed: 2017-03-15].

[71] LoVecchio F, Jacobson S. Approach to generalized weakness and peripheral neuromuscular disease. Emergency Medicine Clinics of North America. 1997; 15: 605–23.

[72] Harris-Love MO. Physical activity and disablement in the idiopathic inflammatory myopathies. Current Opinion in Rheumatology. 2003; 15(6): 679–90.

[73] Atay S, Kırdı N, Kılınç M, Yakut Y, Yıldırım SA, Tan E. Eriskin Nöromusküler Hastalıklarda Farklı Mobilite Değerlendirme Yöntemlerinin Karsılastırılması. Fizyoterapi ve rehabilitasyon. 2005; 16: 10–16.

[74] Saperstein DS, Amato AA, Barohn RJ. Clinical and genetic aspects of distal myopathies. Muscle and Nerve. 2001; 24(11): 1440–50.

[75] Pieterse AJ, Cup EH, Knuijt S, Hendricks HT, van Engelen BG, van der Wilt GJ, et al.

Development of a tool to guide referral of patients with neuromuscular disorders to allied health services. Part One. Disability and Rehabilitation. 2008; 30(11): 855–62.

[76] Kalkman JS, Zwarts MJ, Schillings ML, van Engelen BG, Bleijenberg G. Different types of fatigue in patients with facioscapulohumeral dystrophy, myotonic dystrophy and HMSNI. Experienced fatigue and physiological fatigue. Neurological Sciences. 2008; 29: 238–40.

[77] de Vries JM, Hagemans ML, Bussmann JB, van der Ploeg AT, van Doorn PA. Fatigue in neuromuscular disorders: focus on Guillain-Barré syndrome and Pompe disease. Cellular and Molecular Life Sciences. 2010; 67: 701–13.

[78] Schillings ML, Kalkman JS, Janssen HM, van Engelen BG, Bleijenberg G, Zwarts MJ. Experienced and physiological fatigue in neuromuscular disorders. Clinical Neurophysiology. 2007; 118: 292–300.

[79] Kalkman JS, Schillings ML, van der Werf SP, Padberg GW, Zwarts MJ, van Engelen BG, Bleijenberg G. Experienced fatigue in facioscapulohumeral dystrophy, myotonic dystrophy, and HMSN-I. Journal of Neurology, Neurosurgery, and Psychiatry. 2005; 76: 1406–9.

[80] Krupp LB, Pollina DA. Mechanisms and management of fatigue in progressive neurological disorders. Current Opinion in Neurology, 1996; 9(6); 456–60.

[81] Kalkman JS, Schillings ML, Zwarts MJ, van Engelen BG, Bleijenberg G. The development of a model of fatigue in neuromuscular disorders: a longitudinal study. Journal of Psychosomatic Research. 2007; 62: 571–9.

[82] Appel V, Stewart S, Smith G, Appel S. A rating scale for amyotrophic lateral sclerosis: description and preliminary experience. Annals of Neurology. 1987; 22(3): 328–333.

[83] Emery AE. The muscular dystrophies. The Lancet. 2002; 359(9307): 687–95.

[84] Rozman MB, Anton ZJ. Evaluation of the strength of elbow flexors in patients with neuromuscular diseases. Journal of Medical Engineering and Technology. 2001; 25(6): 235–39.

[85] Zanardi M, Tagliabue A, Orcesi S, Berardinelli A, Uggetti C, Pichiecchio A. Body composition and energy expenditure in Duchenne muscular dystrophy. European Journal of Clinical Nutrition. 2003; 57(2): 273–78.

[86] Bennekom V, Jelles F, Lankhorst GJ. Rehabilitation actives profile: the ICIDH as a framework for a problem – oriented assessment method in rehabilitation medicine. Disability Rehabilitation. 1995; 17: 169–75.

[87] Olsen DB, Orngreen MC, Vissing J. Aerobic training improves exercise performance in facioscapulohumeral muscular dystrophy. Neurology. 200; 64(6): 1064–66.

[88] İrdesel J. Nöromuskuler Hastalıklar Ve Rehabilitasyonu. Bursa: Günes & Nobel Tıp Kitabevleri 2000.

[89] Zebracki K, Drotar D. Pain and activity limitations in children with Duchenne or Becker muscular dystrophy. Developmental Medicine and Child Neurology. 2008; 50(7): 546–52.

[90] Carter GT, Han JJ, Abresch RT, Jensen MP The importance of assessing quality of life in patients with neuromuscular disorders. American Journal of Hospice and Palliative Medicine, 2007; 23(6): 493–97.

[91] Nätterlund B, Ahlström G. Problem-focused coping and satisfaction with activities of daily living in individuals with muscular dystrophy and postpolio syndrome. Scandinavian Journal of Caring Sciences. 1999: 13(1): 26–32.

[92] McNally EM, Pytel P. Muscle diseases: the muscular dystrophies. Annual Review of Pathology Mechanisms of Disease. 2007; 2: 87–109.

[93] Ageing, W.H.O. Unit, LC. WHO global report on falls prevention in older age: World Health Organization, WHO press, Switzerland; 2008.

[94] Al-Aama T. Falls in the elderly spectrum and prevention. Canadian Family Physician. 2011; 57(7): 771–76.

[95] Pollock RD, Martin FC, Newham DJ. Whole-body vibration in addition to strength and balance exercise for falls-related functional mobility of frail older adults: a single-blind randomized controlled trial. Clinical Rehabilitation. 2012; 26(10): 915–23.

[96] Maki BE, Sibley KM, Jaglal SB, Bayley M, Brooks D, Fernie GR, et al. Reducing fall risk by improving balance control: development, evaluation and knowledge-translation of new approaches. Journal of Safety Research. 2011; 42(6): 473–85.

[97] Udell JE, Drahota A, Dean TP, Sander R, Mackenzie H. Interventions for preventing falls in older people: an overview of Cochrane Reviews. Cochrane Database of Systematic Reviews 2011, Issue 4.

[98] Rejeski WJ, Brawley LR. Functional health: innovations in research on physical activity with older adults. Medicine and Science in Sports and Exercise. 2006; 38(1): 93–99.

[99] Lord SR, Sherrington C, Menz HB, Close JC. Falls in older People: Risk factors and strategies for prevention: Cambridge University Press, New York; 2007.

[100] Deandrea S, Bravi F, Turati F, Lucenteforte E, La Vecchia C, Negri E. Risk factors for falls in older people in nursing homes and hospitals. A systematic review and meta-analysis. Archives of Gerontology and Geriatrics. 2013; 56(3); 407–15.

[101] Zijlstra G, Van Haastregt J, Van Eijk JTM, van Rossum E, Stalenhoef PA, Kempen GI. Prevalence and correlates of fear of falling, and associated avoidance of activity in the general population of community-living older people. Age and Ageing. 2007; 36(3): 304–9.

[102] Resnick B, Galik E, Gruber-Baldini AL, Zimmerman S. Falls and fall-related injuries associated with function-focused care. Clinical Nursing Research. 2012; 21(1): 43–63.

[103] Duveneck MJ, Portwood MM, Wicks JJ, Lieberman JS. Depression in myotonic muscular dystrophy. Archives of Physical Medicine and Rehabilitation. 1986; 67(12): 875–77.

[104] Eggers S, Zatz M Social adjustment in adult males affected with progressive muscular dystrophy. American Journal of Medical Genetics. 1998; 81(1): 4–12.

[105] Ahlström G, Sjöden P-O. Coping with illness-related problems and quality of life in adult individuals with muscular dystrophy. Journal of Psychosomatic Research. 1996; 41(4): 365–76.

[106] Gagnon C, Mathieu J, Noreau L. Life habits in myotonic dystrophy type 1. Journal of Rehabilitation Medicine. 2007; 39(7): 560–66.

[107] Morris ME, Perry A, Bilney B, Curran A, Dodd K, Wittwer JE, et al. Outcomes of physical therapy, speech pathology, and occupational therapy for people with motor neuron disease: a systematic review. Neurorehabilitation and Neural Repair. 2006; 20(3): 424–34.

[108] Saguil A. Evaluation of the patient with muscle weakness. American Family Physician. 2005; 71: 1327–36

[109] Mastaglia FL, Laing NG. Distal myopathies: clinical and molecular diagnosis and classification. Journal of Neurology, Neurosurgery, and Psychiatry. 1999; 67: 703–7

[110] Jackson C E A. Clinical approach to muscle diseases. Seminars in Neurology. 2008; 28: 228–40.

[111] Kilmer DD, McCrory MA, Wright NC. Hand-held dynamometry reliability in persons with neuropathic weakness. Archives of Physical Medicine and Rehabilitation. 1997; 78: 1364–8.

[112] Kilmer DD, Abresch TD, Fowler WM Serial manual muscle testing in Duchenne muscular dystrophy. Archives of Physical Medicine and Rehabilitation. 1993; 74(11): 1168–71

[113] Mendell JR, Florence J. Manuel muscle testing. Muscle Nerve. 1990; (Suppl): 16–20.

[114] Griffin JW, McClure MH, Bertorini TE. Sequential isokinetic and manual muscle testing in patients with neuromuscular disease, a pilot study. Physical Therapy. 1986; 66 (1): 32–35.

[115] McDonald CV. Limb contractures in progressive neuromuscular disease and the role of stretching, orthotics and surgery. PM&R Clinics North America. 1995; 9(1): 187–211.

[116] Çıtak Karakaya İE, Yurdalan SU, Fiziksel muayene. Dalkılınç ME, Çıtak Karakaya İ. Yurdalan SU, editor. İstanbul: Hipertıp; 2014.

[117] Berard C, Payan C, Hodgkinson I, Fermanian J, The MFM Collaborative Study Group. A motor function measure scale for neuromuscular diseases. Construction and validation study. Neuromuscular Disorders. 2005; 15: 463–70.

[118] Iannaccone ST, Browne RH, Samaha FJ, Buncher CR, DCN/SMA Group. Prospective

study of Spinal Muscular Atrophy before age 6 years. Pediatric Neurology. 1994; 9: 187–93.

[119] Scott OM, Hyde SA, Goddard C, Dubowitz V. Quantification of muscle function in children: a prospective study in Duchenne muscular dystrophy. Muscle Nerve. 1982; 5: 291–301.

[120] Parlak Demir Y and Aksu Yıldırım S. Reliability and validity of Trunk Control Test in patients with neuromuscular diseases. Physiotherapy Theory and Practice. 2015; 31(1): 39–44.

[121] Parlak DY. Analysis of trunk control assessment methods in adult muscular diseases. Master Thesis. Ankara, 2011.

[122] Brooke MH, et al. Clinical trial in Duchenne dystrophy. I. The design of the protocol. Muscle & Nerve. 1981; 4(3): 186–197.

[123] Vignos PJ, Spencer GE, Archibald KC. Management of progressive muscular dystrophy of childhood. JAMA. 1963; 184(2): 89–96.

[124] Mazzone E, Martinelli D, Berardinelli A, et al. North Star Ambulatory Assessment, 6-minute walk test and timed items in ambulant boys with Duchenne muscular dystrophy. Neuromuscular Disorders 2010; 20: 712–6.

[125] Davis Sears E, Chung KC. Validity and responsiveness of the Jebsen-Taylor Hand Function Test. Journal of Hand Surgery (American volume). 2010; 35: 30–7.

[126] Vandervelde L, et al. ACTIVLIM: A rasch-built measure of activity limitations in children and adults with neuromuscular disorders. Neuromuscular Disorders. 17.6 (2007); 17(6): 459–69.

[127] Fowler WM, Abresch RT, Kimler DD, Measurements of function in Neuromuscular diseases, http://disability.ucdavis.edu/rrtc/publications/research_summaries/measurements_function, 2005.

[128] Smets EM, Garssen B, Bonke B, et al. The multidimensional fatigue inventory (MFI) psychometric quantities of an instrument to assess fatigue. Journal of Psychosomatic Research. 1995; 39(3): 315–25.

[129] Krupp LB, LaRocca NG, Muir-Nash J, Steinberg AD. The fatigue severity scale. Application to patients with multiple sclerosis and systemic lupus erythematosus. Archives of Neurology. 1989; 46(10): 1121–23.

[130] Gledhill JA, Rodary C, Mahe C, Laizet C. French validation of the revised Piper Fatigue Scale Rech. Soins Infirm. 2002; 68: 50–65.

[131] Alberts M, Smets EM, Vercoulen JH, Garssen B, Bleijenberg G. Abbreviated fatigue questionnaire: a practical tool in the classification of fatigue. [Dutch]. Ned Tijdschr Geneeskd. 1997; 141: 1526–30.

[132] Chalder T, Berelowitz G, Pawlikowska T et al. Development of a Fatigue Scale. Journal of Psychosomatic Research. 1993; 37: 147–53.

[133] Fisk JD, Ritvo PG, Ross L, Haase DA, Marrie TJ, Schlech WF. Measuring the functional impact of fatigue: initial validation of the fatigue impact scale. Clinical Infectious Diseases. 1994; 18 (Suppl 1): S79–S83.

[134] Elkins LE, Krupp LB, Scherl W. The measurement of fatigue and contributing neuropsychiatric factors. Seminars in Clinical Neuropsychiatry. 2000; 5(1): 58–61.

[135] Schwartz JE, Jandorf L, Krupp LB. The measurement of fatigue: a new instrument. Journal of Psychosomatic Research. 1993; 37(7): 753–62.

[136] Griggs RC, Donohoe KM, Utell MJ, Goldblatt D, Moxley R. Evaluation of pulmonary function in neuromuscular diseases. Archives of Neurology. 1981; 38: 9–12.

[137] Várdi K. Lung function tests in patients with neuromuscular disorders: how, when and why? Shortness of Breath 2014 July–September; 3(3): 132–39.

[138] Braedley WG, Darof RB, Gerald MH, Jankovic J. Disorders of skeletal muscle disorders of neuromuscular transmission. Neurology in Clinical Practice. Philadelphia: Butterworth-Heinemann, 2004.

[139] Deepak B, William JG. Cardiac function tests in neuromuscular diseases. Neurology Clinic. 2004; 22: 591–617.

[140] Stollberger C, Finsterer J, Keller H. Progression of cardiac involvement in patients with myotonic dystrophy, Becker's muscular dystrophy and mitochondrial myopathy during a 2-year follow-up. Cardiology, 1998; 90: 173–9.

[141] Bachiocco V, Morselli A M, Carli G. Self-control expectancy and postsurgical pain: relationships to previous pain behaviour in past pain, familial pain tolerance models and personality. Journal of Pain and Symptom Management. 1993; 8(4): 205–14.

[142] Collins SL, Moore AR, McQuay HJ. The visual analogue pain intensity scale: what is moderate pain in millimetres? Pain. 1997; 72: 95–7.

[143] Melzack R, Katz J. The MC Gill Pain Questionnaire: Appraised and Current Status, Handbook of Pain Assessment, New York, The Guilford Press, 1992; pp. 152–168.

[144] McCaffery M, Pasero C. Teaching patients to use a numerical pain-rating scale, Am J Nursing. 1999; 99(12): 22.

[145] Ogon M, Krismer M, Söller W, et al. Chronic low back pain measurement with visual analogue scales in different settings. Pain. 1996; 64: 425–28.

[146] Pasero C, Gordon DB. JCAHO on assessing and managing pain. American Journal of Nursing. 1999; 99(7): 22.

[147] Waterhouse M. Why pain assessment must start with believing the patient. Nursing Times. 1996; 92(38): 42–43.

[148] Arena R, Myers J, Williams MA, Gulati M, Kligfield P, Balady GJ, Collins E, Fletcher G. Assessment of functional capacity in clinical and research settings: a scientific statement from the American heart association committee on exercise, rehabilitation, and prevention of the council on clinical cardiology and the council on cardiovascular nursing. Circulation. 2007; 116: 329–43.

[149] Am J. ATS statement: guidelines for the six-minute walk test. ATS Committee on Proficiency Standards for Clinical Pulmonary Function Laboratories. American Journal of Respiratory and Critical Care Medicine. 2002; 166: 111–7.

[150] Solway S, Brooks D, Lacasse Y, Thomas S. A qualitative systematic overview of the measurement properties of functional walk tests used in the cardiorespiratory domain. Chest. 2001; 119: 256–70.

[151] Kierkegaard M, Tollback A. Reliability and feasibility of the six minute walk test in subjects with myotonic dystrophy. Neuromuscular Disorders. 2007; 17: 94–9.

[152] Takeuchi Y, Katsuno M, Banno H, et al. Walking capacity evaluated by the 6 minute walk test in spinal and bulbar muscular atrophy. Muscle & Nerve. 2008; 38: 964–71.

[153] Jain M, Logaraj R, Waite M, Shieh CY, Dastgir J, Donkervoort S, Leach M, Bonnemann C. Validity of 2 min walk test as an outcome measure in individuals with CMD and other neuromuscular diseases. Neuromuscular Disorders. 2013; 23: 738–852.

[154] Parlak DY. The effects of different walk aids on energy expenditure, risk of falling and gait parameters in patients with adult neuromuscular diseases. Hacettepe University, Health Sciences, Physiotherapy and rehabilitation Doctoral Thesis, Ankara, 2015.

[155] Collen FM, Wade DT, Robb GF, Bradshaw CM. The Rivermead Mobility Index: a further development of rivermead motor assessment. International Disability Study. 1991; 13: 50–54.

[156] Kirtley C. Clinical Gait Analysis: Theory and Practice: Elsevier Health Sciences, Philadelphia; 2006.

[157] Shumway-Cook A, Brauer S, Woollacott M. Predicting the probability for falls in community-dwelling older adults using the Timed Up & Go Test. Physical Therapy. 2000; 80: 896–903.

[158] Ganz DA, Bao Y, Shekelle PG, et al. Will my patient fall? JAMA. 2007; 297: 77–86.

[159] Rossiter-Fornoff JE, Wolf SL, Wolfson LI, et al. A cross-sectional validation study of the FICSIT common data base static balance measures. Frailty and Injuries: Cooperative Studies of Intervention Techniques. J Gerontol A Biol Sci Med Sci. 1995; 50: M291–M297.

[160] Vellas BJ, Wayne SJ, Romero L, et al. One-leg balance is an important predictor of injurious falls in older persons. Journal of the American Geriatrics Society. 1997; 45: 735–38.

[161] Oliver D, Britton M, Seed P, Martin FC. Development and evaluation of evidence based risk assessment tool (STRATIFY) to predict which elderly inpatients will fall: case–control and cohort studies. British Medical Journal 1997; 315: 1049–953.

[162] Oliver D, Daly F, Martin FC, Marion ET. Risk factors and risk assessment tools for falls in hospital in patients: a systematic review. Age and Ageing. 2004; 33: 122–30.

[163] Oliver D. Fall risk-prediction tools for hospital inpatients. time to put them to bed? Age and Ageing. 2008; 37: 248–50.

[164] Collin C, Wade DT, Davies S, Home V. The Barthel ADL index: a reliability study. International Disability Study. 1988; 10: 61–3.

[165] Ottenbacher KJ, Hsu Y, Granger CV, Fiedler RC. The reliability of the functional independence measure: a quantitative review. Archives of Physical Medicine Rehabilitation. 1996; 77: 1226–32.

[166] Curatolo M, Petersen-Felix S, and Arendt-Nielsen L. Sensory assessment of regional analgesia in humans: a review of methods and applications. The Journal of the American Society of Anesthesiologists. 2000; 93(6): 1517–30.

[167] Boyer F, Morrone I, Laffont dI, Dizien O, Etienne JC, Novella JL. Health related quality of life in people with hereditary neuromuscular diseases: an investigation of test–retest agreement with comparison between two generic questionnaires, the Nottingham health profile and the short form-36 items. Neuromuscular Disorders. 2006; 16: 99–106.

[168] Carter GT. Rehabilitation management in neuromuscular disease. Journal of Neurological Rehabilitation. 1997; 11: 69–80.

[169] Whittaker R, Ferenczi E, Hilton-Jones D. Myotonic dystrophy: practical issues relating to assessment of strength. Journal of Neurology, Neurosurgery and Psychiatry. 2006; 77(11): 1282–83.

[170] Abresch RT, et al. Exercise in neuromuscular diseases. Physical Medicine and Rehabilitation Clinics of North America 2012; 23(3): 653–73.

[171] Ansved T. Muscle training in muscular dystrophies. Acta Physiologica Scandinavica. 2001; 171: 359–66.

[172] Aksu Yıldırım S, Erden Z, Kılınç M. Nöromusküler hastalıklarda proprioseptif nöromusküler fasilitasyon ve ağırlık eğitiminin etkilerinin karşılaştırılması. Fizyoterapi Rehabilitasyon. 2007; 18(2): 65–71.

[173] Cipriani DJ, Terry ME, Haines MA, et al. Effect of stretch frequency and sex on rate of gain and rate of loss in muscle flexibility during a hamstring stretching program: a randomized single-blind longitudinal study. The Journal of Strength & Conditioning Research. 2012; 26(8): 2119–29.

[174] Nakamura M, Ikezoe T, Takeno Y, et al. Acute and prolonged effect of static stretching on the passive stiffness of the human gastrocnemius muscle tendon unit in vivo. Journal of Orthopaedic Research. 2011; 29(11): 1759–63.

[175] Milner-Brown HS, Miller RG. Muscle strengthening through high-resistance weight training in patients' with neuromuscular disorders. Archives of Physical Medicine an d Rehabilitation. 1998; 69: 14–19.

[176] Fowler WM. Role of physical activity and exercise training in neuromuscular diseases. American Journal of Physical Medicine and Rehabilitation. 2002; 81: 187–95.

[177] Muhammet kılınç et al. Nöromusküler hastalıklar, Fizyoterapi ve Rehabilitasyon, Editör Karaduman A, Tunca Yılmaz Ö, Cilt 3, Bölüm 4, ss 49–61 Hipokrat Kitabevi (Ankara), Pelikan Kitabevi (Ankara),Nisan Kitabevi (Eskisehir), 2016.

[178] Salem Y, Gropack SJ. Aquatic therapy for a child with type III spinal muscular atrophy: a case report. Journal Physical & Occupational Therapy in Pediatrics. 2010; 30(4): 313–24.

[179] Feasson L, Camdessanché JP, El Mhandi L, Calmels P, Millet GY. Fatigue and neuromuscular diseases. In Annales de réadaptation et de médecine physique, 2006; 49(6): 375–384.

[180] American College of Sports Medicine. General principles of exercise prescription. In: Franklin BA, Whaley MH, Howley ET, editors. ACSM's guidelines for exercise testing and prescription. 6th ed. Philadelphia: ACSM; 2000. pp. 137–64.

[181] Cup EH, Pieterse AJ, ten Broek-Pastoor JM, Munneke M, van Engelen BG, Hendricks HT, van der Wilt GJ, Oostendorp RA. Exercise therapy and other types of physical therapy for patients with neuromuscular diseases: a systematic review. Arch Phys Med Rehabil. 2007; 88: 1452–64.

[182] Van der Kooi EL, Lindeman E, Riphagen I. Strength training and aerobic exercise training for muscle disease. Cochrane Database of Systematic Reviews. 2005;(1):CD00 3907.12.

[183] Carpenter MG, Allum JHJ, Honegger F. Directional sensitivity of stretch reflexes and balance corrections for normal subjects in the roll an pitch planes. Experimental Brain Research. 1999; 129: 93–113.

[184] Küng UM, Horlings CG, Honegger F, Allum JH. Incorporating voluntary unilateral knee flexion into balance corrections elicited by multidirectional perturbations to stance. Neuroscience. 2009; 163: 466–81.

[185] Horlings CG, Küng UM, van Engelen BG, Voermans NC, Hengstman GJ, van der Kooi AJ, Bloem BR, Allum JH. Balance control in patients with distal versus proximal muscle weakness. Neuroscience. 2009; 164: 1876–86.

[186] Geiseler J, Karg O. Management of secretion in patients with neuromuscular diseases. Pneumologie 2008; 62(Suppl 1): S43–8.

[187] Kang SW, Bach JR. Maximum insufflation capacity: vital capacity and cough flows in neuromuscular disease. American Journal of Physical Medicine and Rehabilitation. 2000; 79(3): 222–7.

[188] Dohna-Schwake C, Ragette R, Teschler H, et al. IPPB-assisted coughing in neuromuscular disorders. Pediatric Pulmonology. 2006; 41(6): 551–7.

[189] Ishikawa Y, Miura T, Ishikawa Y, et al. Duchenne muscular dystrophy: survival by cardio-respiratory interventions. Neuromuscular Disorders. 2011; 21(1): 47–51.

[190] Kang SW, Kang YS, Moon JH, Yoo TW. Assisted cough and pulmonary compliance in patients with Duchenne muscular dystrophy. Yonsei Medical Journal. 2005; 46: 233–8.

[191] Menotti F, Felici F, Damiani A, et al. Charcot-Marie-Tooth 1A patients with low level of impairment have a higher energy cost of walking than healthy individuals. Neuromuscular Disorders. 2011; 21(1): 52–7.

[192] Maki BE, Holliday PJ, Topper AK. A prospective study of postural balance and risk of falling in an ambulatory and independent elderly population. Journal of Gerontology. 1994; 49(2): M72–M84.

[193] Bateni H, Maki BE Assistive devices for balance and mobility: benefits, demands, and adverse consequences. Archives Physical Medicine and Rehabilitation, 2005; 86(1): 134–45.

[194] Uchikawa K, Liu M, Hanayama K, Tsuji T, Fujiwara T, Chino N. Functional status and muscle strength in people with Duchenne muscular dystrophy living in the community. Journal of Rehabilitation Medicine. 2004; 36: 124–29.

[195] Öksüz Ç. The effect of occupational therapy on activity and community participation in neuromuscular patients, Hacettepe University, Institute of Health Sciences, PhD. Thesis in Occupational Therapy, Ankara, 2009.

[196] Verbrugge LM, Jette AM. The disablement process. Social Science & Medicine. 1994; 38(1): 11–14.

[197] Blake DJ, Bodine C. An overview of assistive technology for persons with multiple sclerosis. Journal of Rehabilitation Research and Development. 2002; 39(2): 299–312.

# 11

# Non-Invasive Brain Stimulation (TMS/ tDCS) and Rehabilitation for Stroke and Parkinson's

Tadamitsu Matsuda, Atsushi Manji, Kazu Amimoto,
Akira Inaba and Yoshiaki Wada

**Abstract**

The aim of this study was to clarify and compare the efficacies of rehabilitation using transcranial direct current stimulation (tDCS) and continuous theta burst stimulation (cTBS), a form of repetitive transcranial magnetic stimulation (rTMS), in convalescing stroke and Parkinson's disease patients. For both types of stimuli, kinetic analysis and performance analysis of upper limb motor paralysis and gait analysis showed an increase in speed of movement, and an improvement in performance was observed. Both stimuli resulted in significant improvement compared with a sham stimulus. Change in speed of movement and performance was observed with both tDCS and cTBS, but there was not a significantly large difference between the stimuli. Improved movement due to reduction of excessive tension caused by spasticity was observed. In patients with Parkinson's disease, gait speed and step length were increased. It is suggested that performance was improved because movement became smoother. The efficacy of tDCS and cTBS in patients with motor disorders caused by stroke or Parkinson's disease will probably be further improved when combined with physical therapy.

**Keywords:** noninvasive brain stimulation, rehabilitation, TMS, tDCS

## 1. Introduction

Cortical plasticity enables modification of functional organization of the cerebral cortex as a result of experience [1]. Facilitation of plasticity whereby cortical excitability is modulated using tDCS and rTMS, which are types of noninvasive brain stimulation (NIBS), is potentially therapeutic for patients recovering from stroke or Parkinson's disease [2–7].

Both rTMS and tDCS can improve motor function, cognitive function, working memory, depression and chronic pain (**Figure 1**). In rTMS, a magnetic field produced by an electric current pulsating through an electromagnetic coil placed on the patient's scalp stimulates the underlying brain tissue by inducing eddy currents in the brain parenchyma. In tDCS, the activity of the brain is transiently changed by altering membrane potential. The equipment used for tDCS is portable and safe, and therefore, in recent years, much research has been carried out into its potential clinical application [8]. Compared with rTMS and epidural stimulation (**Table 1**), tDCS is inexpensive and relatively easy to use without the need for additional holders to maintain coil position, or additional handling after affixing.

Both tDCS and rTMS have been used to up-regulate excitability in the undamaged ipsilesional area and downregulate excitability in the contralesional motor cortex. Neurophysiological

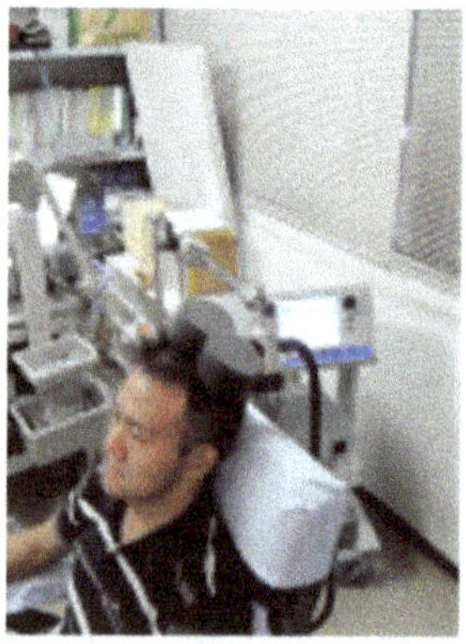

cTBS

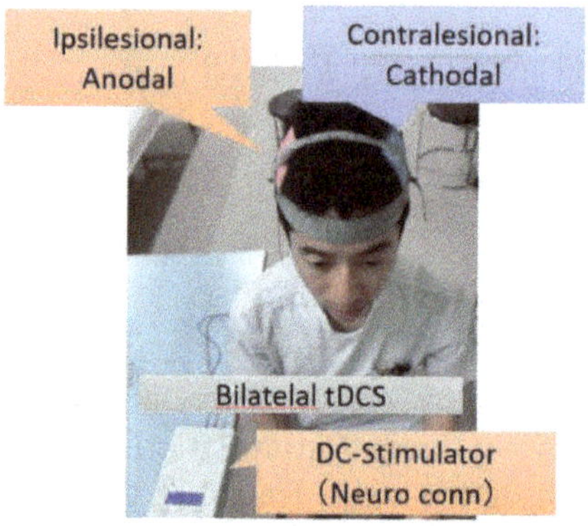


tDCS

**Figure 1.** Participants were seated in a comfortable chair with headrest and armrests. The rTMS of the motor cortex was performed with a 70-mm figure-8 coil attached to a magnetic stimulator. The tDCS of motor cortex tDCS was performed with the anode over the ipsilesional area and the cathode over the contralesional area.

| | **tDCS** | **TMS** |
|---|---|---|
| Mechanism | Change of the resting membrane potential | Induces action potential |
| Sounds during stimulation | Silent | Click |
| Dermal sensation | Tingling | Weak pain |
| Headache | 12% | 23% |
| Epilepsy | No reports | Report by stimulation with high frequency |
| Price of the machine | One million yen | Ten million yen |
| Size | Small | Large |
| Time resolution | Several minutes | Milliseconds |
| Spatial resolution | Several centimeters | 1 cm |

**Table 1.** Comparison tDCS with TMS [8].

studies of these treatments have indicated, poststroke, an imbalance of interhemispheric interactions resulting in disinhibition of the contralesional hemisphere and increased inhibition of the ipsilesional motor cortex (**Figure 2**) [9]. Improvement in motor and language performances has been explained by interhemispheric competition theory. The majority of the clinical studies evaluating the role of NIBS in rehabilitation were performed in patients with subacute or chronic stroke symptoms or with Parkinson's disease.

Recent studies have demonstrated that NIBS treatment can be more effective when combined with physical or occupational therapy, with brain activity changed by NIBS and motor function improved by rehabilitation. Accordingly, there is currently much interest in this combined rehabilitation, and here we will outline the effects of such rehabilitation for patients with stroke symptoms or with Parkinson's disease.

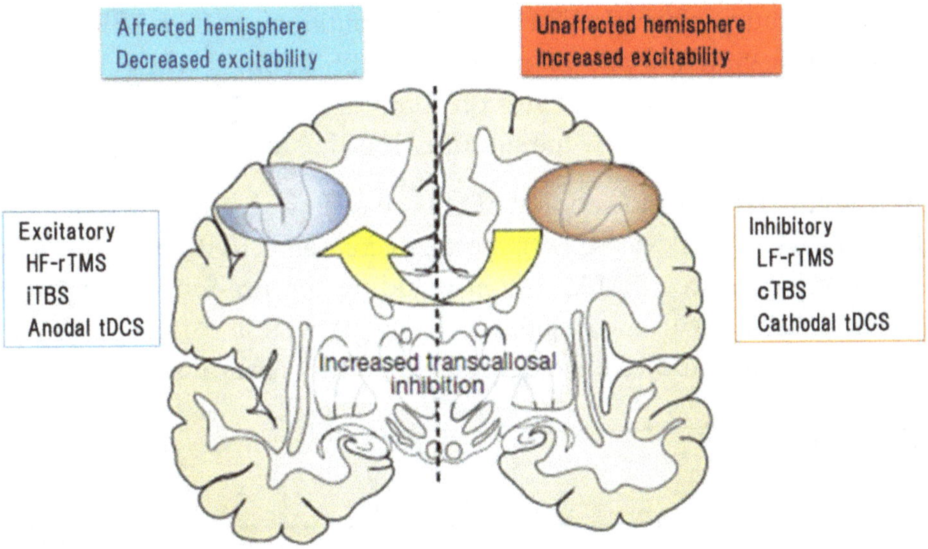


**Figure 2.** Influence of interhemispheric interactions on motor function and point of view on NIBS. Simple repetitive TMS (rTMS) protocols consist of identical stimuli spaced by an identical interval. Effects depend on stimulation frequency: at low frequency (LF-rTMS < 1 Hz). rTMS depresses excitability in the motor cortex, whereas at high frequency (HF-rTMS > 5 Hz), cortical excitability is increased. In addition iTBS and anodal tDCS is increased motor cortex, cTBS and cathodal tDCS is decreased motor cortex [9].

## 2. Noninvasive brain stimulation

Between 1988 and 2012, there were about 1400 publications globally on NIBS studies in humans. The first reported TMS study was by Barker in England in 1985. TMS uses a pulsating magnetic field produced by a current flowing through an electromagnetic coil, and eddy currents flowing in the opposite direction stimulate nerve tissue.

In general, single-pulse TMS (including paired-pulse TMS) is used to explore brain function, whereas rTMS is used to induce changes in brain activity that can last beyond the stimulation period. Noninvasive TMS of the motor cortex causes a twitch in the target muscle, evoking motor-evoked potential (MEP) on electromyography. The MEP is usually used to assess corticospinal tract excitability. Before rTMS is applied, the rest motor threshold (MT) of the contralateral first dorsal interosseous muscle is determined. In the present study, we used the same stimulation parameters with a frequency of 1 Hz on the uninjured hemisphere in six stroke patients with an intensity of 80% MT and located the "hot spot" of the brain area using TMS.

It has been reported that low-frequency rTMS (LF-rTMS) of <1 Hz inhibits local neural activities, while high-frequency rTMS (HF-rTMS) of >5 Hz excites local neural activities [10, 11]. Recent studies indicated that compared with LF-rTMS, HF-rTMS applied to the lesional hemisphere in the early phase of stroke was more beneficial for motor function of the affected upper limb [12].

Theta burst stimulation (TBS) is a modified form of rTMS, but the mechanisms underlying the cortical effect of rTMS and tDCS differ. TBS consists of pulses applied in bursts of three pulses at 50 Hz with an interburst interval at 5 Hz for 2 s. Continuous TBS (cTBS) is when trains of 20 pulses are repeated without a pause. Intermittent TBS (iTBS) is when there are 8 s pauses between the 20 pulse trains. For both, 1 session comprises 600 pulses. cTBS has an inhibitory effect on the brain tissue directly below the stimulus, iTBS has an excitatory effect (**Figure 3**) [13].

A systematic literature review showed that rTMS can exert a significant positive effect on the motor function in Parkinson's disease. In general, decreased activity has been shown around the supplementary motor area (SMA) (often including the pre-SMA) and the dorsolateral prefrontal cortex (DLPFC) with increased activity in parietal and lateral premotor areas in these patients [14]. Animal studies have demonstrated that cortical stimulation can improve

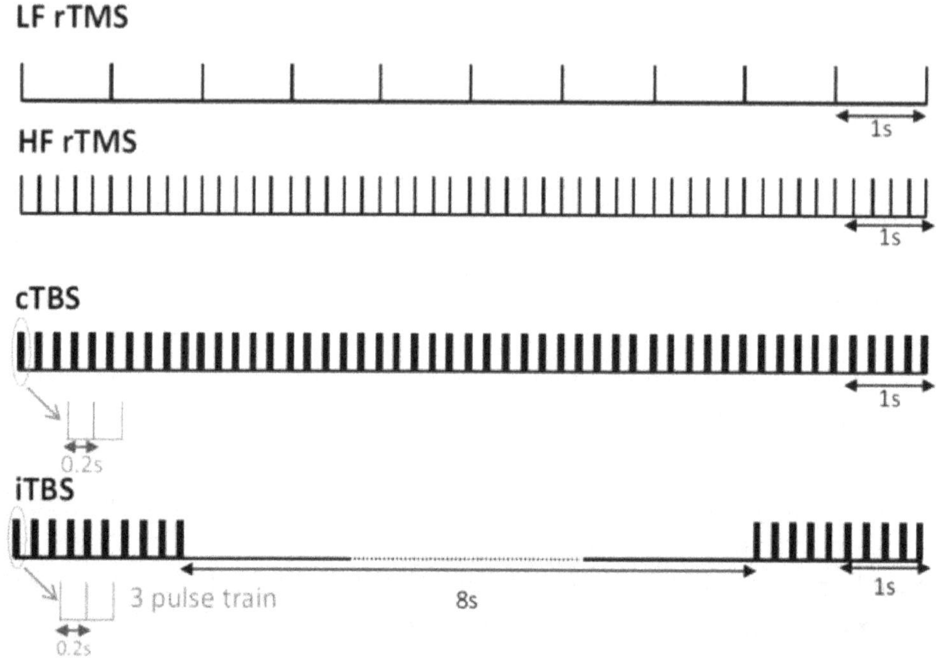


**Figure 3.** Theta burst stimulation (TBS) involves bursts of high-frequency stimulation (3 pulses at 50 Hz) repeated with an inter-stimulus interval (ISI) of 200 ms (5 Hz). In an intermittent TBS (iTBS) protocol, bursts are delivered for 2 s, then repeated every 10 s (2 s of TBS followed by a pause of 8 s). However, in a continuous TBS protocol (cTBS), bursts are repeated for 40 s without any pause [25].

Parkinsonism, and a meta-analysis of clinical studies have shown efficacy of high frequency rTMS, in two clinical trials of SMA rTMS therapy for Parkinson's disease. Therefore, there are reports of NIBS applied to functionally degraded SMA. So if a condition is understood, by considering brain connectivity when applying stimulus, brain activity can be temporarily altered by applying excitatory or suppressive stimulation to the brain localization associated with the condition's localization.

Many researchers have suggested that the underlying mechanism behind rTMS after-effects resembles long-term potentiation (LTP) and long-term depression (LTD) described in animals, where LTP and LTD increases and decreases with synaptic strength, respectively. A short phase (early LTP or LTD) is when changes last for only 30–60 min. A long phase (late LTP or LTD) is when modifications to protein synthesis occur [15].

In TMS, eddy currents generated by a fluctuating magnetic field induce an active potential in mediated nerve cells mainly, whereas in tDCS, the state of the membrane potential is changed. The tDCS reference electrode (7 cm × 5 cm) is placed over the objective area and the stimulation current is 1–2 mA, and the application time is 10–20 min during a motor or cognitive task or rest (**Figure 1**). The anodal electrode may be placed over the presumed area of interest of the brain and the cathodal electrode placed over the contralateral orbit in anodal tDCS and vice versa in cathodal tDCS. In dual tDCS, anodal and cathodal stimulation is applied simultaneously. When positioned over the primary motor cortex in stroke patients, the anodal electrode usually increases cortical excitability, whereas the cathodal electrode decreases cortical excitability. The stimulation effect also varies with intensity and stimulation duration, and may persist up to 1–5 h after 5–10 min of stimulation. In tDCS, cerebral cortical neurons on the brain surface are stimulated and, though not as much as with TMS, the dominant neurons of the lower limbs located in the deep part of the brain are also stimulated. Neuromodulatory effects depend on extrinsic stimulation factors (cortical target, frequency, intensity, duration, number of sessions), intrinsic patient factors (disease process, individual variability and symptoms, state of medication treatment) and outcome measures. Therefore, when reading articles, it is necessary to think about what parameters are responsible for what outcomes.

## 3. tDCS study in post-stroke and Parkinson's disease

The Cochrane database analysis of the ability of rTMS is to improve motor function after stroke has been performed [2]. Many studies were designed to stimulate the inhibition of the contralateral nonaffected primary motor area 3–12 months after a stroke, that is, during the chronic stage [5]. Daily high-frequency rTMS of the ipsilesional M1 is tolerable, and modestly facilitated motor recovery in the paralytic hand of subacute stroke patients [4]. Many studies in Japan found improved motor function of the upper limbs in chronic stroke patients [12, 16]. LF-TMS over the unaffected hemisphere may be more beneficial than rTMS over the affected hemisphere. Most of the individual studies reported clinical improvement of upper-limb motor disorder more commonly found in patients with subcortical lesions, when the rTMS intervention was coupled with traditional rehabilitation, and when the stimulation was applied over the nonlesioned hemisphere [17].

Effects on upper limbs by HF-rTMS stimulating the ipsilesional area and LF-rTMS stimulating the contralesional area have been evaluated using the simple test for evaluating function (STEF) and other evaluation tools. Improvement of patients postinfarction occurs spontaneously within the first 3 months. Many studies on light to moderate paralysis using rTMS, there are no significant improvement that measure tool used in a study [4]. Improvement of patients postinfarction occurs spontaneously within the first 3 months and, in studies of light to moderate paralysis, the effectiveness of rTMS as evaluated by STEF and other such tools was not clear. For both types of stimuli, kinetic analysis and performance analysis of upper limb motor paralysis showed an increase in speed of movement, and a certain improvement in performance was observed in stroke patients.

The aim of our study was to clarify and compare the efficacies of rehabilitation using cTBS, which is a form of rTMS, in convalescing subacute and chronic stroke patients. Newly developed protocols such as TBS present shorter stimulation times and their repeated application can significantly prolong the effects on cortical excitability. We studied effects of inhibition in contralesional areas using kinematic analysis and sitting pressure analysis. Six patients at the first stage of stroke recovery participated.

They received in random order cTBS (40 s intervals, 600 pulses in total) and sham stimulation 1–2 weeks apart. The intensity was set at 80% of active motor threshold. Before and after both cTBS and the sham, the patient was videoed (Sony) performing dorsiflexion of the wrist, abduction of the thumb and abduction of the shoulder in a sitting position. Each movement was performed twice. Kinematic analysis of the video was done using FrameDias IV (DKH Inc.) software, and the maximum angles of movement and mean angular velocity were calculated. Daily rehabilitation consisted of 60 min therapy sessions. Two of the daily sessions were physical and occupational therapy, including gross motor training of the proximal upper extremity, motor training of hand dexterity, training of coordinated movement with both hands and exercises for activities of daily living.

During those exercises, sitting pressure distribution was also measured and the load on the left and right buttocks analyzed. Laterality index was calculated as (buttock load on nonparalytic side − buttock load on paralytic side)/(buttock load on nonparalytic side + buttock load on paralytic side) and deviations in symmetry of the load was investigated.

Comparing pre- and post-stimulation, the improvement rate of the mean angular velocity, shoulder joint abduction on the paralytic side, wrist dorsiflexion and thumb abduction were significantly larger with cTBS than with sham stimulation (**Table 2**). Only for the shoulder joint on the paralyzed side was the joint angle significantly improved compared to when sham stimulation was applied (**Table 2**).

Lager improvements in velocity after the cTBS compared to sham stimulation.

There was not a significantly large difference between the two types of stimuli, but change in speed of movement and performance was observed. Load on the buttock was highly unsymmetrical before stimulation (LI = 0.13 ± 0.10) but nearly symmetrical after cTBS (LI = 0.11 ± 0.05). After sham stimulation, it was changed less (LI = 0.17 ± 0.10 →0.17 ± 0.19). However, the differences

| | Range of motion | | Motor velocity | |
|---|---|---|---|---|
| | cTBS | sham | cTBS | sham |
| Shoulder abduction | 1.27 ± 0.52 | 0.84 ± 0.20* | 1.28 ± 0.45 | 0.89 ± 0.28* |
| Wrist dorsal flexion | 1.03 ± 0.14 | 0.95 ± 0.02 | 1.38 ± 0.1 | 1.03 ± 0.14* |
| Thumb abduction | 1.40 ± 0.30 | 1.35 ± 0.57 | 1.35 ± 0.15 | 1.08 ± 0.20* |

Improvement ratio (post/pre).
*$p < 0.05$.

**Table 2.** Changes in range of motion and motor velocity before and after cTBS and sham stimulation [20].

before and after either stimuli were not statistically significant. Both stimuli resulted in significant improvement compared with the sham stimulus.

Not only upper limb function but also lower limb function and unilateral spatial neglect have been improved by rTMS [18]. Kim et al. found that, compared with a single session, 10 sessions of low-frequency rTMS over the left parietal cortex on hemispatial neglect in stroke patients produced significant improvement in letter cancelation and line bisection tests [19]. The contralesional attentional network in neglect patients by means of rTMS seems to be a viable and effective approach to improving hemispatial attentional deficits related to the disorder. It has been demonstrated recently that low-frequency rTMS over the parietal cortex of the unaffected side transiently reduces the magnitude of neglect **Table 2** [20, 21].

## 4. tDCS study in post-stroke and Parkinson's disease

The tDCS is a method of altering cortical excitability using low-intensity direct current and is used to improve motor and neuropsychological disturbances following stroke and Parkinson's disease. It has mostly been used to treat impairment of upper extremity motor function [22], unilateral spatial neglect (USN) [23], pain [24] and depression [25]. When used to treat hemiplegic arms, a constant direct current of 1–2 mA is given for 10–40 min using a pair of sponge electrodes (5 cm × 7 cm) placed on the scalp overlying the motor cortex and the contralateral supraorbital region. Stimulation parameters include electrode polarity, current intensity and stimulation duration. In particular, bihemispheric stimulation, which involves placement of the source electrode over the damaged motor cortex and placement of the sink electrode over the undamaged motor cortex, may provide additional benefits over stimulation of a single hemisphere by simultaneously increasing excitability in weakened areas and decreasing excitability in regions that inhibit these areas [26]. Previous studies involving individuals with chronic stroke have applied tDCS ranging from 1 to 2 mA delivered for between 10 and 40 min [27], which has been shown to alter excitability of underlying cortical regions for 60–90 min [28]. Therefore, this dosage was used in our study.

In a previous study, we investigated the effects of tDCS on paretic hand function of poststroke patients using kinesiological parameters [29]. Speed and angle of both wrist dorsiflexion and thumb abduction were measured before and after stimulation. Although there was a significant improvement in their speed due to tDCS, no improvement was seen in their angle (**Table 3**). The block box test (BBT) was also used. It assesses manual dexterity by requiring participants to move in one minute as many 2.5 cm blocks as possible over a partition separating two sides of a standardized test box. Normative data on the number of moved blocks for 5-year age groups have been established [30]. BBT results compared before and after stimulation showed significant improvement rates of 1.11 ± 0.03 for tDCS and 1.03 ± 0.02 for sham stimulation ($p < 0.05$).

In another of our studies with five sub-acute post-stroke patients, tDCS and sham stimulation were administered three times per week for two weeks. The stimulation was anodal over the motor area on the ipsilesional side and cathodal on the contralesional side. A direct stimulation current of 1 mA was applied for 20 min at least three times per week. In the BBT, stimulation sessions were continued for 1 week. Improvement rates of results before and after a week, tested using the Wilcoxon signed-rank sum test with $p$ values of 0.05 or less taken as significant, were 133.8 ± 8.3% for tDCS compared with 108.1 ± 6.0% for sham stimulation (**Figure 4**).

| | **Motor velocity** | |
|---|---|---|
| | **tDCS** | **sham** |
| Wrist dorsal flextion | 1.38 ± 0.12 | 1.03 ± 0.05* |
| Thumb abduction | 1.35 ± 1.19 | 1.07 ± 0.06* |

Improvement ratio (post/pre).
*$p < 0.05$ (Wilcoxon signed-rank sum test).

**Table 3.** Changes in motor velocity before and after tDCS and sham stimulation.

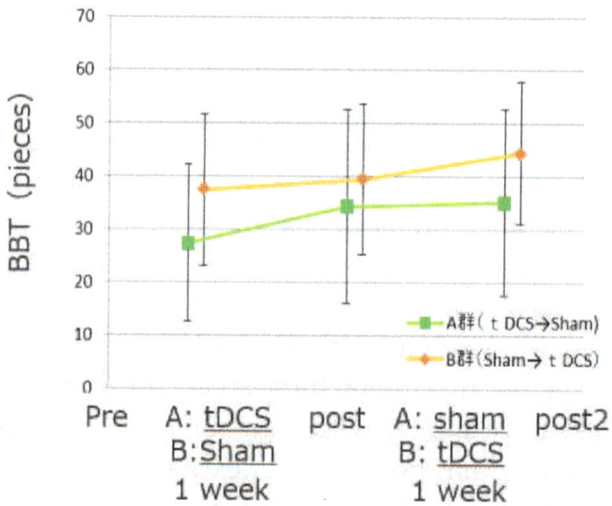


**Figure 4.** tDCS and sham stimulation were performed for 1 week each, and the change in the number of BBT before and after each stimulation. Group A first took tDCS for one week and sham stimulation was given for the following week. Group B was performed in the reverse order of group A.

In another previous study, the gait ability of chronic stroke patients showed a surprising improvement with tDCS. Seven patients at the first stage of stroke recovery (mean age: 61.7 years), who could only walk with supervision participated in a randomized in a double-blind cross-over study. They underwent, in random order, BWSTT (Body Weight Support Treadmill Training) with real tDCS (1 mA, 20 min) on the supplementary motor area (SMA) twice in 1 week and BWSTT with sham stimulation twice in 1 week. We measured the time to complete a 10 m walk test (10MWT) and the timed up and go (TUG) test before and after each BWSTT period. The 10MWT and TUG results are compared in **Table 4**. Comparing before and after stimulation, reduction in time required for the 10MWT was 12.0 ± 10.3% with tDCS and 3.7 ± 8.1% with the sham. For TUG it was 12.9 ± 11.2% with tDCS and 3.3 ± 6.7% with the sham. In both tests, the tDCS results were significant ($p < 0.05$). The findings demonstrated the feasibility and efficacy of tDCS in gait training after stroke. It is possible that the facilitative effects of tDCS on SMA resulted in improvement of postural control during BWSTT. The results indicated implications for the use of tDCS in balance and gait training rehabilitation after stroke.

USN is a common neurological poststroke disorder, with a reported prevalence rate of 43% following right, and 20% following left, hemispheric stroke. Sparing et al. [31] reported that both anodal tDCS over the right posterior parietal cortex (PPC) and cathodal tDCS over the left PPC were effective for left USN. Past studies have shown that some of these cognitive deficits can be improved by tDCS [32]. The effects of tDCS over the left dorsolateral prefrontal cortex (LDLPFC) with 2 mA might be explained by the local increase in the excitability of the dorsolateral prefrontal cortex.

Motor imagery facilitated by tDCS has attracted attention as a conditioning tool. Matsumoto et al. studied the effects of tDCS on motor related areas in six subjects asked to imagine their hand grasping an object [33]. Their study suggested that anodal tDCS stimulation to the motor-related areas promoted brain activity and enhanced motor imagery.

Corticospinal excitability of the motor cortex is usually reduced in Parkinson's disease [7]. Studies have investigated whether tDCS over M1 improves bradykinesia of the upper and lower limb in Parkinson's disease. tDCS produced modest improvements in gait in Parkinson's disease [34]. We studied the effects of tDCS on the gait of six patients with Parkinson's disease when it was applied to the left motor cortex for 20 min and found that, compared to sham stimulation, tDCS improved gait speed and step length. We also showed that posture can be improved with tDCS alone during simple gait tasks. Comparing before and after stimulation for both tDCS and the sham, tDCS significantly improved gait speed and step length but not

| | tDCS | | Sham | |
|---|---|---|---|---|
| | Pre | Post | Pre | post |
| 10MWT (s) | 21.9 ± 11.7 | 19.3 ± 11.1* | 20.8 ± 11.1 | 19.5 ± 9.3 |
| TUG (s) | 25.0 ± 12.5 | 21.9 ± 12.1* | 22.0 ± 11.0 | 21.3 ± 11.0 |

*$p < 0.05$ (Wilcoxon signed-rank sum test).

**Table 4.** Changes in 10 m walking test and TUG (timed up and go test) before and after tDCS and sham stimulation.

the number of steps per minute ($p < 0.05$; **Table 5**). Therefore, the increase in gait speed is thought to be due to increased step length (see **Figure 5**) [9].

Gait and balance in patients with Parkinson's disease may be further improved by combining anodal tDCS with physical training. Electroconvulsive therapy (ECT) may also have a significant effect on motor function in Parkinson's disease [35]. In conclusion, rTMS and tDCS are promising noninvasive cortical stimulation tools for movement disorders [36].

| | tDCS | | Sham | |
|---|---|---|---|---|
| | **Pre** | **Post** | **Pre** | **Post** |
| Gait speed (m/min) | 25.9 ± 12.5 | 30.8 ± 11.8* | 29.1 ± 11.2 | 26.2 ± 12.5 |
| Cadence (steps/min) | 105.5 ± 21.1 | 113.6 ± 24.5 | 99.9 ± 23.1 | 103.7 ± 25.4 |
| Step length (cm) | 24.9 ± 12.5 | 27.4 ± 10.7* | 29.9 ± 12.1 | 25.2 ± 11.8 |

*$p < 0.05$ (Wilcoxon signed-rank sum test).

**Table 5.** Comparison of 10 m walking test before and after tDCS and sham stimulation for Parkinson's disease patients.

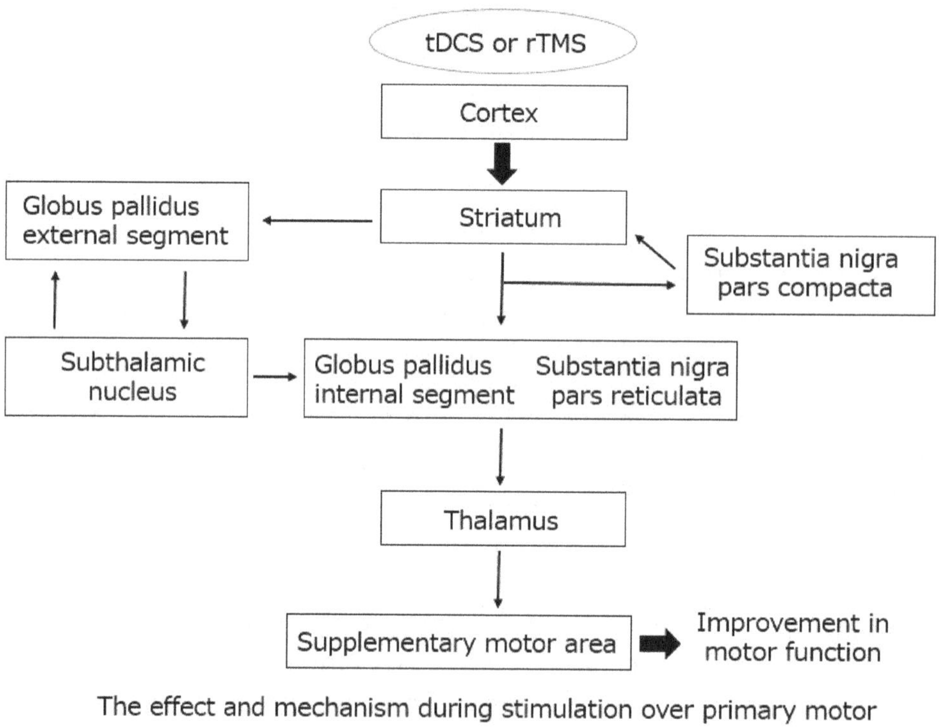


**Figure 5.** The effect and mechanism during stimulation over primary motor. Stimulation of the motor cortex by tDCS is thought to improve Parkinson's disease through input stimulus from the primary motor cortex increasing input into the basal ganglia. The stimulus spreads from the stimulation position (electrode contact position) to the supplementary motor cortex ahead of the motor cortex itself, and activation through an exercise program may be involved [9].

## 5. Combined approaches

Therapy is started in most cases within 1 hour of the completion of rTMS sessions. NIBS, using either rTMS or tDCS, may be combined with physical therapy [23], occupational therapy

Kakuda et al. [16], BWSTT training, robotic therapy [32], constraint-induced (CI) therapy [3] and simultaneous percutaneous neuromuscular stimulation. Lee et al. [29] investigated the effects of cathodal tDCS combined with visual reality (VR) therapy for upper extremity training in patients with subacute stroke. The changes in manual function test (MFT) and Fugl-Meyer Scale (FMS) scores were significantly higher in the combination therapy group than in the control group. However, further research is needed to give definitive conclusions as to the efficacy of combination therapy. Preconditioning with tDCS is a powerful tool for modulating the behavioral effect of 1 Hz rTMS over the primary motor cortex in PD [6]. This combined stimulation was reported to improve motor function.

There have only been a few reports on the combination of LF-rTMS and physical therapy including gait training. In one study, 38 patients with post stroke hemiparesis, LF-rTMS (20 min) was combined with physical exercise during 15 days of hospitalization [17] and scores of the TUG test, dynamic gait index and the functional balance scale were significantly improved.

Few studies have used NIBS techniques combined with physical therapy as an antispastic approach, though rTMS combined with PT can be beneficial in reducing poststroke spasticity [20]. In a study by Middleton et al., 5 participants with chronic stroke completed 24 sessions of upper extremity physical therapy combined with tDCS over the motor cortex [23], and improvements on the UE Fugl-Meyer assessment (FMA), BBT and robotic measures were largely sustained at 6 months. Kakuda et al. [16] studied combination protocol for poststroke upper limb hemiparesis in inpatients as part of a multiinstitutional study. The protocol was two sessions of 20 min rTMS and 120 min occupational therapy daily, except Sundays and admission and discharge days for 15 days. At discharge, increase in FMA score, shortening in performance time of the Wolf motor function test (WMFT), and increase in the functional ability scale (FAS) score of WMFT were significant (FMA score 46.8 ± 12.2–50.9 ± 11.4 points, $p < 0.001$; performance time of WMFT 2.57 ± 1.32–2.21 ± 1.33, $p < 0.001$; FAS score of WMFT 47.4 ± 14–51.4 ± 14.3 points, $p < 0.001$).

However, more studies are needed to clarify the clinical changes underlying the reduction in spasticity induced by NIBS [20]. NIBS, depending on whether it is applied before, during or after neuromodulation, might interfere with the motor task and have opposite and invalidating effects. Therefore, stimulation from a physical and occupational therapy program may be necessary, and more research on stimulation is required.

## 6. Conclusion

We investigated improvement of movement speed due to the reduction of excessive tension caused by spasticity in poststroke. In addition, patients with Parkinson's disease improved gait speed and step length after tDCS, probably due to smoother movement. NIBS of the motor and prefrontal cortices may have therapeutic potential in Parkinson's disease. NIBS could be a useful therapeutic rehabilitation tool for stroke and Parkinson's disease. Both methods may enhance the neuroplasticity in the injured area and re-establish the balance between different regions of the brain. However, better stimulation parameters and rehabilitation methods after NIBS need to be established to make the technique clinically viable.

Such noninvasive stimulation therapy seems effective against central nervous system disease. Temporary transformations of the neural circuit of the brain are seen from the recovery stage to even the chronic stage. It is thought that spastic tension in stroke patients is reduced by inhibitory stimulation of the noninjured side, in accordance with interhemispheric inhibition theory, thereby directly influencing mobility. Furthermore, the gait of patients with Parkinson's disease can be improved by stimulation of the left motor cortex. The effect of noninvasive brain stimulation-induced brain plasticity—has a relatively long duration (over 30 min), but appropriate rehabilitation is necessary at the time the effect is continued. The effect of the stimulation alone and in combination with effective rehabilitation leave questions unanswered about rehabilitation programs. It is thought important to put into practice issue-specific approaches employing the changes induced by noninvasive brain stimulation. From the present findings on brain stimulation, it is suggested that further research is warranted to develop applicable approaches.

## Author details

Tadamitsu Matsuda*, Atsushi Manji, Kazu Amimoto, Akira Inaba and Yoshiaki Wada

*Address all correspondence to: funwavesurfgogo@yahoo.co.jp

Josai International University, Chiba, Japan

## References

[1] Nudo, RJ, Plasticity. NeuroRx, 2006, 3: pp. 420–427.

[2] Hao, Z, Wang, D, Zeng, Y, Liu, M, Repetitive transcranial magnetic stimulation for improving function after stroke. Cochrane Database Syst Rev, 2013, 5: CD008862. doi:10.1002/14651858.cd008862

[3] Malcolm, MP, Triggs, WJ, Light, KE, Gonzalez, Rothi LJ. Wu, S, Reid, K, Nadeau, SE, Repetitive transcranial magnetic stimulation as an adjunct to constraint-induced therapy: an exploratory randomised controlled trial. Am J Phys Med Rehab, 2007, 86: pp. 707–715.

[4] Hosomi, K, Morris, S, Sakamoto, T, Taguchi, J, Maruo, T, Kageyama, Y, Kinoshita, Y, Goto, Y, Shimokawa, T, Koyama, T, Saitoh, Y, Daily repetitive transcranial magnetic stimulation for poststroke upper limb paresis in the subacute period. J Stroke Cerebrovasc Dis, 2016, 25(7): pp. 1655–1664.

[5] Emara, TH, Moustafa, RR, Elnahas, NM, Elganzoury, AM, Abdo, TA, Mohamed, SA, Eletribi, MA, Repetitive transcranial magnetic stimulation at 1 Hz and 5 Hz produces sustained improvement in motor function and disability after ischaemic stroke. Eur J Neurol, 2010, 17: pp. 1203–1209.

[6] Grüner, U, Eggers, C, Ameli, M, Sarfeld, AS, Fink, GR, Nowak, DA. 1 Hz rTMS preconditioned by tDCS over the primary motor cortex in Parkinson's disease: effects on bradykinesia of arm and hand. J Neural Transm, 2010, 117(2): pp. 207–216.

[7] Lefaucheur, JP. Motor cortex dysfunction revealed by cortical excitability studies in Parkinson's disease: influence of antiparkinsonian treatment and cortical stimulation. Clin Neurophysiol, 2005, 116: pp. 244–253.

[8] Tanaka, S, Watanabe, K, Transcranial direct current stimulation—a new tool for human cognitive neuroscience. Brain Nerve, 2009, 61(1): pp. 53–64.

[9] Fregni, F, Pascual-Leone, A, Technology insight: noninvasive brain stimulation in neurology-perspectives on the therapeutic potential of rTMS and tDCS. Nat Clin Pract Neurol, 2007, 3(7): pp. 383–393.

[10] Ward, NS, Mechanisms underlying recovery of motor function after stroke. Postgrad Med J, 2005, 81(895): pp. 510–514.

[11] Butler, AJ, Wolf, SL, Putting the brain on the map: use of transcranial magnetic stimulation to assess and induce cortical plasticity of upper-extremity movement. Phys Ther, 87(6): pp. 719–736.

[12] Sasaki, N, Mizutani, S, Kakuda, W, Abo, M, Comparison of the effects of high- and low-frequency repetitive transcranial magnetic stimulation on upper limb hemiparesis in the early phase of stroke. J Stroke Cerebrovasc Dis, 2013, 22(4): pp. 413–418.

[13] Klomjai, W, Katz, R, Lackmy-Vallée, A, Basic principles of transcranial magnetic stimulation (TMS) and repetitive TMS (rTMS). Ann Phys Rehabil Med, 2015, 58(4): pp. 208–213.

[14] Haslinger, B, Erhard, P, Kämpfe, N, Boecker, H, Rummeny, E, Schwaiger, M, Conrad, B, Ceballos-Baumann, AO, Event-related functional magnetic resonance imaging in Parkinson's disease before and after levodopa. Brain, 2001, 124: pp. 558 –570.

[15] Hoogendam, JM, Ramakers, GM, Di Lazzaro, V, Physiology of repetitive transcranial magnetic stimulation of the human brain. Brain Stimul, 2010, 3: pp. 95–118.

[16] Kakuda, W, Abo, M, Sasanuma, J, Shimizu, M, Okamoto, T, Kimura, C, Kakita, K, Hara, H, Combination protocol of low-frequency rTMS and intensive occupational therapy for post-stroke upper limb hemiparesis: a 6-year experience of more than 1700 Japanese patients. Transl Stroke Res, 2016, 7(3): pp. 172–179.

[17] Cha, HK, Ji, SG, Kim, MK, Chang, JS, Effect of transcranial direct current stimulation of function in patients with stroke. J Phys Ther Sci, 2014, 26(3): pp. 363–365.

[18] Yoshida, Y, Watanabe, S, Kakuda, W, Yokoi, A, Fukuda, A, Ito, H, Tominaga, A, Umemori, T, Kameda, Y, Clinical effect of combined protocol of low-frequency repetitive transcranial magnetic stimulation and an intensive rehabilitative program on gait and lower-limb motor function in patients with poststroke hemiparesis. Tokyo Jikeikai Med J, 2011, 126: pp. 177–185 (in Japanese).

[19] Kim YK, Jung JH, Shin SH. A comparison of the effects of repetitive transcranial magnetic stimulation (rTMS) by number of stimulation sessions on hemispatial neglect in chronic stroke patients. Exp Brain Res. 2015, 233(1): pp. 283–289.

[20] Yi, YG, Chun, MH, Do, KH, Sung, EJ, Kwon, YG, Kim, DY, The effect of transcranial direct current stimulation on neglect syndrome in stroke patients. Ann Rehabil Med, 2016, 40(2): pp. 223–229.

[21] Manji, A, Matsuda, T, Amimoto, K, Inaba, A, Wada, Y, Kinesiological evaluation after cTBS to contralesional motor cortex in restorative stage stroke patients. The XXI World Congress of Neurology, 2013 (congress).

[22] Hyun, KC, San, GJ, Myoung, KK, Effect of transcranial direct current stimulation of function in patients with stroke. J Phys Ther Sci, 2014, 26: pp. 363–365.

[23] Luvizutto, GJ, Rizzati, GR, Fogaroli, MO, Rodrigues, RT, Ribeiro, PW, de, Carvalho, Nunes, HR, Braga, GP, da, Costa, RD, Bazan, SG, de, Lima, Resende, LA, Conforto, AB, Bazan, R, Treatment of unilateral spatial neglect after stroke using transcranial direct current stimulation (ELETRON trial): study protocol for a randomized controlled trial. Trials, 2016, 17(1): p. 479.

[24] Concerto, C, Al Sawah, M, Chusid, E, Trepal, M, Taylor, G, Aguglia, E, Battaglia, F, Anodal transcranial direct current stimulation for chronic pain in the elderly: a pilot study. Aging Clin Exp Res, 2016, 28(2): pp. 231–237.

[25] Shiozawa, P, Fregni, F, Benseñor, IM, Lotufo, PA, Berlim, MT, Daskalakis, JZ, Cordeiro, Q, Brunoni, AR, Transcranial direct current stimulation for major depression: an updated systematic review and meta-analysis. Int J Neuropsychopharmacol, 2014, 17(9): pp. 1443–1452.

[26] Vines, BW, Cerruti, C, Schlaug, G, Dual-hemisphere tDCS facilitates greater improvements for healthy subjects' non-dominant hand compared to uni-hemisphere stimulation. BMC Neurosci, 2008, 9: p. 103.

[27] Ang, KK, Guan, C, Phua, KS, Wang, C, The, I, Chen, CW, Chew, E, Transcranial direct current stimulation and EEG-based motor imagery BCI for upper limb stroke rehabilitation. Conf Proc IEEE Eng Med Biol Soc, 2012, 2012: pp. 4128–4131.

[28] Nitsche, MA, Paulus, W, Sustained excitability elevations induced by transcranial DC motor cortex stimulation in humans. Neurology, 2001, 57(10): pp. 1899–1901.

[29] Manji, A, Matsuda, T, Amimoto, K, Inaba, A, Wada, Y, Effects of tanscranial direct current stimulation on paretic arm function in restorative and chronic stage stroke patients. 9th World Congress of the International Society of Physical and Rehabilitation Medicine (ISPRM), June 19–23, Berlin, Germany, 2015 (congress).

[30] Mathiowetz, V, Volland, G, Kashman, N, Weber, K, Adult norms for the box and block test of manual dexterity. Am J Occup Ther, 1985, 39(6): pp. 386–391.

[31] Sparing, R, Thimm, M, Hesse, MD, Küst, J, Karbe, H, Fink, GR, Bidirectional alterations of interhemispheric parietal balance by non-invasive cortical stimulation. Brain, 2009, 132: pp. 3011–3020.

[32] Boggio, PS, Ferrucci, R, Rigonatti, SP, Covre, P, Nitsche, M, Pascual-Leone, A, Fregni, F, Effects of transcranial direct current stimulation on working memory in patients with Parkinson's disease. J Neurol Sci, 2006, 249(1): pp. 31–38.

[33] Matsumoto, J, Fujiwara, T, Takahashi, O, Liu, M, Kimura, A, Ushiba, J, Modulation of mu rhythm desynchronization during motor imagery by transcranial direct current stimulation. J Neuroeng Rehabil, 2010, 7: p. 27.

[34] Benninger, DH, Lomarev, M, Lopez, G, Wassermann, EM, Li, X, Considine, E, Hallett, M, Transcranial direct current stimulation for the treatment of Parkinson's disease. J Neurol Neurosurg Psychiatry, 2010, 81: pp. 1105–1111.

[35] Fregni, F, Simon, DK, Wu, A, Pascual-Leone, A, Non-invasive brain stimulation for Parkinson's disease: a systematic review and meta-analysis of the literature. J Neurol Neurosurg Psychiatry, 2005, 76(12): pp. 1614–1623.

[36] Wu, AD, Fregni, F, Simon, DK, Deblieck, C, Pascual-Leone, A, Noninvasive brain stimulation for Parkinson's disease and dystonia. Neurotherapeutics, 2008, 5(2): pp. 345–361.

12

# Relationship Between Excitability of Spinal Motor Neurons in Remote Muscles and Voluntary Movements

Naoki Kado, Yuki Takahashi, Satoshi Fujiwara and Masanori Ito

**Abstract**

In physical therapy, it is important to understand the influence of the contraction of a particular muscle on other muscles. The mechanism of the facilitation effect of muscle contraction in healthy subjects has been analyzed in previous studies. These studies indicated that muscle contraction with voluntary movement enhances the excitability of spinal motor neurons and motor areas in the cerebral cortex that are not directly associated with the contracting muscle. Furthermore, it has been reported that the facilitation effects on remote muscles not related to movement are affected by the elapsed time since the start of the movement, the strength of muscle contraction, the number of muscle spindles, and the difficulty of the movement. In addition, the facilitation effects of difficult voluntary movements of the unilateral upper limbs on spinal motor neurons in the contralateral upper limb decrease with motor learning. We expect that these findings will be useful not only for physical therapy evaluation but also for patient treatment.

**Keywords:** F-wave, spinal motor neuron, arm movement, motor learning

## 1. Introduction

In physical therapy, it is necessary to understand the influence of the muscle contraction accompanying a movement on the muscles not involved in the movement. For instance, associative reactions observed in patients with hemiplegia due to cerebrovascular disorders (CVDs) are tonic reflexes that originate in the muscles of one limb and act on the muscles of another limb. Associative reactions usually occur prior to or during a behavior and lead to enhancement of muscle tone on the affected side. This phenomenon makes selective movement of the upper limb or the lower limb on the affected side more difficult.

When using exercise and therapy, we have to evaluate the movements responsible for the appearance of associative reactions. It is thus important to understand the neurophysiological effects of the voluntary contraction of a particular muscle on the muscles not involved in the movement.

The mechanism of the facilitation effect on the muscles not involved in the movement (i.e., remote muscles) has been analyzed in studies of motor-evoked potentials (MEPs) evoked by transcranial magnetic stimulation (TMS), H-reflexes, and F-waves [1–6]. These studies indicate that muscle activation enhances the excitability of motor areas in the cerebral cortex and spinal motor neurons that are not directly associated with the activating muscle. Furthermore, it has been reported that the facilitation effects on remote muscles not related to voluntary contraction are affected by the elapsed time since the start of movement [2], the strength of the muscle contraction [5–7], the number of muscle spindles [8], and the difficulty of the movement [9].

One of the objectives of physical therapy is the recovery of reduced function and the relearning of previously learned movement patterns. Various plastic changes occur in the central nervous system during motor learning. Practicing complex movements leads to notable reorganization in the primary motor cortex [10, 11]. Spinal reflexes are reduced following exercise training requiring accurate movements [12]. The performance of exercises requiring high levels of skill involves strong control of the spinal cord from the cortex. Therefore, the gain of spinal reflexes is estimated to decrease in the spinal cord. However, when performing difficult movements, muscles that are not directly involved in the intentional movement may be moved involuntarily. Such a phenomenon is rarely observed in the automatization phase of motor learning. A previous study reported that the facilitation effects of difficult voluntary movements of the unilateral upper limb on spinal motor neurons in the contralateral upper limb decrease with motor learning [13]. These findings will be useful for physical therapy evaluation. In addition, they may help to establish an important index for evaluating the effects of a particular task of different difficulties on muscle groups that are not directly involved in the movement.

## 2. The mechanism of the facilitation effect of muscle contraction on contralateral spinal motor neurons

It has been reported that the activity of muscle spindles associated with a particular movement may play a role in the facilitation effect of muscle contraction. Delwaide and Toulouse [14] reported that the facilitation effect is not observed after movement attempts when the radial nerve that innervates the muscles of the upper limb involved in the movement is blocked. Hayashi et al. [8] reported the remote facilitation of the soleus H-reflex during contractions of the finger, jaw, and tongue muscles, which have numerous muscle spindles. In contrast, Bussel et al. [1] reported that the H-reflex is facilitated even when the muscle spindle afferent input is blocked by lower limb ischemia. Hess et al. [15] reported the involvement of the facilitation effect in intracortical mechanisms, noting that MEPs following TMS increase in the contralateral limb of amputee patients with phantom limbs when muscle contractions in the amputated limb are imaged. These studies enable us to explain the facilitation of spinal motor neurons following unilateral arm movement as follows. The excitability of contralateral spinal motor neurons is enhanced when unilateral arm movement is executed. This phenomenon may be attributed to proprioceptive input during unilateral arm movements and the facilitation effect generated by activation of brain regions involved in the planning and execution of movement. We believe that the facilitation effect occurs via commissural fibers and/or uncrossed projections from the ipsilateral brain hemisphere.

The facilitation effects of muscle contraction on muscles other than the contracting muscle are affected by the strength of the muscle contraction. Suzuki et al. [5] reported that as the F/M amplitude ratio for the contralateral F-wave of the opponens pollicis muscle gradually increases with increasing strength of contraction. In particular, F-waves generated at 75 and 100% contraction of the elbow flexor muscles are significantly higher than those generated during relaxation. Muellbacher et al. [6] reported that the F-wave amplitude of the contralateral abductor pollicis brevis (APB) increases at the time of maximum contraction. In contrast, Stinear et al. [7] reported that the maximum contraction of the APB does not alter the F-wave amplitude of the contralateral APB. Therefore, facilitation effects on contralateral spinal motor neurons may occur during contractions of greater than 75%.

## 3. The influence of movement difficulty on contralateral spinal motor neurons

A few reports have evaluated the effects of qualitative differences in movements, such as task difficulty, on the spinal motor neurons of muscles other than the contracting muscle. We thus evaluated the influence of the difficulty of movement performed with one arm on the excitability of spinal motor neurons in the contralateral arm using F-wave data obtained via electromyography (EMG) [9]. There are only a few reports regarding changes in the facilitation effects of unilateral upper limb movements on spinal motor neurons in the contralateral upper limb associated with motor learning. Therefore, we used F-waves to examine changes in the excitability of spinal motor neurons in the contralateral upper limb following difficult movements performed with the unilateral upper limb [13]. The F-waves measured in these studies are considered to be generated when antidromic impulses induced by motor nerve fiber stimulation excite $\alpha$-motor neurons in the anterior horn of the spinal cord, and the recurrent discharge generates orthodromic impulses that induce myopotentials [16]. They are used as an index of motor neuron pool excitability in the anterior horn of the spinal cord. The parameters used for analysis were latency, persistence, and F/M amplitude ratio. Latency was the mean time from stimulus pulse to F-wave onset. Persistence was calculated for all ratios that were distinguished on the display. The F/M amplitude ratio was calculated as the ratio of the average peak-to-peak F-wave amplitude to the maximum M-wave amplitude. Latency measures the conduction in motor axons, persistence reflects the state of excitability in the neuronal pool that is examined, and the F/M amplitude ratio represents the percentage of motor neurons activated by antidromic stimulation [17]. F-waves were recorded using a Viking Quest EMG system (Nicolet Biomedical, WI, USA).

### 3.1. Experiment 1: excitability of spinal motor neurons in the contralateral arm during voluntary arm movements with various levels of difficulty

In this study, we evaluated the influence of movement difficulty in tasks performed with one arm on the excitability of spinal motor neurons in the contralateral arm using F-wave data obtained via EMG (**Figure 1**). Twenty right-handed healthy volunteers (mean age, 26.6±4 years) with no orthopedic or neurological abnormalities were enrolled in this study. The Edinburgh handedness inventory [18] was used to determine the dominant hands of the subjects. The subjects were seated on a chair during the test. The F-waves were recorded from the right APB during the movement tasks and the control task. Movement tasks were executed with the left arm. The F-waves were analyzed for latency, persistence, and F/M amplitude ratio. The index of difficulty was defined by the movement distance and target width [19]. As distance and/or speed of movement can affect the excitability of contralateral spinal motor neurons, tasks with different levels of difficulty were established by altering the target width. Each subject held a pen in his or her left hand and executed repetitive movements between two targets placed on a desk during the movement task (**Figure 2**). The targets were 5 × 15 cm (width × length) for task 1, 0.5 × 15 cm for task 2, and 0.25 × 15 cm for task 3, and were 20 cm

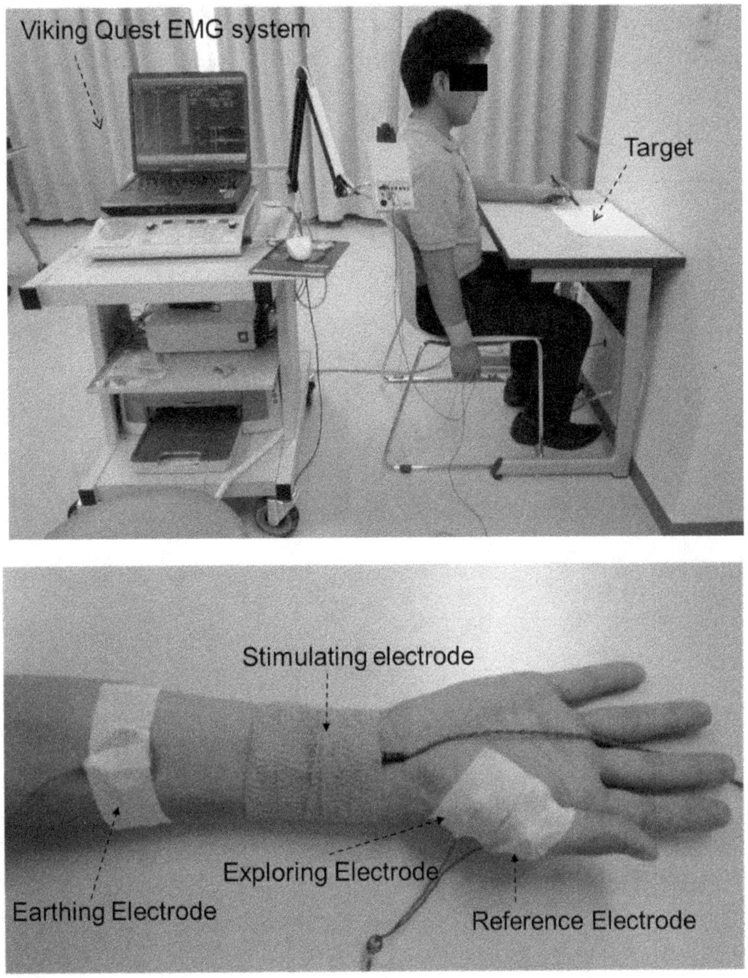


**Figure 1.** Measurement of the F-wave.

apart for all tasks. The subjects were instructed to accurately touch the target area with the tip of a pen. Each movement task was performed at a frequency of 1 Hz. The tasks were performed in random order. During each task, electrical stimulations were administered when the arm was moving toward the right target (i.e., internal rotation of the left shoulder joint) in order to induce F-waves. The number of times the pen tip deviated from the target was counted and the success rate was calculated after each movement task. The control task comprised remaining in the sitting posture without executing arm movements.

The F-wave parameters (persistence, F/M amplitude ratio, and latency) during the control and movement tasks were compared using Dunnett's tests. The results are shown in **Figures 3–6.** Persistence significantly increased during tasks 1, 2, and 3 compared to the control task. The F/M amplitude ratio also significantly increased during tasks 2 and 3 compared to the control task. The F/M ratio was comparable between task 1 and the control task. There were no significant differences in latency between the control task and any of the movement tasks. The success rates were 100.0% for task 1, 83.3% for task 2, and 52.8% for task 3. The success rates suggested that the tasks had different difficulty levels.

The persistence data suggest that the excitability of spinal motor neurons during movements of the contralateral arm was enhanced during unilateral arm movement. This phenomenon may be attributable to the proprioceptive input during the left arm movement and the facilitation effect generated by the activation of the regions of the brain involved in the planning and

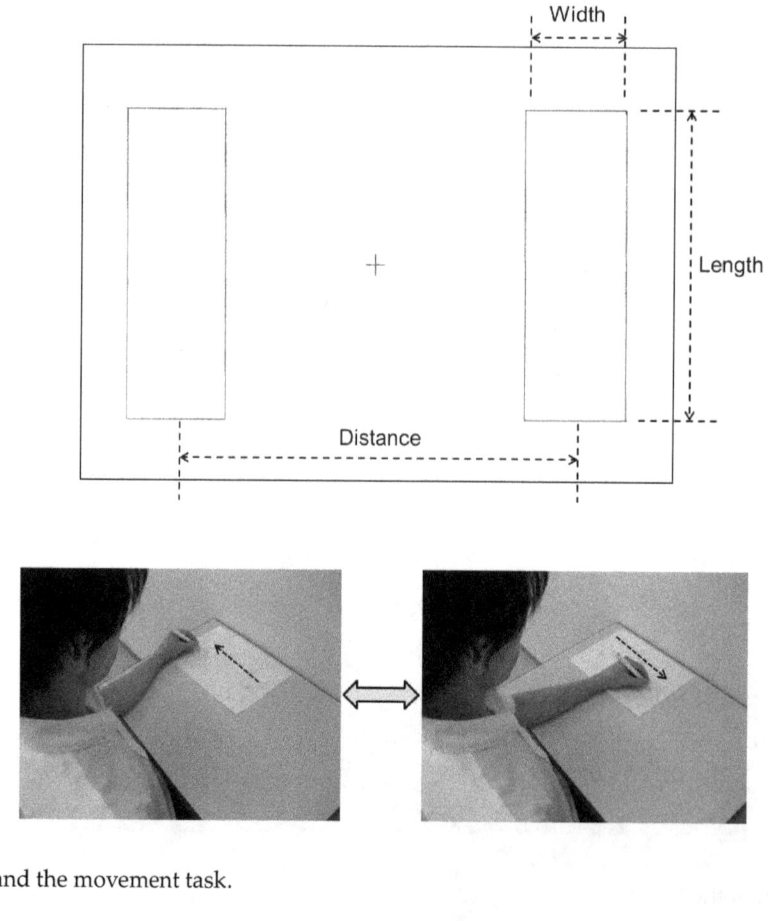


**Figure 2.** The target and the movement task.

execution of movements. We believe that the facilitation effect occurs via commissural fibers and/or uncrossed projections from the ipsilateral hemisphere.

On the basis of the F/M amplitude ratio data and the success rates, we speculate that task difficulty may have been responsible for the differences observed in the excitability of spinal motor neurons. As the movement speed and range were the same in each movement task, it is unlikely that there were differences in proprioceptive input among the

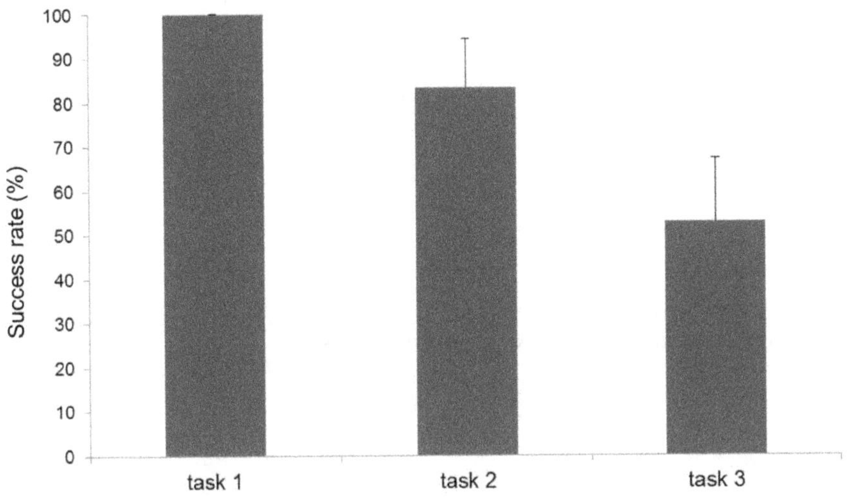


**Figure 3.** Success rates of the movement tasks.

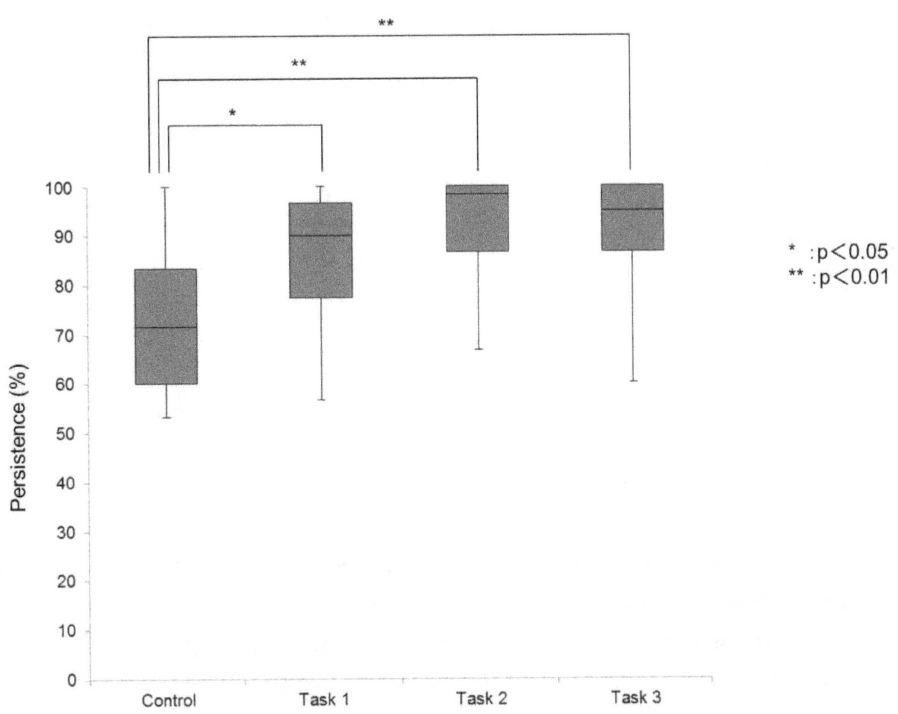


**Figure 4.** Persistence during the control and movement tasks.

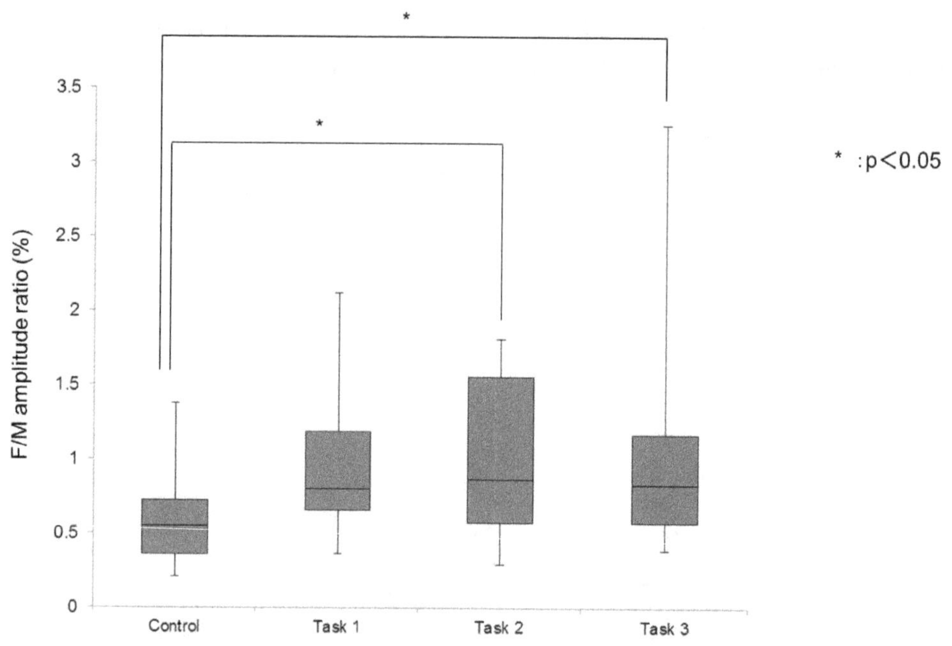


**Figure 5.** F/M amplitude ratios during the control and movement tasks.

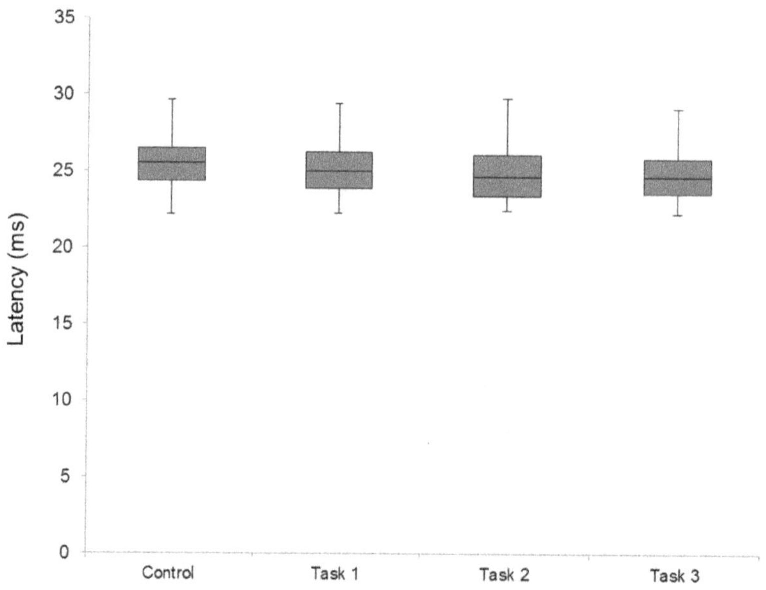


**Figure 6.** Latency during the control and movement tasks.

tasks. In addition, the success rates indicate that tasks 2 and 3 were more difficult than task 1. According to Shibasaki et al. [20], both the contralateral sensorimotor cortex and the ipsilateral sensorimotor area are activated during the execution of complex sequential finger movements. Winstein et al. [21] examined the relationship between task difficulty and brain activity and reported that activities in areas related to complex movement planning requiring visual motion processing, such as the ipsilateral dorsal premotor area increase with increased task difficulty. Here, we considered that the excitability of contralateral spinal motor neurons increases during tasks 2 and 3, which have high levels of difficulty and require more accurate movements than task 1. It is possible that the motor-related areas ipsilateral to the movement are activated when difficult movements are performed. This may have led to enhanced excitability of the contralateral spinal motor neurons via projection fibers. Furthermore, although unilateral limb movements are adjusted for by the contralateral motor area, it has been reported that the activation of this contralateral motor area affects the excitability of the ipsilateral motor area via the corpus callosum [22, 23]. We also believe that when difficult movements are performed, motor-related areas contralateral to the movement are strongly activated. This may enhance the excitability of spinal motor neurons contralateral to the movement via commissural fibers. The facilitation effect is described in **Figure 7**. These results suggest that possible differences in the facilitation effects of muscle contraction arising from task difficulty should be considered when evaluating the effects of the contraction of a particular muscle on other muscles.

While we only studied healthy subjects, Eisen and Odusote [24] reported that F-wave amplitudes of patients with spasticity were larger than those in healthy subjects. This result suggests that the influence of the facilitation effect is more remarkable in patients with hemiplegia due to CVDs. Further studies are thus required to investigate the effects of difficult movements of the unilateral limb on the excitability of contralateral spinal motor neurons in patients with hemiplegia.

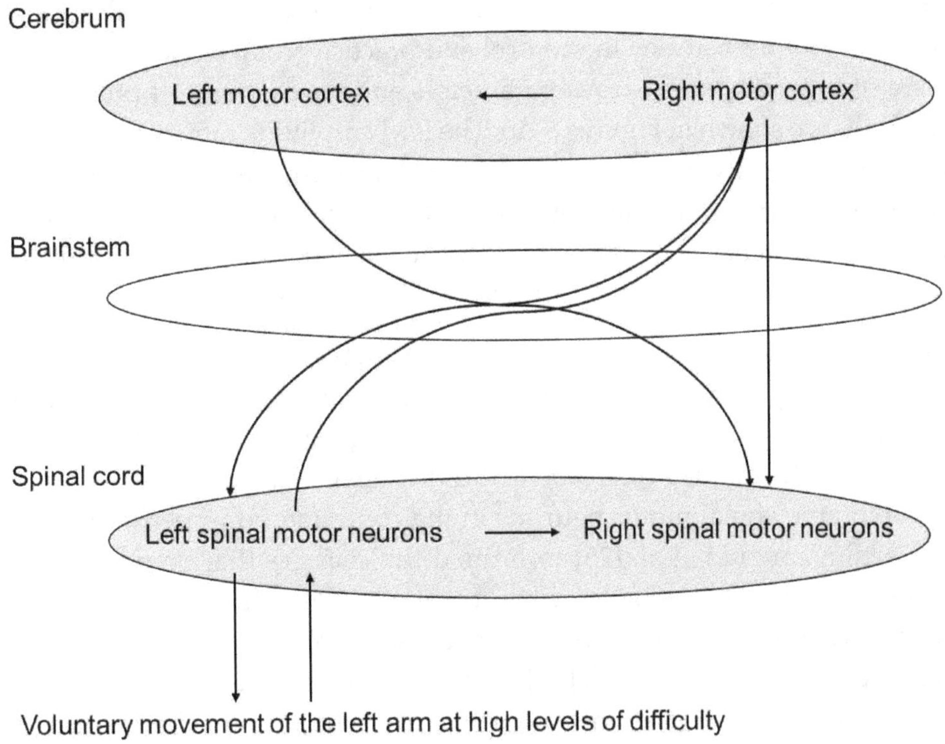


**Figure 7.** The facilitation effect during voluntary movements with high levels of difficulty.

### 3.2. Experiment 2: effects of practicing difficult movements with the unilateral arm on the excitability of spinal motor neurons in the contralateral arm

In this study, we used F-waves to evaluate changes in the excitability of spinal motor neurons in the contralateral upper limb caused by practicing high-difficulty movements with the unilateral upper limb. Sixteen right-handed healthy adults (12 men and 4 women; mean age, 26.1 ± 6.0 years) with no orthopedic or neurological abnormalities participated in the study. The subjects were randomly assigned equally to either a control group (6 men and 2 women; mean age, 26.4 ± 7.2 years) or a practice group (6 men and 2 women; mean age, 26.0 ± 4.9 years). The Edinburgh handedness inventory [18] was used to determine the subjects' dominant hands. F-waves were recorded from the right APB during motor tasks performed with the left upper limb before and after the practice task. The subjects were seated on a chair during the test. The limb position was the same as that in experiment 1. The subjects were instructed to not move any body parts other than the left arm throughout the study. The motor tasks used when recording the F-waves were the same as those used in experiment 1. The target width used in the motor task was 0.5 × 15 cm (width × length), as this target size led to facilitation effects on spinal nerve function in the contralateral upper limb in a previous study [9]. The number of times the tip of the pen touched a location outside of the target was counted. The practice task consisted of repetitive movements at a frequency of 1 Hz. The practice group performed repetitive movements using the same targets when recording the F-waves, and the control group performed repetitive movements without the targets. The practice task was performed for five sessions with each session consisting of 30 movements. One-minute breaks were provided between successive sessions. F-waves were analyzed to determine latency and the F/M amplitude ratio.

Mann-Whitney tests were used to compare F-wave parameters (F/M amplitude ratio and latency) and the number of failures between the control and practice groups. The Wilcoxon-signed rank sum tests were used to compare F-wave parameters and the numbers of pre- and postpractice failures. The results are shown in **Figures 8–10**. The F/M amplitude ratio during the post-practice session was significantly lower than the pre-practice value. In addition, the postpractice values in the practice group were significantly lower than those in the control group. There were no significant differences in latency pre- versus postpractice in either group. The numbers of failures during the postpractice session were significantly lower than the pre-practice values.

We speculated that the facilitation effects on spinal motor neurons in the contralateral upper limb while performing high-difficulty unilateral upper limb movements could be reduced by practicing the movements. Motor learning is thought to depend on plasticity in motor and sensory areas of the brain. Therefore, facilitation effects during movements of the unilateral upper limb on the spinal motor neurons in the contralateral upper limb can be reduced with motor learning. Suzuki et al. [25] examined the changes that occur in the brain while learning the task of rotating two balls by hand using MEPs induced by TMS. They reported that the excitability of the primary motor cortex ipsilateral to the movements is reduced as performance improves. Winstein et al. [21] examined the relationship between the efficiency of motor tasks and brain activity, and reported that activation of the ipsilateral premotor area is related to motor task difficulty. In addition, Nelson et al. [26] recorded somatosensory evoked potentials (SEPs) during motor tasks, such as adjusting the angle of the joint

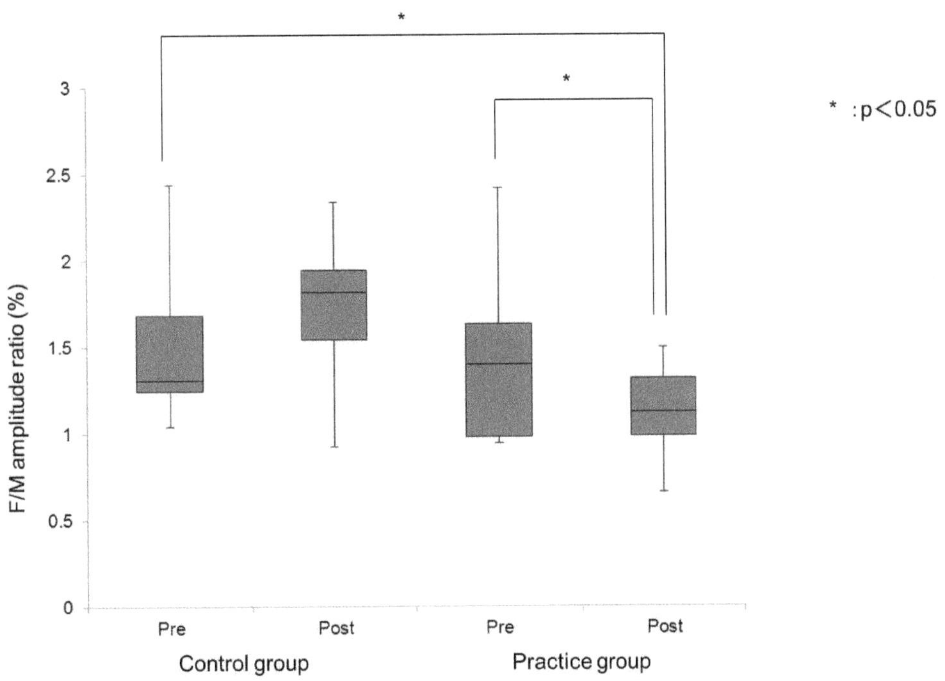


**Figure 8.** Prepractice and postpractice F/M amplitude ratios in the control and practice groups.

to the correct position. They reported that the input of sensory information to the cerebrum in the central nervous system is reduced when motor tasks are acquired by motor learning. This was reflected in the shorter latency of SEP amplitude decreases with increasing familiarity with the tasks. The results of the present study suggest that the facilitation effects of the sensory input and the upper central nervous system associated with voluntary movements of the upper limb on spinal motor neurons in the contralateral upper limb decrease

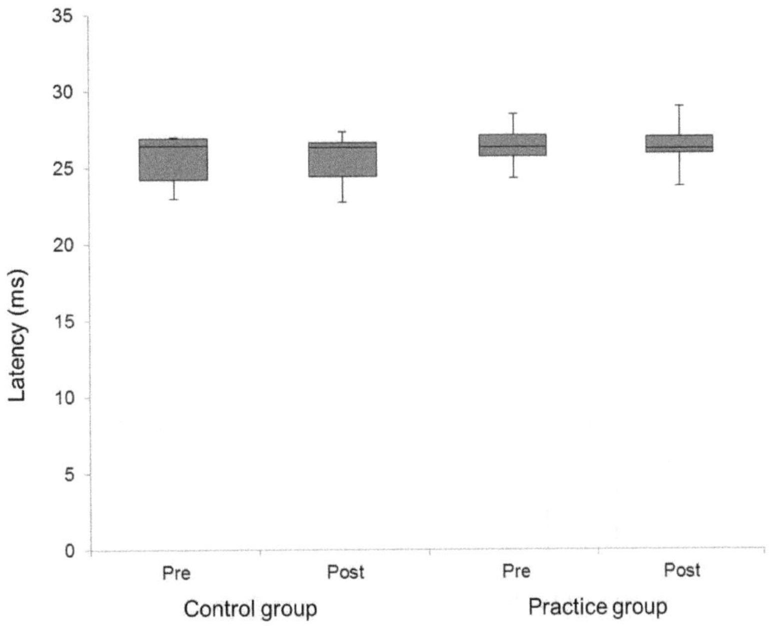


**Figure 9.** Pre- and postpractice latencies in the control and practice groups.

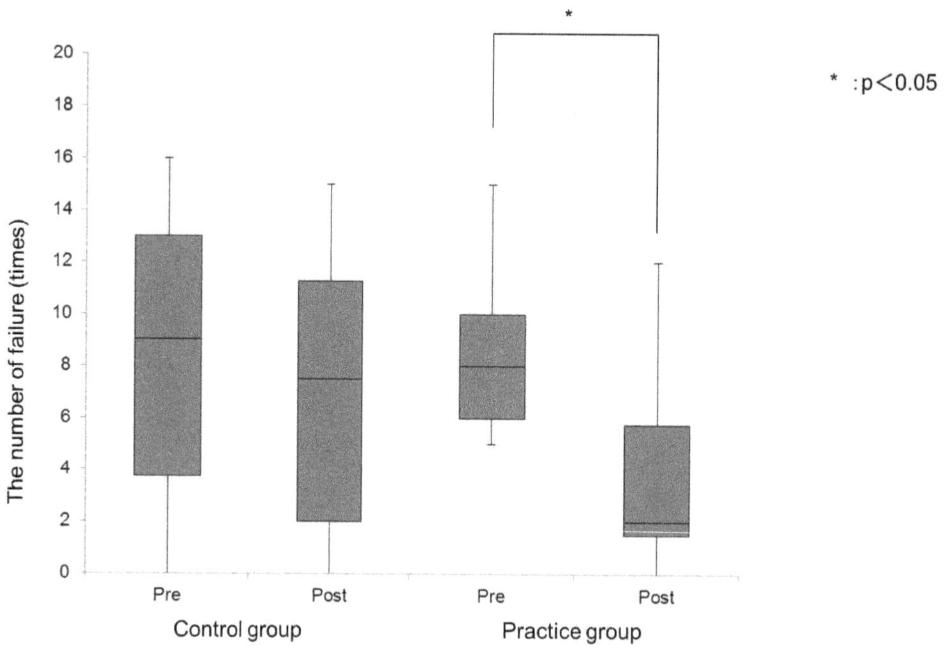


**Figure 10.** Failures pre- and postpractice in the control and practice groups.

with familiarity with the tasks due to practice. Changes in facilitation effects are described in **Figure 11**. Thus, the facilitation effects of difficult voluntary movements of the unilateral upper limb on spinal motor neurons in the contralateral upper limb decrease with motor learning.

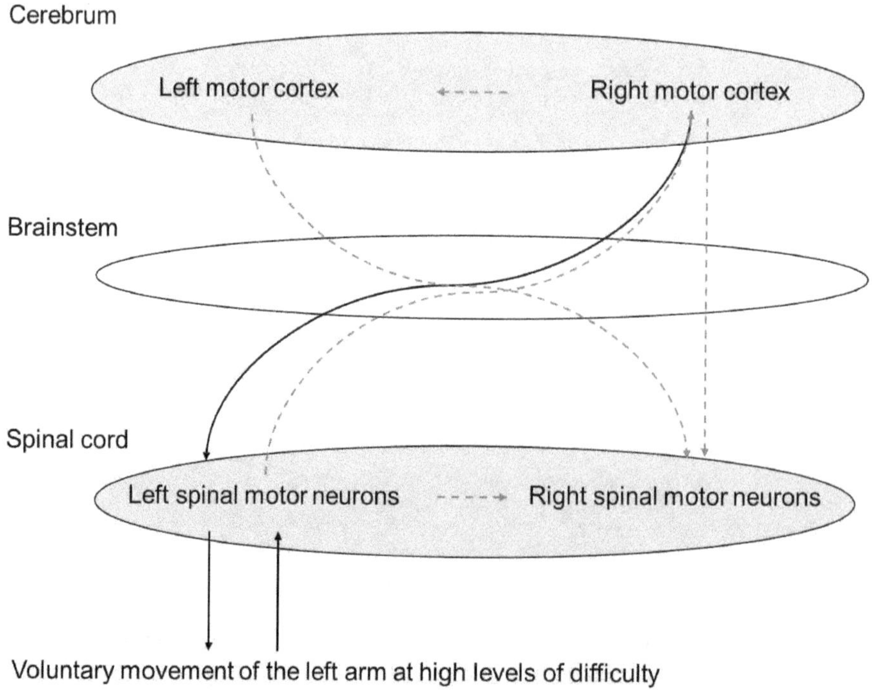


**Figure 11.** Change in the facilitation effects of voluntary movements after practice.

## 4. Clinical suggestion

We examined the relationship between the excitability of spinal motor neurons in the upper limb on the affected side and voluntary movements of the lower limb in patients with CVDs and healthy subjects. The voluntary movement performed in this study was simple and consisted of maintaining a straight-leg-raising test position with 30° flexion in the hip joint. No significant differences were observed in healthy subjects, while the excitability of spinal motor neurons in the upper limb on the affected side during voluntary movement was significantly higher than that during rest in patients with CVDs. Patients with CVDs thus experience an increase in the excitability of spinal motor neurons due to the collapse of the regulatory mechanism in the central nervous system. In brief, patients with CVDs are more susceptible to the facilitation effect than are healthy subjects.

In physical therapy, there is a need to evaluate facilitation effects due to the contractions of remote muscles. For example, in hemiplegic patients with CVDs, the associated reaction may disrupt accurate voluntary movement. Neurophysiological interpretations of the facilitation effects of postures and movements are necessary during these evaluations. The facilitation effect may increase with high muscle strength, high movement speed, activity of numerous muscle spindles, and difficult movements, and during the first stages of motor learning. Therapies for patients with hemiplegia with the associated reactions should begin with slow movements requiring low muscle strength. While practicing difficult movements, it is necessary to attenuate the facilitation effect by exercise.

Finally, we will present a related case report. We examined the influence of one physical therapy sessions for trunk muscle function on the function of the affected arm muscles in a patient with left hemiplegia and CVD using surface EMG and H-reflex-evoked EMG [27]. In this study, we compared the H/M amplitude ratio and muscle action potential in the sitting position after physical therapy to those in the sitting position before physical therapy. The H-reflex was recorded from the left APB and muscle action potentials were recorded from both the obliquus abdominis and the iliocostalis lumborum. Physical therapy was performed to improve the alignment of the trunk and the hip joint in a sitting position. We did not perform therapy on the affected arm. The sitting posture improved after physical therapy. The surface EMGs of the obliquus abdominis on the affected side and those of both the iliocostalis lumborum muscles after physical therapy were lower than those before physical therapy (**Figure 12**). The H/M amplitude ratio after physical therapy was also lower than that before physical therapy (**Figure 13**). The results of this study indicate that the excitability of spinal neural function in the affected arm might be decreased after physical therapy for trunk and lower extremity muscles in patients with CVD. The results also suggest that physical therapy on the affected arm in patients with CVD should account for the effects of the contraction of the trunk muscles and the low back muscles. Therefore, evaluation of the facilitation effect due to the contraction of remote muscles requires neurophysiological knowledge. The facilitation effect cannot be interpreted only using knowledge of the kinematic chain. Neurophysiological understanding of the influence of the contraction of a particular muscle on other muscles can be useful not only for evaluation, but also for therapy.

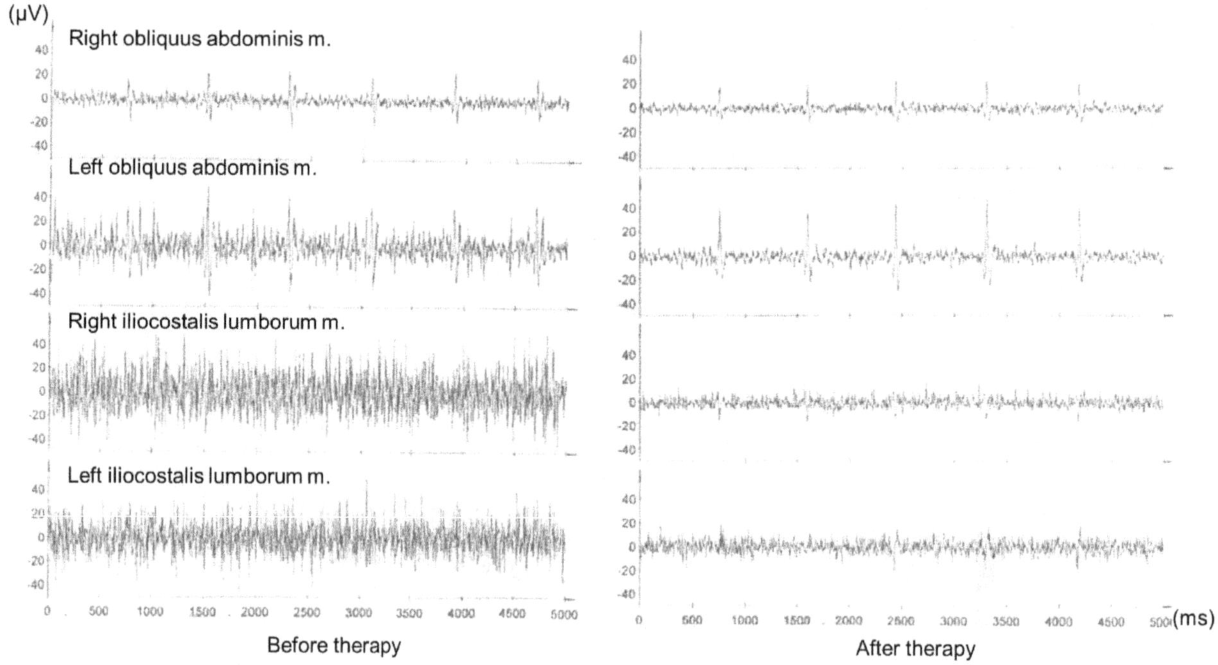


**Figure 12.** Change in the EMG waveforms before and after therapy.

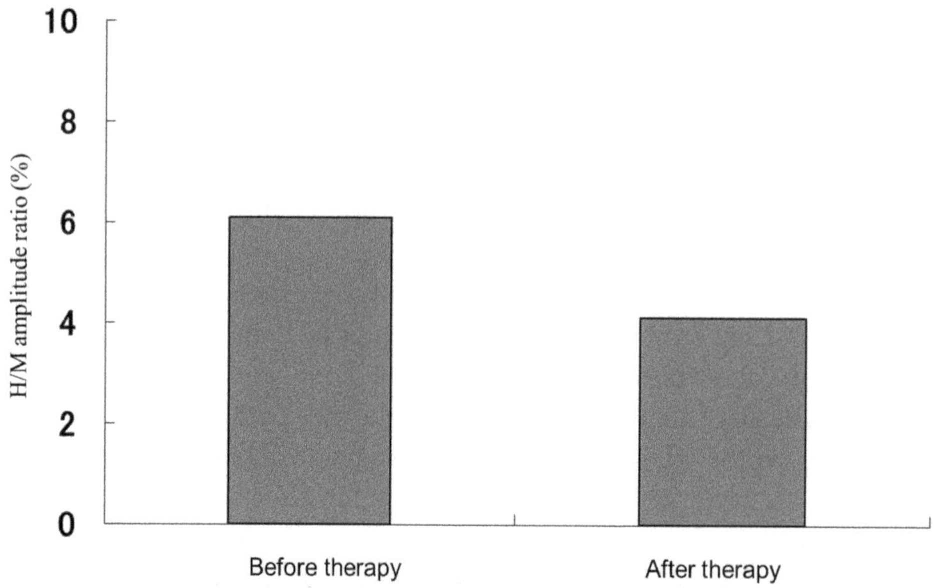


**Figure 13.** Change in the H/M amplitude ratios before and after therapy.

## Author details

Naoki Kado*, Yuki Takahashi, Satoshi Fujiwara and Masanori Ito

*Address all correspondence to: kado@sumire-academy.ac.jp

Department of Physical Therapy, Kobe College of Rehabilitation and Welfare, Hyogo, Japan

## References

[1] Bussel B, Morin C, Pierrot-Deseilligny E. Mechanism of monosynaptic reflex reinforcement during Jendrassik maneuver in man. Journal of Neurology, Neurosurgery, and Psychiatry. 1978;41(1):40–44. DOI: 10.1136/jnnp.41.1.40

[2] Kawamura T, Watanabe S. Timing as a prominent factor of the Jendrassik maneuver on the H reflex. Journal of Neurology, Neurosurgery, and Psychiatry. 1975;38(5):508–516. DOI: 10.1136/jnnp.38.5.508

[3] Boroojerdi B, Battaglia F, Muellbacher W, Cohen LG. Voluntary teeth clenching facilitates human motor system excitability. Clinical Neurophysiology. 2000;111(6):988–993. DOI: 10.1016/S1388-2457(00)00279-0

[4] Sugawara K, Kasai T. Facilitation of motor evoked potential and H-reflexes of flexor carpi radialis muscle induced by voluntary teeth clenching. Human Movement Science. 2002;21(2):203–212. DOI: 10.1016/S0167-9457(02)00099-4

[5] Suzuki T, Fujiwara T, Takeda I. Influence of voluntary isometric contraction in elbow flexor muscle on contralateral spinal motor neuron function: F-wave study (in Japanese). The Journal of Japanese Physical Therapy Association. 1992;19(4):359–363.

[6] Muellbacher W, Facchini S, Boroojerdi B, Hallett M. Changes in motor cortex excitability during ipsilateral hand muscle activation in humans. Clinical Neurophysiology. 2000;111(2):344–349. DOI: 10.1016/S1388-2457(99)00243-6

[7] Stinear CM, Walker KS, Byblow WD. Symmetric facilitation between motor cortices during contraction of ipsilateral hand muscles. Experimental Brain Research. 2001;139(1):101–105. DOI: 10.1007/s002210100758

[8] Hayashi A, Konopacki RA, Hunker CJ. Remote facilitation of H-reflex during voluntary contraction of orofacial and limb muscles. In: Stelmach GE, Requin J, editors. Tutorials in Motor Behavior II. Amsterdam: Elsevier; 1992. p. 960.

[9] Kado N, Ito M, Suzuki T, Ando H. Excitability of spinal motor neurons in the contralateral arm during voluntary arm movements of various difficulty levels. Journal of Physical Therapy Science. 2012;24(10):949–952. DOI: 10.1589/jpts.24.949

[10] Karni A, Meyer G, Jezzard P, Adams MM, Turner R, Ungerleider LG. Functional MRI evidence for adult motor cortex plasticity during motor skill learning. Nature. 1995;377(6545):155–158. DOI: 10.1038/377155a0

[11] Pascual-Leone A, Nguyet D, Cohen LG, Brasil-Neto JP, Cammarota, Hallett M. Modulation of muscle responses evoked by transcranial magnetic stimulation during the acquisition of new fine motor skills. Journal of Neurophysiology. 1995;74(3):1037–1045.

[12] Nielsen J, Crone C, Hultborm H. H-reflexes are smaller in dancers from The Royal Danish Ballet than in well-trained athletes. European Journal of Applied Physiology. 1993;66(2):116–121.

[13] Kado N, Ito M, Fujiwara S, Takahashi Y, Nomura M, Suzuk T. Effects of practicing difficult movements of the unilateral arm on the excitability of spinal motor neurons in the contralateral arm. Journal of Novel Physiotherapies. 2017;7(1):330. DOI: 10.4172/2165-7025.1000330

[14] Delwaide PJ, Toulouse P. Facilitation of monosynaptic reflexes by voluntary contraction of muscle in remote parts of the body. Brain. 1981;104(Pt 4):701–719. DOI: 10.1093/brain/104.4.701

[15] Hess CW, Mills KR, Murray NMF. Magnetic stimulation of the human brain: facilitation of motor responses by voluntary contraction of ipsilateral and contralateral muscles with additional observations on an amputee. Neuroscience Letters. 1986;71(2):235–240. DOI: 10.1016/0304-3940(86)90565-3

[16] Kimura J. Electrodiagnosis in Diseases of Nerves and Muscles: Principles and Practice. 2nd ed. Philadelphia: F. A. Davis Company; 2001. p. 997.

[17] Mesrati F, Vecchierini MF. F-waves, neurophysiology and clinical value. Neurophysiologic Clinique. 2005;34(5):217–243. DOI: 10.1016/j.neucli.2004.09.005

[18] Oldfield RC. The assessment and analysis of handedness: the Edinburgh inventory. Neuropsychologia. 1971;9(1):97–113. DOI: 10.1016/0028-3932(71)90067-4

[19] Fitts PM. The information capacity of the human motor system in controlling the amplitude of movement. Journal of Experimental Psychology. 1954;47(6):381–391. DOI: 10.1037/h0055392

[20] Shibasaki H, Sadato N, Lyshkow H, Yonekura Y, Honda M, Nagamine T, et al. Both Primary motor cortex and supplementary motor area play an important role in complex finger movement. Brain. 1993;116(Rt 6):1387–1398. DOI: 10.1093/brain/116.6.1387

[21] Winstein CJ, Grafton ST, Pohl PS. Motor Task Difficulty and Brain Activity: Investigation of Goal-Directed Reciprocal Aiming Using Positron Emission Tomography. Journal of Neurophysiology. 1997;77(3):1581–1594.

[22] Liang N, Murakami T, Funase K, Narita T, Kasai T. Further evidence for excitability changes in human primary motor cortex during ipsilateral voluntary contraction. Neuroscience Letters. 2008;433(2):135–140. DOI: 10.1016/j.neulet.2007.12.058

[23] Kobayashi M, Hutchinson S, Schlaug G, Pascual-Leone A. Ipsilateral motor cortex activation on functional magnetic resonance imaging during unilateral hand movements is related to interhemispheric interactions. NeuroImage. 2003;20(4):2259–2270. DOI: 10.1016/S1053-8119(03)00220-9

[24] Eisen A, Odusote K. Amplitude of the F wave: A potential means of documenting spasticity. Neurology. 1979;29(9):1306–1309. DOI: 10.1212/WNL.29.9_Part_1.1306

[25] Suzuki T, Higashi T, Takagi M, Sugawara K. Hemispheric asymmetry of ipsilateral motor cortex activation in motor skill learning. Neuroreport. 2013;24(13):693–697. DOI: 10.1097/WNR.0b013e3283630158

[26] Nelson AJ, Brooke JD, Mcllroy WE, Bishop DC, Norrie RG. The Gain of Initial Somatosensory Evoked Potentials Alters with Practice of an Accurate Motor Task. Brain Research. 2001;890(2):272–279. DOI: 10.1016/S0006-8993(00)03136-X

[27] Kado N. Function of the affected arm improved by Physical Therapy for function of trunk and lower extremity muscles in patient with cerebrovascular disease: A case report (In Japanese). Journal of Kansai Physical Therapy. 2002;2:109–112. DOI: 10.11542/icpt.1.155

# Permissions

All chapters in this book were first published in NPT, by InTech Open; hereby published with permission under the Creative Commons Attribution License or equivalent. Every chapter published in this book has been scrutinized by our experts. Their significance has been extensively debated. The topics covered herein carry significant findings which will fuel the growth of the discipline. They may even be implemented as practical applications or may be referred to as a beginning point for another development.

The contributors of this book come from diverse backgrounds, making this book a truly international effort. This book will bring forth new frontiers with its revolutionizing research information and detailed analysis of the nascent developments around the world.

We would like to thank all the contributing authors for lending their expertise to make the book truly unique. They have played a crucial role in the development of this book. Without their invaluable contributions this book wouldn't have been possible. They have made vital efforts to compile up to date information on the varied aspects of this subject to make this book a valuable addition to the collection of many professionals and students.

This book was conceptualized with the vision of imparting up-to-date information and advanced data in this field. To ensure the same, a matchless editorial board was set up. Every individual on the board went through rigorous rounds of assessment to prove their worth. After which they invested a large part of their time researching and compiling the most relevant data for our readers.

The editorial board has been involved in producing this book since its inception. They have spent rigorous hours researching and exploring the diverse topics which have resulted in the successful publishing of this book. They have passed on their knowledge of decades through this book. To expedite this challenging task, the publisher supported the team at every step. A small team of assistant editors was also appointed to further simplify the editing procedure and attain best results for the readers.

Apart from the editorial board, the designing team has also invested a significant amount of their time in understanding the subject and creating the most relevant covers. They scrutinized every image to scout for the most suitable representation of the subject and create an appropriate cover for the book.

The publishing team has been an ardent support to the editorial, designing and production team. Their endless efforts to recruit the best for this project, has resulted in the accomplishment of this book. They are a veteran in the field of academics and their pool of knowledge is as vast as their experience in printing. Their expertise and guidance has proved useful at every step. Their uncompromising quality standards have made this book an exceptional effort. Their encouragement from time to time has been an inspiration for everyone.

The publisher and the editorial board hope that this book will prove to be a valuable piece of knowledge for researchers, students, practitioners and scholars across the globe.

# List of Contributors

**Takayuki Kodama and Hideki Nakano**
Department of Physical Therapy, Faculty of Health Sciences, Kyoto Tachibana University, Kyoto, Japan

**Yoshinori Yamamoto**
Department of Rehabilitation, Sakakibara Hakuho Hospital, Mie, Japan

**Yoshibumi Bunno and Yuki Fukumoto**
Graduate School of Health Sciences, Graduate School of Kansai University of Health Sciences, Osaka, Japan
Clinical Physical Therapy Laboratory, Faculty of Health Sciences, Kansai University of Health Sciences, Wakaba, Kumatori, Sennan, Osaka, Japan

**Todo Marina and Chieko Onigata**
Clinical Physical Therapy Laboratory, Faculty of Health Sciences, Kansai University of Health Sciences, Osaka, Japan

**Julio Plata-Bello**
Department of Neurosurgery, Hospital Universitario de Canarias, Spain Magnetic Resonance Imaging Service for Biomedical Research, University of La Laguna, Spain

**Akiyoshi Matsugi**
Faculty of Rehabilitation, Shijonawate Gakuen University, Osaka, Japan

**Tsubasa Kawasaki**
Department of Physical Therapy, Faculty of Health Science, Ryotokuji University, Urayasu, Chiba, Japan

**Yasuhiko Hatanaka, Kazuki Yamaguchi, Koichi Saito and Satomi Tada**
Suzuka University of Medical Science, Suzuka, Mie, Japan

**Yasemin Parlak Demir**
Hacettepe University, Physiotherapy and Rehabilitation, Ankara, Turkey

**Tadamitsu Matsuda, Atsushi Manji, Kazu Amimoto, Akira Inaba and Yoshiaki Wada**
Josai International University, Chiba, Japan

**Naoki Kado, Yuki Takahashi, Satoshi Fujiwara and Masanori Ito**
Department of Physical Therapy, Kobe College of Rehabilitation and Welfare, Hyogo, Japan

# Index

www.ingramcontent.com/pod-product-compliance
Lightning Source LLC
LaVergne TN
LVHW060602210926
848485LV00005B/1357
* 9 7 8 1 6 3 9 8 9 4 1 5 4 *